ARRHYTHMIAS IN WOMEN

Diagnosis and Management

MAYO CLINIC SCIENTIFIC PRESS

Mayo Clinic Atlas of Regional Anesthesia and Ultrasound-Guided Nerve Blockade
Edited by James R. Hebl, MD, and Robert L. Lennon, DO

Mayo Clinic Preventive Medicine and Public Health Board Review
Edited by Prathibha Varkey, MBBS, MPH, MHPE

Mayo Clinic Challenging Images for Pulmonary Board Review
Edward C. Rosenow III, MD

Mayo Clinic Gastroenterology and Hepatology Board Review, Fourth Edition
Edited by Stephen C. Hauser, MD

Mayo Clinic Infectious Diseases Board Review
Edited by Zelalem Temesgen, MD

Mayo Clinic Antimicrobial Handbook: Quick Guide, Second Edition
Edited by John W. Wilson, MD, and Lynn L. Estes, PharmD

Just Enough Physiology
James R. Munis, MD, PhD

Mayo Clinic Cardiology: Concise Textbook, Fourth Edition
Edited by Joseph G. Murphy, MD, and Margaret A. Lloyd, MD, MBA

Mayo Clinic Internal Medicine Board Review, Tenth Edition
Edited by Robert D. Ficalora, MD

Mayo Clinic Internal Medicine Board Review: Questions and Answers
Edited by Robert D. Ficalora, MD

Mayo Clinic Electrophysiology Manual
Edited by Samuel J. Asirvatham, MD

Mayo Clinic Gastrointestinal Imaging Review, Second Edition
C. Daniel Johnson, MD

ARRHYTHMIAS IN WOMEN

Diagnosis and Management

EDITORS-IN-CHIEF

Yong-Mei Cha, MD
Consultant and Co-Director, Implantable Cardiac Device Service,
Division of Cardiovascular Diseases
Mayo Clinic, Rochester, Minnesota
Professor of Medicine
Mayo Clinic College of Medicine

Margaret A. Lloyd, MD, MBA
Consultant, Division of Cardiovascular Diseases
Mayo Clinic, Rochester, Minnesota
Assistant Professor of Medicine
Mayo Clinic College of Medicine

Ulrika M. Birgersdotter-Green, MD
Director, Pacemaker and ICD Services
UC–San Diego Health Sciences, San Diego, California
Professor of Medicine
UC–San Diego School of Medicine

MAYO CLINIC SCIENTIFIC PRESS   OXFORD UNIVERSITY PRESS

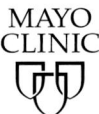

MAYO CLINIC

The triple-shield Mayo logo and the words MAYO, MAYO CLINIC, and MAYO CLINIC SCIENTIFIC PRESS
are marks of Mayo Foundation for Medical Education and Research.

OXFORD
UNIVERSITY PRESS

Oxford University Press is a department of the University of Oxford.
It furthers the University's objective of excellence in research, scholarship,
and education by publishing worldwide.

Oxford   New York
Auckland   Cape Town   Dar es Salaam   Hong Kong   Karachi
Kuala Lumpur   Madrid   Melbourne   Mexico City   Nairobi
New Delhi   Shanghai   Taipei   Toronto

With offices in
Argentina   Austria   Brazil   Chile   Czech Republic   France   Greece
Guatemala   Hungary   Italy   Japan   Poland   Portugal   Singapore
South Korea   Switzerland   Thailand   Turkey   Ukraine   Vietnam

Oxford is a registered trademark of Oxford University Press
in the UK and certain other countries.

Published in the United States of America by
Oxford University Press
198 Madison Avenue, New York, NY 10016

© Mayo Foundation for Medical Education and Research 2014

All rights reserved. No part of this publication may be reproduced, stored in a
retrieval system, or transmitted, in any form or by any means, without the prior
permission in writing of Mayo Clinic, or as expressly permitted by law,
by license, or under terms agreed with the appropriate reproduction rights organization.
Inquiries concerning reproduction outside the scope of the above should be sent to
Scientific Publications, Mayo Clinic, 200 First Street SW, Rochester, MN, 55905.

You must not circulate this work in any other form
and you must impose this same condition on any acquirer.

Library of Congress Cataloging-in-Publication Data
Arrhythmias in women : diagnosis and management / edited by Yong-Mei Cha, Margaret A. Lloyd,
Ulrika M. Birgersdotter-Green.
p. ; cm.—(Mayo Clinic scientific press)
Includes bibliographical references.
ISBN 978–0–19–932197–1 (alk. paper)
I. Cha, Yong-Mei, editor of compilation.   II. Lloyd, Margaret A., editor of compilation.   III. Birgersdotter-Green, Ulrika M.,
editor of compilation.   IV. Series: Mayo Clinic scientific press (Series)
[DNLM: 1. Arrhythmias, Cardiac—diagnosis.   2. Arrhythmias, Cardiac—therapy.   3. Women's Health. WG 330]
RC685.A65
616.1′280082—dc23
2013047125

Mayo Foundation does not endorse any particular products or services, and the reference to any products or services in this book
is for informational purposes only and should not be taken as an endorsement by the authors or Mayo Foundation. Care has been
taken to confirm the accuracy of the information presented and to describe generally accepted practices. However, the authors,
editors, and publisher are not responsible for errors or omissions or for any consequences from application of the information
in this book and make no warranty, express or implied, with respect to the contents of the publication. This book should not be
relied on apart from the advice of a qualified health care provider.

The authors, editors, and publisher have exerted efforts to ensure that drug selection and dosage set forth in this text are in
accordance with current recommendations and practice at the time of publication. However, in view of ongoing research, changes
in government regulations, and the constant flow of information relating to drug therapy and drug reactions, readers are urged to
check the package insert for each drug for any change in indications and dosage and for added wordings and precautions. This is
particularly important when the recommended agent is a new or infrequently employed drug.

Some drugs and medical devices presented in this publication have US Food and Drug Administration (FDA) clearance for
limited use in restricted research settings. It is the responsibility of the health care providers to ascertain the FDA status of each
drug or device planned for use in their clinical practice.

1 3 5 7 9 8 6 4 2
Printed in China on acid-free paper

With this book, the editors wish to honor Doris J. W. Escher, MD, Nora F. Goldschlager, MD, Anne B. Curtis, MD, and Anne M. Gillis, MD—past presidents of the North American Society of Pacing and Electrophysiology and its successor, the Heart Rhythm Society—who have provided inspirational leadership with integrity, compassion, and good cheer.

Foreword

SEX MATTERS

Sex matters—more and differently than was ever believed, especially as it relates to cardiovascular disease. But the fact that sex should be considered when caring for patients with arrhythmias is a relatively new concept and one for which there is a substantial gap between its recognition and the realization of health benefits. The Institute of Medicine in its landmark 2001 report, *Exploring the Biological Contributions to Human Health: Does Sex Matter?*, answered its own question with a resounding yes; sex must be taken into consideration "from womb to tomb" when it comes to the science of medicine and caring for women and men. Evidence of important sex differences affecting every aspect of cardiovascular disease is mounting, and arrhythmias are no exception. Aside from the obvious differences associated with gonadal hormones, differences in natural history, symptoms, accuracy of diagnostic tests, response to therapy, prevalence and relative risk of risk factors, and social and behavioral issues have been identified, each of which has the potential to impact treatment and outcomes.

Therein is the challenge. While discoveries and advances in the diagnosis and treatment of heart disease have come at apparent lightning speed over the past few decades, compared with men, women have not experienced the same decrease in cardiovascular mortality, and until the past decade, they were largely ignored as a population worthy of separate study or consideration. Previously, women and their physicians were told that heart disease did not develop in women, or if it did, it did not develop until women were elderly. When and if women ultimately received a diagnosis of heart disease, it was not felt to be as serious a health threat as it was in men. Women's symptoms are sometimes challenging to address, and both women and their physicians can be quick to attribute manifestations of cardiovascular disease to menopause, mental health issues, or aging. In studies of several arrhythmias and related conditions, compared with men, women have received a diagnosis and treatment at a more advanced stage of disease and received delayed or less-intensive therapy. These practices have likely contributed to women's higher cardiovascular-related total mortality.

Compounding these historical practices, physicians and patients have been faced with insufficient sex-specific scientific evidence to confidently manage women with cardiac arrhythmias. The lack of relevant cardiovascular research on women and inadequate enrollment of women in clinical trials, compounded by the absence of sex-specific data analysis or reporting, have led to a substantial and persistent sex-based knowledge gap in care for women with suspected or diagnosed arrhythmias. These care and knowledge gaps include key issues such as symptoms and the effects, side effects, risks, and benefits of commonly used diagnostic tests and therapies.

Without sex-specific evidence to guide them, clinicians are left with the option of either withholding therapies from women when there is no sex-specific proof of benefit, or alternatively, treating women in a "sex-blind" manner using data from studies on men as a means to guide their treatment. Neither approach is evidence-based, and both have the potential for harm, overtreatment, or undertreatment.

While cardiac arrhythmias continue to be responsible for substantial morbidity and mortality in women, progress is being made. Over the past decade there has been exponential growth in the availability of evidence-based and sex-specific data and strategies for optimal arrhythmia diagnosis, risk assessment and modification, and clinical management. Many of these discoveries have informed important changes in recommended practice and have affirmed the need for a sex-based approach to arrhythmia management in order to optimize practice and outcomes for women.

An important next step in bridging the sex gap in care is to provide to medical practitioners and the women they care for a practical, comprehensive, and accessible source of this new information. For that reason, I celebrate the publication of this superb textbook, in which the very experts who have made the most significant contributions to the field of electrophysiology in women synthesize their knowledge into a practical work that will be a valuable reference for anyone who provides medical care to women. On behalf of women who are living with or are at risk for heart disease, I wish to thank the editors and authors for providing this resource to the health care community.

Sharonne N. Hayes, MD
Consultant, Division of Cardiovascular Diseases
Founder, Women's Heart Clinic
Professor of Medicine, Mayo Clinic College of Medicine
Mayo Clinic, Rochester Minnesota

Preface

Discoveries in human biology have demonstrated that both normal physiologic function and pathophysiologic function are directly influenced by sex-based biology. For example, lifetime cardiac automaticity and rhythm may not be the same between sexes. A better understanding of the physiologic differences in rhythm generation and arrhythmogenesis between women and men is essential, as is the translation of these differences into clinical practice.

Increasing evidence shows that sex matters in understanding and recognizing the differences between men and women in the fundamental electrophysiologic properties of the cardiac myocardium, the effects of female sex hormones, and the dynamic effects of hormonal regulation that occur throughout the life cycle. It matters in clinical practice as well, where there are clear sex differences in both clinical presentation and management.

Since women have longer QT intervals and less repolarization reserve than men, women are particularly prone to either QT-interval prolongation or antiarrhythmic drug–mediated proarrhythmia. Specific attention and knowledge are required for diagnosis and management when women have these genetic predispositions or mutations.

Supraventricular tachycardia is more common in women than in men. Although mortality increases only modestly among patients with supraventricular tachycardia, morbidity increases considerably. In particular, quality of life for women with supraventricular tachycardia is significantly impaired. The prevalence of atrial fibrillation at all ages is higher among men than women, but, because women live longer than men, more than half of all elderly patients with atrial fibrillation are women. Furthermore, women with atrial fibrillation have a higher risk of stroke than men, yet advanced therapies such as catheter ablation are offered to women later in the course of therapy, often only after more antiarrhythmic drug options have failed.

Cardiovascular disease (and sudden cardiac death secondary to life-threatening ventricular arrhythmias) is the leading killer of women. The incidence of sudden cardiac death among women doubles with each decade of life, although the rate increase lags behind men's by more than a decade. Women are also less likely than men to have left ventricular dysfunction at the time of sudden death, underscoring the difficulty in risk prediction for sudden death prevention in women.

Historically, women have been underrepresented in state-of-the-art device trials and other clinical trials relating to managing arrhythmias. As a result, questions remain as to whether women will benefit from the therapies to the same extent as men. The truth is that fewer women than men receive appropriate device therapy based on current guidelines. Among patients who undergo pacemaker, defibrillator, and resynchronization device implantation, as well as lead extraction when indicated, the complication risks are higher for women than for men.

The scope of diagnosing and managing arrhythmia disorders in women has implications throughout the world. The prevalence of arrhythmia may vary on different continents as a result of many factors, including geography, socioeconomics, ethnicity, culture, and environmental risks. In developing countries, women have less access to medical care and more often receive conservative management.

Arrhythmias and implantable cardiac devices during pregnancy present another set of clinical challenges. The presence of structural or congenital heart diseases, the aggravation of supraventricular tachycardia or ventricular tachycardia recurrence, the selection of antiarrhythmic drugs for the safety of mother and fetus, the careful management of anticoagulation, and the dilemmas related to implantable cardioverter-defibrillator shocks all need to be addressed, guided by knowledge of the hemodynamic, physiologic, and pharmacokinetic changes caused by pregnancy.

This book is not intended to be a comprehensive review of the overall concepts, mechanisms, pathophysiology, diagnoses, and therapies of cardiac electrophysiology and cardiac implantable electronic devices, all of which have been extensively covered by many talented authors. Instead, the following chapters review the unique biologic features of cardiac rhythm and dysrhythmia in women, a subject that has been overlooked in other books. Each chapter draws on the expertise of the coauthors, who have had a lifelong dedication to the investigation of the related subjects, especially in women. Their extensive contributions to the cardiology literature in their specific subjects prove their substantial track records. We cannot thank these pioneer female electrophysiologists enough for their significant contributions to this book. We hope the book will be a useful resource for electrophysiologists, cardiologists, internists, clinicians, and allied professionals who seek to better manage arrhythmias in female patients.

We greatly appreciate the editorial support from the Mayo Clinic Section of Scientific Publications and the design support from the Mayo Clinic Division of Media Support Services in the preparation of this book.

Yong-Mei Cha, MD
Margaret A. Lloyd, MD, MBA
Ulrika M. Birgersdotter-Green, MD

Contents

Contributors   xvii

Names of Clinical Trials, Studies, and Registries   xxi

1. Sex Bias or Sex Disparities Among Women With Arrhythmias?   1
   Jodie L. Hurwitz, MD

2. Women in Clinical Trials   17
   Jeanne E. Poole, MD

3. Genetic and Hereditary Considerations for Arrhythmias in Women   35
   Ohad Ziv, MD, and Elizabeth S. Kaufman, MD

4. Sex-Specific Electrophysiologic Properties   47
   Christine Tanaka-Esposito, MD, and Mina K. Chung, MD

5. Supraventricular Arrhythmias   59
   Cevher Ozcan, MD, and Anne B. Curtis, MD

6. Atrial Fibrillation in Women   79
   Susan J. Eisenberg, MD, and Taya V. Glotzer, MD

7. Drug Treatment in Women   103
   Katherine T. Murray, MD

8. Sudden Cardiac Death in Women　113
Laura M. Gravelin, MD, and Rachel J. Lampert, MD

9. Implantable Cardioverter-Defibrillator Therapy in Women　129
Andrea M. Russo, MD

10. Pacing and Cardiac Resynchronization Therapy in Women　153
Judith A. Mackall, MD, and Yong-Mei Cha, MD

11. Syncope and POTS: Are Women Really Faint of Heart?　177
Celina M. Yong, MD, MSc, MBA, and Karen J. Friday, MD

12. The Road to a Successful Women's Heart Clinic　191
Darcy H. Theisen, MSN, CNP, and Bobbi L. Hoppe, MD

13. Taking a Look Around the World　209
Uma N. Srivatsa, MBBS, MAS, and Amparo C. Villablanca, MD

14. Pregnancy and Arrhythmias　227
Lynda E. Rosenfeld, MD

15. Lead Extraction in Women　243
Ulrika M. Birgersdotter-Green, MD, and Margaret A. Lloyd, MD, MBA

Index　259

Contributors

Ulrika M. Birgersdotter-Green, MD
Director, Pacemaker and ICD Services, University of California–San Diego Health Sciences, San Diego, California; Professor of Medicine, UC–San Diego School of Medicine

Yong-Mei Cha, MD
Consultant and Co-Director, Implantable Cardiac Device Service, Division of Cardiovascular Diseases, Mayo Clinic, Rochester, Minnesota; Professor of Medicine, Mayo Clinic College of Medicine

Mina K. Chung, MD
Staff, Department of Cardiovascular Medicine, Heart and Vascular Institute and Department of Molecular Cardiology, Lerner Research Institute, Cleveland Clinic, Cleveland, Ohio; Professor of Medicine, Cleveland Clinic Lerner College of Medicine, Case Western Reserve University, Cleveland, Ohio

Anne B. Curtis, MD
Charles and Mary Bauer Professor, UB Distinguished Professor, and Chair, Department of Medicine, State University of New York at Buffalo, Buffalo, New York

Susan J. Eisenberg, MD
Medical Director, Cardiac Rhythm Center, John Muir Medical Center, Concord, California

Karen J. Friday, MD
Staff Physician, Palo Alto VA Medical Center, Palo Alto, California; Clinical Professor of Medicine (Affiliated), Stanford School of Medicine, Stanford University, Stanford, California

Taya V. Glotzer, MD
Director of Cardiac Research, Hackensack University Medical Center, Hackensack, New Jersey; Clinical Assistant Professor of Medicine, Rutgers University Medical School, Rutgers, New Jersey

Laura M. Gravelin, MD
Cardiac Electrophysiologist, Delaware Heart and Vascular, PA, Dover, Delaware

Bobbi L. Hoppe, MD
North Memorial Heart and Vascular Clinic, Robbinsdale, Minnesota

Jodie L. Hurwitz, MD
Director of Electrophysiology, Medical City Hospital and North Texas Heart Center, Dallas, Texas

Elizabeth S. Kaufman, MD
Director, Familial Heart Rhythm Program, MetroHealth Medical Center, Cleveland, Ohio; Professor of Medicine, Case Western Reserve University School of Medicine, Cleveland, Ohio

Rachel J. Lampert, MD
Associate Professor of Medicine, Yale University School of Medicine, New Haven, Connecticut

Margaret A. (Peg) Lloyd, MD, MBA
Consultant, Division of Cardiovascular Diseases, Mayo Clinic, Rochester, Minnesota; Assistant Professor of Medicine, Mayo Clinic College of Medicine

Judith A. Mackall, MD
Section Chief, Electrophysiology, University Hospitals Case Medical Center, Cleveland, Ohio; Associate Professor of Medicine, School of Medicine, Case Western Reserve University

Katherine T. Murray, MD
Associate Professor of Medicine and of Pharmacology, Divisions of Cardiovascular Medicine and Clinical Pharmacology, Vanderbilt University School of Medicine, Nashville, Tennessee

Cevher Ozcan, MD
Assistant Professor of Medicine, Clinical and Translational Research Center, State University of New York at Buffalo, Buffalo, New York

Jeanne E. Poole, MD
Director, Electrophysiology Section and Clinical Cardiac Electrophysiology Fellowship Program, University of Washington Medical Center, Seattle, Washington; Professor of Medicine, University of Washington School of Medicine

Lynda E. Rosenfeld, MD
Associate Professor of Medicine (Cardiology) and of Pediatrics, Yale University School of Medicine, New Haven, Connecticut

Andrea M. Russo, MD
Director, Electrophysiology and Arrhythmia Services, Director, Cardiac Electrophysiology Fellowship, Cooper University Hospital, Camden, New Jersey; Professor of Medicine, Cooper Medical School of Rowan University

Uma N. Srivatsa, MBBS, MAS
Cardiovascular Services, Lawrence J. Ellison Ambulatory Care Center, Sacramento, California; Associate Professor of Medicine, School of Medicine, University of California—Davis

Christine Tanaka-Esposito, MD
Associate Staff, Cardiovascular Medicine, Cleveland Clinic, Cleveland, Ohio

Darcy H. Theisen, MSN, CNP
North Memorial Heart and Vascular Clinic, Robbinsdale, Minnesota

Amparo C. Villablanca, MD
Director, Women's Cardiovascular Medicine Program, UC Davis Medical Group, Sacramento, California; Professor of Medicine and Lazda Endowed Chair, Women's Cardiovascular Medicine, School of Medicine, University of California—Davis

Celina M. Yong, MD, MSc, MBA
Instructor in Cardiovascular Medicine, Stanford School of Medicine, Stanford University, Stanford, California

Ohad Ziv, MD
Director, Cardiac Electrophysiology, MetroHealth Medical Center, Cleveland, Ohio; Assistant Professor of Medicine, Case Western Reserve University School of Medicine, Cleveland, Ohio

Names of Clinical Trials, Studies, and Registries

ADVANCENT	National Registry to Advance Heart Health
AFFIRM	Atrial Fibrillation Follow-up Investigation of Rhythm Management
ANDROMEDA	Antiarrhythmic Trial With Dronedarone in Moderate to Severe CHF Evaluating Morbidity Decrease
ARISTOTLE	Apixaban for Reduction in Stroke and Other Thromboembolic Events in Atrial Fibrillation
ATRIA	Anticoagulation and Risk Factors in Atrial Fibrillation
AVERROES	Apixaban Versus Acetylsalicylic Acid to Prevent Stroke in Atrial Fibrillation Patients Who Have Failed or Are Unsuitable for Vitamin K Antagonist Treatment
AVID	Antiarrhythmics Versus Implantable Defibrillators
BWHHS	British Women's Heart and Health Study
CABG-Patch	Coronary Artery Bypass Graft Surgery With/Without Simultaneous Epicardial Patch for Automatic Implantable Cardioverter Defibrillator
CAMIAT	Canadian Amiodarone Myocardial Infarction Arrhythmia Trial
CANRACE	Canadian Registry of Acute Coronary Events
CARAF	Canadian Registry of Atrial Fibrillation
CARE-HF	Cardiac Resynchronization—Heart Failure

CASS	Coronary Artery Surgery Study
CAST	Cardiac Arrhythmia Suppression Trial
CHF-STAT	Congestive Heart Failure: Survival Trial of Antiarrhythmic Therapy
CHS	Cardiovascular Health Study
CIDS	Canadian Implantable Defibrillator Study
COMET	Carvedilol or Metoprolol European Trial
COMPANION	Comparison of Medical Therapy, Pacing, and Defibrillation in Heart Failure
CONTAK CD	Cardiac Resynchronization Therapy Combined With Implantable Cardioverter Defibrillator Therapy
CONTAK CD 2	Cardiac Resynchronization Therapy Defibrillator for the Treatment of Heart Failure
CREATE	Treatment and Outcomes of Acute Coronary Syndromes in India
DEFINITE	Defibrillators in Nonischemic Cardiomyopathy Treatment Evaluation
DIAMOND-CHF	Danish Investigations of Arrhythmia and Mortality on Dofetilide in Congestive Heart Failure
DIG	Digitalis Investigation Group
DINAMIT	Defibrillator in Acute Myocardial Infarction Trial
EMIAT	European Myocardial Infarct Amiodarone Trial
FOLLOWPACE	Cost-Effectiveness of Routine Follow-up Visits in Patients With a Pacemaker
FRACTAL	Fibrillation Registry Assessing Costs, Therapies, Adverse Events, and Lifestyle
GESICA	Grupo de Estudio de la Sobrevida en la Insuficiencia Cardiaca en Argentina
GRACE	Global Registry of Acute Coronary Events
HERS	Heart and Estrogen/Progestin Replacement Study
HPFS	Health Professionals Follow-up Study
ICD-LABOR	Implantable Cardioverter-Defibrillator Latin American Bioelectronic Ongoing Registry
IMPROVE HF	Registry to Improve the Use of Evidence-Based Heart Failure Therapies in the Outpatient Setting
INSYNC	InSync Implantable Cardioverter-Defibrillator Registry: Cardiac Resynchronization Therapy

INTRINSIC RV	Inhibition of Unnecessary Right Ventricular Pacing With Atrioventricular Search Hysteresis in Implantable Cardioverter-Defibrillators
IRIS	Immediate Risk-Stratification Improves Survival
ISSUE-3	Third International Study on Syncope of Uncertain Etiology
LExICon	Lead Extraction in the Contemporary Setting
MADIT	Multicenter Automatic Defibrillator Implantation Trial
MADIT II	Multicenter Automatic Defibrillator Implantation Trial II
MADIT-CRT	Multicenter Automatic Defibrillator Implantation Trial With Cardiac Resynchronization Therapy
MESA	Marshfield Epidemiologic Study Area
MIRACLE	Multicenter InSync Randomized Clinical Evaluation
MIRACLE-ICD	Multicenter InSync ICD Randomized Clinical Evaluation
MIRACLE-ICD II	Multicenter InSync ICD Randomized Clinical Evaluation II
MUSTT	Multicenter Unsustained Tachycardia Trial
MUSTIC-SR	Multisite Stimulation in Cardiomyopathy—Sinus Rhythm
NCDR	National Cardiovascular Data Registry
NHS	Nurses' Health Study
Oregon SUDS	Oregon Sudden Unexpected Death Study
PALLAS	Permanent Atrial Fibrillation Outcome Study Using Dronedarone on Top of Standard Therapy
PATH-CHF	Pacing Therapies in Congestive Heart Failure
RACE	Rate Control Versus Electrical Cardioversion for Persistent Atrial Fibrillation
RACE II	Rate Control Efficacy in Permanent Atrial Fibrillation: A Comparison Between Lenient and Strict Rate Control II
RAFT	Resynchronization/Defibrillation for Ambulatory Heart Failure Trial
RE-LY	Randomized Evaluation of Long-term Anticoagulant Therapy: Dabigatran vs Warfarin
REVERSE	Resynchronization Reverses Remodeling in Systolic Left Ventricular Dysfunction
ROCKET AF	Rivaroxaban Once Daily Oral Direct Factor Xa Inhibition Compared With Vitamin K Antagonism for Prevention of Stroke and Embolism Trial in Atrial Fibrillation

SAFIRE-D	Symptomatic Atrial Fibrillation Investigative Research on Dofetilide
SCD-HeFT	Sudden Cardiac Death in Heart Failure Trial
SEARCH-MI	Survey to Evaluate Arrhythmia Rate in High-Risk Myocardial Infarction Patients
SPAF I	Stroke Prevention in Atrial Fibrillation I
SPAF II	Stroke Prevention in Atrial Fibrillation II
SPAF III	Stroke Prevention in Atrial Fibrillation III
SPORTIF	Stroke Prevention Using an Oral Thrombin Inhibitor in Atrial Fibrillation
SWORD	Survival With Oral D-Sotalol
VALIANT	Valsartan in Acute Myocardial Infarction Trial
WHI	Women's Health Initiative
WHS	Women's Health Study: A Randomized Trial of Low-Dose Aspirin and Vitamin E in the Primary Prevention of Cardiovascular Disease and Cancer
WISE	Women's Ischemia Syndrome Evaluation

CHAPTER ONE

Sex Bias or Sex Disparities Among Women With Arrhythmias?

JODIE L. HURWITZ, MD

INTRODUCTION

Is there more sex bias than sex disparity in the diagnosis and management of arrhythmias in women? *Sex bias* implies that it is incorrectly believed that women do not have the disease or that they will not benefit from treatment; therefore, they are not included in studies and they are not encouraged to participate. *Sex disparity* implies that women do not have the disease in question; therefore, fewer women are included in clinical trials.

According to 2009 data from the Centers for Disease Control and Prevention Morbidity and Mortality Weekly Report, women represent the majority of patients treated for heart rhythm disorders, yet there is widespread agreement that electrophysiology clinical trials have enrolled predominantly men. In this chapter, sex bias and sex disparity are addressed in relation to the general topics of basic and clinical electrophysiology, long QT syndrome (LQTS), atrial fibrillation (AF), supraventricular tachycardias, pacemaker mode selection, sudden cardiac death (SCD), and implantable cardioverter-defibrillator (ICD)–cardiac resynchronization therapy (CRT).

SEX DIFFERENCES IN BASIC AND CLINICAL ELECTROPHYSIOLOGY

Prolongation of repolarization in women compared with men has been well documented. In experimental models, estrogen affects potassium channel protein synthesis, which in turn can alter repolarization and increase atrial refractory periods. Female hearts show decreased expression for various potassium channel subunits that are thought to be potentially important in cardiac repolarization. Physiologic concentrations of estrogen can also act like calcium channel antagonists and prolong repolarization.

Male and female gonadal steroid receptors are found in cardiac muscle bundles and in isolated cardiomyocytes. These receptors can modulate gene expression through various signaling pathways. Estradiol-17β has been shown to work on the cellular level and is thought to exert an antiarrhythmic effect through inhibition of the calcium channel.

Sex differences also exist in ion channel subunit composition but are poorly categorized, in part because of a lack of experimental data from healthy human myocytes. In addition, the available models are built on experimental data obtained predominantly from myocytes acquired from men. Sex-related differences in subunit composition may be involved in the genesis of ventricular arrhythmias.

The average duration of systole is longer in women than in men. Women have higher heart rates at rest than men by about 3 to 5 beats per minute. This heart rate differential holds true even after autonomic blockade with propranolol and atropine. Potential mechanisms for this observation include differences in the quantity of individual ion channels or in the hormonal effects on ion channel expression and function. Sex differences in autonomic tone, 3-dimensional myocyte architecture, cell-to-cell coupling, and heart size and function may be responsible. Nuclear and cytosolic receptors for sex hormones in myocytes may also be involved. It is not known whether this heart rate disparity is inherited or acquired.

Other clinical electrophysiologic differences between the sexes have been established:

1. Women normally have a narrower QRS complex and lower QRS voltage than men.

2. Women are less likely to have premature ventricular contractions than men (5%-7% of women compared with 7%-8% of men).
3. Women have less orthostatic tolerance than men. The mechanism for this finding is not known, but it is thought that reduced stroke volume in women results in a lower basal systolic blood pressure. Estrogen given to perimenopausal women decreased systolic and diastolic blood pressure by enhancing the basal levels of nitric oxide, yet normal fluctuations of sex hormones, as occur during the menstrual cycle, have no or minimal effect on blood pressure or orthostatic stress during tilt-table testing.

Understanding these basic and clinical electrophysiologic differences may yield better sex-specific treatment recommendations. If cellular responses are specific for age and sex, it would be beneficial to control for the sex and hormonal status of persons included in clinical studies.

LONG QT SYNDROME

At birth, the length of the corrected QT interval (QTc) is similar between the sexes. As male sex hormone levels increase in boys during puberty, the QTc shortens. The QTc then lengthens as testosterone levels slowly decrease with age until, when men are about 50 years old, the length of the QTc approaches that of women. Generally, the QT interval in adult premenopausal women is approximately 10 to 20 ms longer than in adult men. The QT interval lengthens during menstruation; hypotheses include the effect of female hormones on calcium and potassium channel function, on the fast and persistent sodium current, and on the sodium-calcium exchanger. Sex differences are also present in the activity of membrane transporters and myocardial cytochrome P450 enzymes. Novel nongenomic actions of gonadal steroids have been identified.

Before puberty, boys with congenital LQTS have a 3- to 4-fold higher risk of cardiac events; after puberty, the sex risk reverses. Even so, an unexplained female prevalence of congenital LQTS exists, and female sex is considered an independent risk factor for the development of arrhythmias in patients with congenital LQTS. Compared with men, adult women (aged 18–40) who have LQTS have a 2.7-fold higher risk and a higher cumulative probability of aborted cardiac arrest and SCD (11% vs 3%). In addition, LQTS alleles are more frequently transmitted to daughters than to sons.

In a relatively small study of antiarrhythmic medication–induced torsades de pointes, 70% of patients were women even though only 44% of the drug prescriptions were registered to women. Torsades de pointes is more likely to develop in women not only from antiarrhythmic drugs but also from other medications. In 1 study, for example, QT interval prolongation due to erythromycin caused 67% more life-threatening ventricular arrhythmias in women than in men. The slower drug clearance in women could result in higher myocyte concentrations of blockers of the rapid component of the delayed rectifier potassium current and may explain the predisposition of women to drug-induced LQTS and torsades de pointes.

All these observations support the idea that pharmacologic trial data should be not only sex specific but also controlled for the hormonal status of enrolled women.

PAROXYSMAL SUPRAVENTRICULAR TACHYCARDIA

Women have more paroxysmal supraventricular tachycardia (PSVT) episodes than men and are more symptomatic with these episodes. Variation in PSVT inducibility is cyclic: PSVT episodes tend to be more inducible during the luteal phase of the menstrual cycle and during pregnancy, times when progesterone levels are elevated. A molecular basis for the proarrhythmic effects of progesterone has not been identified. Some authors suggest that there are changes associated with body temperature and increased sympathetic activity, which independently may be responsible for the increased incidence of PSVT. If PSVT is noninducible in a woman at her midcycle, it might thus be appropriate to repeat the electrophysiology study during menstruation. It has been suggested that higher levels of circulating progesterone influence the refractory period of both the slow pathway and the atrioventricular node.

A 2:1 female to male predominance of atrioventricular nodal reentrant tachycardia is known to exist. The 2 general times in a woman's life when a higher incidence of atrioventricular nodal reentrant tachycardia occurs relate to times of increased hormonal changes: during the third decade, when female sex hormone production peaks, and during menopause. In contrast, atrioventricular reentrant tachycardia occurs half as often in women as in men.

Does treatment differ between men and women? By the time women undergo ablation, they typically have had a longer history of tachyarrhythmias and have taken more antiarrhythmic medications than men. Yet studies on ablation document comparable efficacy, complications, and recurrences between the sexes. Dagres et al studied 894 patients undergoing radiofrequency ablation for supraventricular tachycardia and found that women presented at a mean (SD) of 185 (143) months after onset of symptoms, compared with 157 (144) months for men. In another study, the time from first onset of palpitations to invasive treatment was a mean of 5 years longer for women compared with men.

The delay in ablation for women might be related to the timing of the onset of symptomatic PSVT in women. Onset typically corresponds to the childbearing years; thus, radiation exposure may be delayed. Sometimes the symptoms of PSVT are attributed to anxiety attacks, which occur more frequently in younger women. Symptoms in menopausal women may be attributed to hot flashes. Physicians need to be aware of the efficacy of ablative procedures in women, the times when PSVT is most likely to be inducible, and the optimal timing of studies to ensure diagnostic accuracy and ablation success.

ATRIAL FIBRILLATION

In the Framingham study, men had a 1.5-fold higher risk of AF than women; however, since women live longer than men, the absolute number of women with AF was greater. About half of all patients with AF are women, and about 60% of patients with AF who are older than 75 years are women. The presence of AF tends to be an equalizer between men and women in terms of risk of death. AF diminishes a woman's survival advantage, with a 1.9-fold increased risk of death compared with women without AF; the comparable risk increase for men is 1.5-fold. Women with congestive heart failure (CHF) have a 14-fold increased risk of AF, compared with an 8.5-fold risk among men.

Women with AF tend to be more symptomatic than men with AF: Women with AF have higher mean heart rates and longer episodes, and they are more likely to have embolic strokes. The Euro Heart Survey on Atrial Fibrillation showed that at 1 year, women with AF had a higher stroke rate than men (2.2% vs 1.2%) and more major bleeding events (2.2% vs 1.3%). Reasons for the increased stroke risk in women are still unknown, but women have been shown to have a procoagulant milieu (eg, higher levels of prothrombin and von Willebrand factor).

In the ATRIA study, which prospectively followed 13,559 adults for 2.4 years, the annual rate of thromboembolism in patients not taking anticoagulant therapy was 3.5% in women and only 1.8% in men. Thus, women would most likely benefit more from appropriate anticoagulation than men. However, in the CARAF study, women were 54% less likely to receive warfarin compared with men but were twice as likely as men to receive aspirin. It is thought that women were treated less aggressively with anticoagulation because of their older age at presentation and the sense that the elderly are at higher risk of bleeding with anticoagulation, resulting in bias since there are no good supporting data against careful anticoagulation in the elderly.

A difference between the sexes seems apparent for rhythm control as well. Men are more likely to undergo cardioversion, although the documented success rate for cardioversion is the same for men and women. Recurrence of AF after successful direct current cardioversion is higher in women than in men (75.8% vs 67% at 2 years) perhaps because of the chronicity of AF in women by the time they are actually treated.

The Euro Heart Survey on Atrial Fibrillation showed that women tended to be treated less aggressively with fewer cardioversions and fewer catheter ablations, but men and women were treated similarly with anticoagulation (in contrast to the CARAF study). Women were usually older and had a longer history of AF and more comorbidities when they presented for ablation, yet the acute success rates and complications were no different between the sexes. Women who were referred for ablation had more concomitant structural heart disease, they were significantly older, and they were more symptomatic than their male counterparts.

The AF ablation success rates for men and women are similar (83.1% for women and 82.7% for men). Yet in 1 series of 3,477 AF ablation patients, only 939 (27%) were women. Among patients who had persistent AF, only 19% were women. In several studies that looked at referral for AF ablation, the women who were referred were older and had more comorbidities than the men.

Patel et al evaluated 3,265 patients who had pulmonary vein antrum isolation and noted that the referral rate for women was lower than for men. Women were more likely to have persistent AF and, most interestingly, were more likely to have nonpulmonary vein sites of firing than men (50.4% vs 16.3%) (Figure 1.1). The increased prevalence of nonpulmonary vein sites noted at ablation could be assumed to result from the chronicity of the AF in these women. Lee et al, however, showed that female sex was an independent predictor of nonpulmonary vein ectopic beats and a strong predictor of superior vena cava firing. Some studies have shown that female sex appears to be an independent predictor of catheter ablation complications for AF, with an increased incidence of hematomas and pseudoaneurysms. Although sex referral bias may have a role, operators should be aware of these observations during AF ablation procedures in women.

Earlier referral for ablation is appropriate because of the increased risk of drug-induced QT prolongation in women and the increased efficacy of early ablation. A substudy of the RACE trial showed that women randomly assigned to the rhythm-control group had more complications than men, a result likely due to the increased risk to women posed by QT-prolonging drugs.

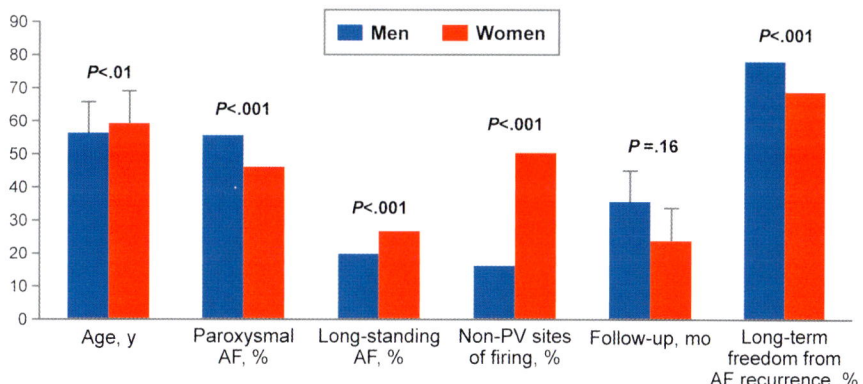

FIGURE 1.1. Differences Between Men and Women in Baseline Characteristics and Catheter Ablation Outcomes After Pulmonary Vein Isolation for Atrial Fibrillation. Patient age and follow-up data are mean values; error bars indicate standard deviations. AF indicates atrial fibrillation; PV, pulmonary vein. (Adapted from Santangeli P, di Biase L, Pelargonio G, Natale A. Outcome of invasive electrophysiological procedures and gender: are males and females the same? J CardiovascElectrophysiol. 2011 May;22[5]:605–12. Epub 2010 Oct 11. Used with permission.)

PACEMAKER IMPLANTATION AND MODE SELECTION

Considerable sex bias appears to be present in the pacemaker implantation literature. Women have a lower incidence of atrioventricular block and a higher incidence of sinus node dysfunction then men. This suggests that women would more likely benefit from dual-chamber pacing than men; however, Medicare data from 31,913 patients (1988–1990) showed that male sex was an independent predictor of dual-chamber and rate-responsive pacemaker implantations.

In a large 2010 study of 17,826 patients receiving pacemakers, 47.2% were women and 52.8% were men. Compared with similarly aged men, women aged 80 to 89 were more likely to receive VVI devices. Women were more likely to have acute complications, including pocket hematoma and pneumothorax (rates were more than double those for men); this finding was thought to reflect the smaller size of women compared with men. Women had longer hospital stays than men; the comments suggested that this finding was either from procedural complications or from "social situations."

In an editorial associated with the publication of that study, "gender bias" was noted in the older patient population by decreased appropriateness of device and mode selection. The editorial suggested that older women tend to prefer to avoid travel and are therefore more frequently treated in smaller, low-volume clinics closer to home, where pacemaker model and mode selection are not always optimal. Interestingly, after pacemakers were placed, women had better outcomes than men.

SUDDEN CARDIAC DEATH

The Framingham data showed that, compared with men, women have a lower incidence of SCD in all age groups—in fact, the incidence was less than half that of men. Women seem to have a 10- to 20-year delay in SCD events that then catches up to the rates for men. Women who have SCD tend to have less coronary artery disease (CAD) and present later in life. These sex differences can cause challenges in risk stratification and prevention for women if generalized SCD data are applied.

Women who present with SCD are more likely to have structurally normal hearts (10% compared with 3% in men). Women who have out-of-hospital cardiac arrest present more commonly with asystole and pulseless electrical activity

(PEA) rather than ventricular tachycardia (VT) or ventricular fibrillation. The success rate for resuscitation from PEA is less than 7%, while the success rate for resuscitation from VT or ventricular fibrillation can be as high as 40%. One suggested explanation for the increased rate of PEA in women is that there is a delay in obtaining life-supporting help for women who present with SCD. However, a study from Seattle and King County, Washington, showed that there were no sex-related differences in response time. Some data suggest that a history of syncope correlates with future PEA; this finding should be further evaluated to consider any clinical relevance for improved treatment and risk stratification for women.

In a retrospective study of out-of-hospital cardiac arrest survivors, left ventricular (LV) ejection fraction less than 40% was the strongest independent predictor of total and cardiac mortality for men but not for women. The SCD risk factors for women appear to be different from those for men, confirming the need to evaluate women separately from men and not to generalize SCD study findings across the sexes.

ICD STUDIES

The most obvious instances of sex bias and sex disparity appear to be related to ICD implantation. The proportion of women in ICD implantation studies has been remarkably low (Figure 1.2). In the first MADIT, only 8% of

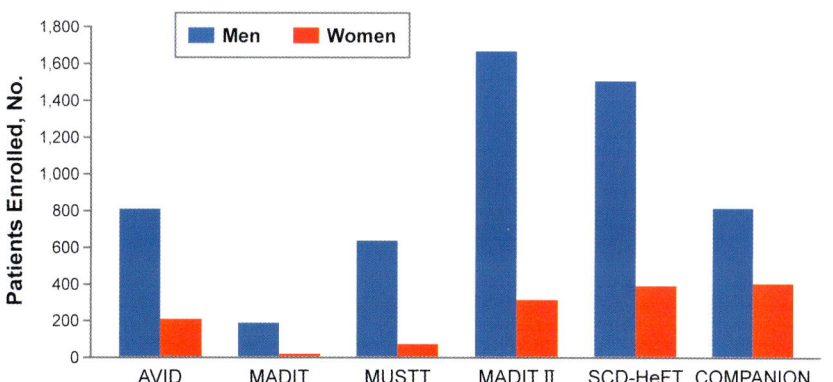

FIGURE 1.2. Total Enrollment of Men and Women in Implantable Cardioverter-Defibrillator Trials. (Adapted from Lampert R. Implantable cardioverter-defibrillator use and benefit in women. Cardiol Rev. 2007 Nov-Dec;15[6]:298–303. Used with permission.)

the enrolled patients were women; in MADIT-II, 16% were women. In the COMPANION trial, 32% were women, but in the CABG-Patch trial, only 10% were women.

Santangeli et al performed a meta-analysis of studies of ICD use in primary prevention that included 7,229 patients; of these patients, only 23% were women. The women had more severe CHF, they were less likely to receive renin-angiotensin system blockers, and they were less likely to undergo coronary revascularization procedures. This meta-analysis showed that there was a significant mortality reduction with ICD implantation in men but that the mortality reduction in women was inconclusive. One suspected cause for this inconclusive mortality reduction was late referral of women for implantation of an ICD for primary prevention.

The trend observed in these clinical trials—decreased use of an ICD for primary prevention in women—occurs in clinical practice. In the United States, about 2.4 million women and 2.5 million men have CHF. Thus, one would expect that relatively equal numbers of men and women with CHF would be enrolled in ICD trials, but that is not the case. In a study of Medicare beneficiaries, men were 3.2 times more likely than women to receive an ICD for primary prevention and 2.4 times more likely to receive an ICD for secondary prevention.

Women represent about 45% of the total prevalence of CAD and 41% of those with a history of myocardial infarction and fatal CAD in the United States, but they account for only about 20% of the study populations in ICD clinical trials of patients with CAD. In a review of the Medicare database from 1995 to 2005, Lampert et al found that 4 times as many men as women received ICDs. This bias was seen as early as the AVID study, in which male sex appeared to correlate with the decision to implant an ICD. In the Medicare database the number of ICDs implanted for primary prevention was 8.6 per 1,000 women and 32.3 per 1,000 men.

Do women benefit as much as men from ICD implantation? After ICD implantation, women have been shown to have significantly fewer appropriate shocks than men. This association has held true even though women have more aneurysmal and left anterior descending CAD. The difference in appropriate shocks appears likely to be related to VT substrate. Analysis of ICD shocks shows that VT, not ventricular fibrillation, is the more frequently treated arrhythmia. VT is more likely to occur with an anatomically stable VT circuit associated with structural heart disease, which occurs less frequently in women. Autonomic differences in arrhythmia triggering may be involved as well. Sex differences in the inducibility of sustained VT during an electrophysiology study have been identified; in the electrophysiology laboratory, VT was more likely to be inducible in men than in women (73% vs 39%) according to data from the University of Pennsylvania.

Lampert et al, in an evaluation of stored diagnostic information from 650 patients who had ICDs implanted, showed that 52% of men compared with 34% of women had VT or ventricular fibrillation requiring ICD therapy. The authors looked at potentially protective factors, commenting that although women had less diabetes mellitus and higher ejection fractions, sex remained an independent risk factor for appropriate ICD therapy. They also noted that women were more likely to have ventricular aneurysms, yet again ventricular arrhythmias occurred less often in women. These differences were not identified in patients who received ICD after cardiac arrest (secondary prevention).

The MUSTT data showed no differences in ICD therapy between sexes; however, only 10% of the randomly assigned patients and 16% of patients in the registry were women. Women were less likely to have inducible ventricular arrhythmias even after they were singled out for this study. Any real differences in sex outcome could have been missed because of the small sample size.

In the SCD-HeFT, mortality significantly decreased among men but not women. Women represented only 23% of the patients in this study, although the study was adequately powered to compare men and women for ICD benefit. An interesting potential bias in this study should be noted: Patients who had class III CHF did not show a benefit with the ICD, and this subgroup had a higher percentage of women than the others.

The use of ICDs in appropriate populations is surprisingly low for men and women. In a study that looked at 13,000 patients who had been admitted with systolic CHF and participated in the American Heart Association "Get With the Guidelines" program, only 35.4% had ICDs or planned ICDs, whether male or female. Apparently, CHF in women is not the same clinical disease as CHF in men. In the Medicare population, 79% of heart failure patients with preserved

LV function (ie, diastolic dysfunction) were women. This group has not been studied in terms of benefit for ICD implantation, suggesting both bias and disparity related to women's enrollment in ICD trials and treatment in clinical practice. In the past, physicians were less inclined to advise women to participate in ICD trials; to be fair, though, women may have refused trial participation more often than men. Nonetheless, the issue of ICDs being protective in patients with diastolic heart failure (more likely in women with CHF) has not been well evaluated.

CHRONIC RESYNCHRONIZATION PACING AND DEFIBRILLATOR THERAPY

Many of the sex bias and disparity issues with CRT in combination with defibrillator implantation are the same issues with ICD implantation, as noted earlier in this chapter. Women with CHF tend to present at an older age than men, and women are more likely to have heart failure with preserved LV function (ie, diastolic heart failure). Little or no data have been reported on the benefit of CRT for diastolic heart failure; nevertheless, a sex difference in the response to CRT appears to favor women.

The MIRACLE-ICD showed a significant difference in primary end points, with a decreased likelihood of reaching the combined end point of first CHF hospitalization or death for women but not for men. It may be that the higher prevalence of ischemic cardiomyopathy with scar in men complicates ideal LV lead placement. Of interest is that 32% of the patients enrolled in this study were women. This proportion is higher than in the primary prevention ICD trials with patients who had CAD most likely because patients with nonischemic cardiomyopathies were included.

For any given prolonged QRS duration, women seem to have more mechanical cardiac dyssynchrony than men. When sex differences in LV reverse remodeling were evaluated, female sex was independently associated with a better response to CRT: Women had a greater reduction in LV end-systolic volume. This observation may explain why women fare better than men in some CRT studies. While neither the CARE-HF nor the COMPANION trial showed a better response in women, a substudy of the MADIT-CRT trial did. When the use of CRT in combination with an ICD was compared with the use of an ICD alone in asymptomatic

CHF patients, the combination therapy was associated with a greater benefit in women (hazard ratio, 0.37; 95% CI, 0.22–0.61).

CONCLUSIONS

Both sex bias and sex disparities are apparent in the diagnosis and treatment of arrhythmias in women. Table 1.1 summarizes sex differences in clinical outcomes for some of the arrhythmias that have been discussed.

TABLE 1.1 Sex Differences in Clinical Outcomes

Invasive Procedure	Women	Men	Details
Catheter ablation of SVT	=	=	Similar outcome Higher incidence of AVNRT in women and of AVRT in men
Catheter ablation of atrial fibrillation	−	+	Better outcome in men Women present for catheter ablation when older, with a higher incidence of long-standing persistent atrial fibrillation and of nonpulmonary vein sites of firing
ICD therapy for the primary prevention of sudden cardiac death	−	+	No significant survival benefit with prophylactic ICD in women owing to a smaller impact of sudden cardiac death on overall mortality in women with severe left ventricular dysfunction
Cardiac resynchronization therapy	=/+	=/−	No significant sex differences in survival Women have a greater degree of left ventricular reverse remodeling after CRT

Abbreviations: AVNRT, atrioventricular nodal reentrant tachycardia; AVRT, atrioventricular reentrant tachycardia; CRT, cardiac resynchronization therapy; ICD, implantable cardioverter-defibrillator; SVT, supraventricular tachycardia; +, better outcome; −, worse outcome; =, similar outcome.

Adapted from Santangeli P, di Biase L, Pelargonio G, Natale A. Outcome of invasive electrophysiological procedures and gender: are males and females the same? J Cardiovasc Electrophysiol. 2011 May;22(5):605–12. Epub 2010 Oct 11. Used with permission.

Disparities in diagnosing and treating arrhythmias in women are real. Heart disease in women develops later than in men, and women have different kinds of heart disease than men. Women have less structural heart disease, more diastolic heart failure, and more sinus node disease. Perhaps it is not appropriate to consider the diagnosis and treatment of arrhythmias in men and women together. Perhaps some of these perceived differences are not bias but dissimilarity. Perhaps it is time to have studies of women only.

Evidence of bias exists. Women are often not encouraged to enroll in clinical trials; thus, they do not have the opportunity to benefit from the positive outcomes possible with new treatment options. It is important to remember that women do benefit from appropriate ICD implantation; from ablation for supraventricular tachycardia and, importantly, atrial fibrillation; and from pacemaker placement. Women are often older when they present with at least some arrhythmias, and therefore they may not be given appropriate treatment options—this observation may represent age bias as well as sex bias. Women tend to stay closer to home, perhaps to take care of their families, and they tend to go to smaller, closer, and potentially less sophisticated clinics, putting themselves at a disadvantage when it comes to health care.

What can physicians do? As physicians, we can remember that age, sex, and hormone status are important in arrhythmia diagnosis and treatment. As physicians, we can remember that women can have different drug responses. As physicians, we can offer similar arrhythmia diagnostic and treatment options to women and men. We can educate women to take care of themselves. Women tend to have mammograms, Papanicolaou tests, and even colonoscopies performed, and they should also be encouraged to have palpitations evaluated. We can abolish the idea that older women will not benefit from available treatment options. We can encourage women to go to high-volume centers for their procedures and support their involvement in clinical studies. Perhaps most importantly, we can change our current clinical paradigm and encourage more single-sex clinical studies.

SUGGESTED READING

Cook NL, Orav EJ, Liang CL, Guadagnoli E, Hicks LS. Racial and gender disparities in implantable cardioverter-defibrillator placement: are they due to overuse or underuse? Med Care Res Rev. 2011 Apr;68(2):226–46. Epub 2010 Sep 9.

Dagres N, Nieuwlaat R, Vardas PE, Andresen D, Levy S, Cobbe S, et al. Gender-related differences in presentation, treatment, and outcome of patients with atrial fibrillation in Europe: a report from the Euro Heart Survey on Atrial Fibrillation. J Am Coll Cardiol. 2007 Feb 6;49(5):572–7. Epub 2007 Jan 22.

Ghani A, Maas AH, Delnoy PP, Ramdat Misier AR, Ottervanger JP, Elvan A. Sex-based differences in cardiac arrhythmias, ICD utilisation and cardiac resynchronisation therapy. Neth Heart J. 2011 Jan;19(1):35–40.

Hu X, Wang J, Xu C, He B, Lu Z, Jiang H. Effect of oestrogen replacement therapy on idiopathic outflow tract ventricular arrhythmias in postmenopausal women. Arch Cardiovasc Dis. 2011 Feb;104(2):84–8. Epub 2011 Feb 17.

Jonsson MK, Vos MA, Duker G, Demolombe S, van Veen TA. Gender disparity in cardiac electrophysiology: implications for cardiac safety pharmacology. Pharmacol Ther. 2010 Jul;127(1):9–18. Epub 2010 May 10.

Lampert R. Implantable cardioverter-defibrillator use and benefit in women. Cardiol Rev. 2007 Nov-Dec;15(6):298–303.

Lampert R, McPherson CA, Clancy JF, Caulin-Glaser TL, Rosenfeld LE, Batsford WP. Gender differences in ventricular arrhythmia recurrence in patients with coronary artery disease and implantable cardioverter-defibrillators. J Am Coll Cardiol. 2004 Jun 16;43(12):2293–9.

Lee SH, Tai CT, Hsieh MH, Tsao HM, Lin YJ, Chang SL, et al. Predictors of nonpulmonary vein ectopic beats initiating paroxysmal atrial fibrillation: implication for catheter ablation. J Am Coll Cardiol. 2005 Sep 20;46(6):1054–9.

Michelena HI, Powell BD, Brady PA, Friedman PA, Ezekowitz MD. Gender in atrial fibrillation: ten years later. Gend Med. 2010 Jun;7(3):206–17.

Patel D, Mohanty P, Di Biase L, Sanchez JE, Shaheen MH, Burkhardt JD, et al. Outcomes and complications of catheter ablation for atrial fibrillation in females. Heart Rhythm. 2010;7(2):167–72. Epub 2009 Oct 23.

Santangeli P, di Biase L, Pelargonio G, Natale A. Outcome of invasive electrophysiological procedures and gender: are males and females the same? J Cardiovasc Electrophysiol. 2011 May;22(5):605–12. Epub 2010 Oct 11.

CHAPTER TWO

Women in Clinical Trials

JEANNE E. POOLE, MD

INTRODUCTION

Women have been underrepresented in every major randomized clinical trial examining arrhythmia management in patients with advanced cardiovascular disease. In 1986, the National Heart, Lung, and Blood Institute established a policy encouraging the inclusion of women in clinical trials. The mandate to include women in clinical research became public law through a section in the National Institutes of Health (NIH) Revitalization Act of 1993 (Public Law 103–43).

The NIH Department of Health and Human Services established the Office of Research on Women's Health in 1990. The goal of this office is to promote research on women's health and sex differences in NIH-funded studies and to promote and partner with women's health research in studies funded through alternate agencies and sources. Important in this effort is a mandate to provide sex-specific results and communicate the results of women's health research to the public.

NIH clinical trial applications must include a plan for ensuring the enrollment of women into the proposed clinical trial. This plan is an important aspect in determining the priority score given to the proposal. After the trial is approved and initiated, principal investigators must demonstrate ongoing efforts to reach a targeted enrollment of women (generally, 25%) and have plans to remedy recruitment into the trial if the target is not being reached. The NIH has provided information to assist investigators in achieving the goal of adequate female (and racial minority) enrollment.

Despite these efforts, the enrollment of women remains low. The reasons for this sex disparity are not entirely clear, although many explanations have been suggested, ranging from smaller proportions of women who are eligible for these trials to socioeconomic or psychosocial reasons.

Three decades of randomized clinical trials examining the role of antiarrhythmic drugs (AADs), implantable cardioverter-defibrillators (ICDs), and cardiac resynchronization therapy (CRT) have clarified the appropriate use of these interventions in broad populations of patients. Many of these studies are discussed in this chapter and summarized in Table 2.1 and Table 2.2. Hazard ratios and relative risk benefits are noted if they were provided in the trial publication.

RANDOMIZED CLINICAL TRIALS OF ANTIARRHYTHMIC DRUGS

CAST was one of the first important, large randomized clinical trials in complex arrhythmia management. It was conducted when ICD technology was in its infancy and limited to open thoracotomy procedures. AAD therapy was still considered the first line of treatment for ventricular arrhythmias and for prevention of sudden cardiac death (SCD). In the open-label CAST, 1,727 patients with prior myocardial infarction (MI) and asymptomatic or mildly symptomatic ventricular premature beats or nonsustained ventricular tachycardia (VT) were randomly assigned to receive flecainide, encainide, or moricizine. In the subsequent CAST II, 1,325 patients who also had reduced left ventricular function were randomly assigned to receive moricizine in a double-masked design. Women represented only 18% of all patients enrolled. Active drug therapy with flecainide or encainide was associated with increased all-cause mortality when the CAST study was terminated early, and no benefit was seen in patients treated with encainide in CAST II, which was also terminated early. In a subanalysis of covariables, an interaction between sex and mortality was not identified. Five other large, randomized clinical trials exploring the use of AAD therapy as a primary prevention strategy to reduce all-cause or SCD mortality were conducted over the following decade, 1 with D-sotalol and 4 with amiodarone.

In the double-blind, placebo-controlled SWORD trial, 3,121 patients (14% women) with left ventricular ejection fraction (EF) of 40% or less and either recent MI (within 6–42 days) or symptomatic heart failure (HF) were randomly assigned to receive D-sotalol. The study was terminated early because of

TABLE 2.1. Women in Antiarrhythmic Drug Randomized Clinical Trials

Trial (Mean or Median Follow-up)	Enrollment Population	Randomized Therapy	Patient Enrollment Total, No.	Patient Enrollment Women, %	Primary Outcome End Point	Primary Outcome	Interaction With End Point by Sex
CAST (10 mo) and CAST II (18 mo)	Prior MI; EF <40% if >90 d after MI (otherwise <55%); VPBs or NSVT	Placebo-controlled; flecainide, encainide, or moricizine	CAST: 1,725 CAST II: 1,325	18	All-cause mortality	Increased mortality with flecainide and encainide; 2.5-fold relative risk reduction (95% CI, 1.6–4.5; P<.001)	No significant interaction by sex
EMIAT (21 mo)	Acute MI (5–21 d); EF ≤40%	Placebo-controlled, double-blind; amiodarone	1,486	16	All-cause mortality	No significant difference (risk ratio, 0.99; P=.96)	No data on sex
CAMIAT (1.79±0.44 y[a])	Acute MI (6–45 d); ≥10 VPBs/h or VT	Placebo-controlled, double-blind; amiodarone	1,202	18	Resuscitated VF or arrhythmic death	Relative risk benefit with amiodarone, 48.5% (95% CI, 4.5–72.2; P=.016)	No significant interaction by sex
SWORD (148 d)	Acute MI (6–42 d) or symptomatic HF and MI >42 d; EF ≤40%	Placebo-controlled, double-blind; D-sotalol	3,121	14	All-cause mortality	Excess risk with D-sotalol (HR, 1.65; 95% CI, 1.15–2.36; P=.006)	Risk of death increased with dofetilide Women: 4.7-fold increased mortality (95% CI, 1.4–16.5) Men: 1.4-fold increased mortality (95% CI, 1.0–2.1)

(*continued*)

TABLE 2.1. (Continued)

Trial (Mean or Median Follow-up)	Enrollment Population	Randomized Therapy	Patient Enrollment Total, No.	Women, %	Primary Outcome End Point	Primary Outcome	Interaction With End Point by Sex
CHF-STAT (45 mo, 0–54 mo[b])	Moderate HF, CAD, or NIDCM; EF ≤40%; ≥10 VPBs/h	Placebo-controlled, double-blind; amiodarone	674	1.0	All-cause mortality	2-y actuarial survival: amiodarone, 69.4% (95% CI, 64.2–74.6); placebo, 70.8 (95% CI, 65.7–75.9; P=.6)	No data on sex
GESICA (13 mo)	CAD or NIDCM; EF ≤35%; NYHA class II-IV	Open-label; amiodarone	516	22	All-cause mortality	Relative risk benefit with amiodarone, 28% (95% CI, 4-45; P=.002)	No significant interaction by sex Men: relative risk reduction, 26% (95% CI, 2–46; P=.10) Women: relative risk reduction, 48% (95% CI, 0–75; P=.076)
SCD-HeFT (amiodarone or placebo patients, 45.5 mo)	CAD or NIDCM; EF ≤35%; NYHA class II or III	Placebo-controlled, double-blind; amiodarone	1,692	24	All-cause mortality	No significant difference (HR, 0.85; 95% CI, 0.65–1.11; P=.17)	No significant interaction by sex Men: HR, 1.04 (95% CI, 0.72–1.90) Women: HR, 1.17 (95% CI, 0.83–1.30)
COMET[c] (58 mo)	NYHA class II-IV	Double-blind; carvedilol vs metoprolol	3,029	20	All-cause mortality	Reduced mortality with carvedilol (HR, 0.83; 95% CI, 0.74–0.93; P=.002)	No significant interaction by sex Men: HR, 0.80 (95% CI, 0.70–0.91) Women: HR, 0.97 (95% CI, 0.73–1.27)

Study	Population	Design	N	Follow-up (mo)	Primary outcome	Results	Sex-specific findings
VALIANT amiodarone substudy[c] (24.7 mo)	12 h to 10 d after acute MI; HF; EF ≤35% or 40%	Double-blind, active-control; captopril or valsartan or captopril + valsartan Substudy analyzed amiodarone use in the randomized groups	14,700 analyzed in amiodarone substudy	31	All-cause mortality	Increased mortality with amiodarone use over the majority of the follow-up time	Adverse effect of amiodarone observed in both sexes; effect in women was limited to later follow-up
SAFIRE-D (12 mo)	AF or Aflutter	Placebo-controlled, dofetilide (3 doses)	273	14	Maintenance of SR at 1 y	Dofetilide associated with significant improvement in maintenance of SR compared with placebo	No data on sex
DIAMOND-CHF (18 mo)	NYHA class III or IV with recent new or worsened HF	Placebo-controlled, double-blind; dofetilide	1,518	27	All-cause mortality	No significant difference (HR, 0.95; 95% CI, 0.81–1.11)	No significant interaction by sex Men: HR, 1.00 (95% CI, 0.83–1.20) Women: HR, 0.85 (95% CI, 0.62–1.15)
ANDROMEDA (2 mo)	Symptomatic HF	Double-blind, placebo-controlled; dronedarone	627	25	All-cause mortality or HF hospitalization	Study terminated for increased risk with dronedarone (HR, 2.13; 95% CI, 1.07–4.25; P=.03)	No data on sex

(*continued*)

TABLE 2.1. (Continued)

Trial (Mean or Median Follow-up)	Enrollment Population	Randomized Therapy	Patient Enrollment Total, No.	Women, %	Primary Outcome End Point	Primary Outcome	Interaction With End Point by Sex
PALLAS (3.5 mo)	Permanent AF; age ≥65 y; major CV risk factors	Placebo-controlled, double-blind; dronedarone	3,236	35	1) Stroke, MI, systemic embolism, CV death *and* 2) Unplanned CV hospitalization or death	Study terminated for increased risk with dronedarone 1) HR, 2.29 (95% CI, 1.34–3.94; $P=.002$) 2) HR, 1.95 (95% CI, 1.34–2.62; $P<.001$)	No data on sex

Abbreviations: AF, *atrial fibrillation*; Aflutter, *atrial flutter*; CAD, *coronary artery disease*; CV, *cardiovascular*; EF, *ejection fraction*; HF, *heart failure*; HR, *hazard ratio*; MI, *myocardial infarction*; NIDCM, *nonischemic dilated cardiomyopathy*; NSVT, *nonsustained ventricular tachycardia*; NYHA, *New York Heart Association*; SR, *sinus rhythm*; VF, *ventricular fibrillation*; VPB, *ventricular premature beat*; VT, *ventricular tachycardia*.

[a] *Mean ± SD.*

[b] *Median and range.*

[c] *See text for discussion of amiodarone substudies.*

TABLE 2.2. Women in Implantable Cardiac Defibrillator Randomized Clinical Trials

Trial (Mean or Median Follow-up)	Enrollment Population	Randomized Therapy	Patient Enrollment Total, No.	Patient Enrollment Women, %	Primary Outcome End Point	Primary Outcome	Interaction With End Point by Sex
AVID (18.2±12.2 mo[a])	Cardiac arrest or syncopal VT if EF ≤40%	ICD or class III AADs	1,016	21	All-cause mortality	3.32-fold increased survival with ICD vs AAD (P=.02)	Substudy showed no significant difference by sex
CIDS (amiodarone patients, 2.9 y; ICD patients, 3.0 y)	Cardiac arrest or syncopal VT or symptomatic VT if EF ≤35%	ICD or amiodarone	659	15	All-cause mortality	Nonsignificant decrease with ICD; relative risk reduction, 19.7% (95% CI, 27.7–40; P=.142)	No significant interaction by sex
MADIT II (21 mo)	Prior remote MI; EF ≤30%	ICD or conventional therapy	1,232	15	All-cause mortality	Lower mortality with ICD (HR, 0.69; 95% CI, 0.51–0.93; P=.016)	No significant interaction by sex
DEFINITE (29.0±14.4 mo[a])	Nonischemic CM, EF ≤35%, VPBs or NSVT, NYHA class I-III	ICD or conventional medical therapy	916	29	All-cause mortality	ICD vs optimal medical therapy (HR, 0.65; 95% CI, 0.40–1.06; P=.08)	No significant interaction by sex
SCD-HeFT (45.5 mo)	Ischemic and nonischemic CM, EF ≤35%, NYHA class II or III	ICD or optimal HF medical therapy	1,676 randomly assigned to ICD or placebo	23	All-cause mortality	Lower mortality with ICD vs placebo (HR, 0.77; 95% CI, 0.62–0.96; P=.007)	No significant interaction by sex Women: HR, 0.96 (95% CI, 0.58–1.61) Men: HR, 0.73 (95% CI, 0.57–0.93)

(*continued*)

TABLE 2.2. (Continued)

Trial (Mean or Median Follow-up)	Enrollment Population	Randomized Therapy	Patient Enrollment Total, No.	Patient Enrollment Women, %	Primary Outcome End Point	Primary Outcome	Interaction With End Point by Sex
DINAMIT (30±13 mo[a])	Recent MI (6–40 d), EF <35%, depressed HRV or elevated heart rate	ICD or conventional medical therapy	674	24	All-cause mortality	No significant difference for primary end point (HR, 1.08; 95% CI, 0.76–1.44; P=.66)	No significant interaction by sex
IRIS (37 mo)	Recent MI (5–31 d), EF ≤40% and heart rate ≥90 bpm and/or NSVT at ≥150 bpm during Holter monitoring	ICD or conventional medical therapy	898	24	All-cause mortality	No significant difference for primary end point (HR, 1.04; 95% CI, 0.81–1.35; P=.78)	No significant interaction by sex
COMPANION (range, 11.9–16.2 mo)	Ischemic or nonischemic CM, NYHA class III or IV, EF ≤35%, QRS ≥120 ms	CRT-P, CRT-ICD, or optimal HF medical therapy	1,520	33	All-cause mortality and hospitalization for any cause	Improved outcome with CRT-ICD vs optimal HF medical therapy (HR, 0.80; P=.01) and with CRT-P vs optimal HF medical therapy (HR, 0.81; P=.014)	No significant interaction by sex
CARE-HF (29.4 mo)	Ischemic CM or NIDCM, NYHA class III or IV, EF ≤35%, QRS ≥120 ms	CRT-P or optimal medical therapy	813	27	All-cause mortality and unplanned CV hospitalization	Improved outcome with CRT-P (HR, 0.63; 95% CI, 0.51–0.77; P<.001)	No significant interaction by sex Men: HR, 0.62 (95% CI, 0.49–0.79) Women: HR, 0.64 (95% CI, 0.42–0.97)

Study	Inclusion criteria	Intervention	N	Women, %	Primary end point	Main results	Sex-specific results
MADIT-CRT (2.4 y)	Ischemic or nonischemic CM, NYHA class I or II, EF ≤30%, QRS ≥130 ms	CRT-ICD or ICD	1,820	26	All-cause mortality or nonfatal HF event	CRT-ICD associated with improved outcome (HR, 0.66; 95% CI, 0.52–0.84; P=.001)	Significant interaction by sex Women: HR, 0.37 (95% CI, 0.22–0.61) Men: HR, 0.76 (95% CI, 0.59–0.97) (P=.01 for the interaction)
REVERSE (12 mo)	NYHA class I or II, LVEDD 0.55 mm, EF ≤40%, QRS ≤120 ms	CRT-ICD: active CRT (n=419) or control (n=191)	610	21	1) HF clinical composite response 2) LV end-systolic volume index	Active CRT not associated with a significant difference in the primary end point compared with control (P=.10)	No significant interaction by sex Men: HR, 0.69 (95% CI, 0.43–1.11) Women: HR, 0.75 (95% CI, 0.26–2.19)
RAFT (40 mo)	NYHA class II or III, EF ≤30%, QRS ≥120 ms	ICD alone or ICD plus CRT	1,798	17	All-cause mortality or HF hospitalization	CRT-ICD associated with improved primary outcome (HR, 0.75; 95% CI, 0.64–0.87; P<.001)	No significant interaction by sex (P=.09)

Abbreviations: AAD, antiarrhythmic drug; *bpm*, beats per minute; *CM*, cardiomyopathy; *CRT*, cardiac resynchronization therapy; *CRT-P*, cardiac resynchronization therapy pacemaker; *CV*, cardiovascular; *EF*, ejection fraction; *HF*, heart failure; *HR*, hazard ratio; *HRV*, heart rate variability; *ICD*, implantable cardioverter-defibrillator; *LV*, left ventricular; *LVEDD*, left ventricular end-diastolic dimension; *MI*, myocardial infarction, *NIDCM*, nonischemic dilated cardiomyopathy; *NSVT*, nonsustained ventricular tachycardia; *NYHA*, New York Heart Association; *VPB*, ventricular premature beat; *VT*, ventricular tachycardia.

[a] *Mean ± SD.*

excess mortality (accounted for entirely by arrhythmic mortality) among the patients receiving D-sotalol. Mortality was highest among patients with EF of 31% to 40% (compared with <30%). In a subanalysis of this study, D-sotalol was associated with a 4.7-fold increased risk of death for women (95% CI, 1.4–16.5) compared with a 1.4-fold increased risk of death for men (95% CI, 1.0–2.1).

Two trials evaluated amiodarone as a primary prevention AAD in patients after recent MI: the CAMIAT and the EMIAT. In the double-blind, placebo-controlled CAMIAT, 1,202 patients who were survivors of MI with frequent or repetitive ventricular premature beats or VT were randomly assigned to receive amiodarone. The use of amiodarone was associated with a significant 48.5% relative risk reduction in the primary end point of resuscitated ventricular fibrillation or arrhythmic death. Only 213 women (18% of the total enrollment) were enrolled in the CAMIAT study. The risk reduction by sex was 45% for male patients and 51% for female patients, a difference that was not statistically significant. In the double-blind, placebo-controlled EMIAT, 1,486 survivors of MI with left ventricular EF of 40% or less were randomly assigned to receive amiodarone. The primary end point was all-cause mortality, and the secondary end point was cardiac mortality and arrhythmic death. Amiodarone was associated with a 35% relative risk reduction for arrhythmic death, but no significant difference was observed for all-cause mortality or cardiac mortality. The 232 enrolled women represented 16% of the patient population; an interaction between the outcomes and sex was not reported.

Two large, randomized trials studied amiodarone therapy as a primary prevention strategy for reducing all-cause mortality among patients with moderate HF: the CHF-STAT and the GESICA trial. In the double-blind, placebo-controlled CHF-STAT, 674 patients who had EF of 40% or less, frequent premature ventricular beats, and ischemic or nonischemic moderate HF were randomly assigned to receive a moderate dose of amiodarone. All patients were treated with optimal HF medication therapy. Amiodarone use was not associated with a difference in the primary end point of overall mortality or in SCD, but amiodarone was significantly more effective at reducing ventricular arrhythmias when compared with placebo drug and optimal HF medication therapy alone. Only 1.0% of the patients (7 of 674) enrolled in the CHF-STAT were women, which is not surprising, given that this trial was conducted at US Veterans Administration Hospitals. In the open-label GESICA study, 516 patients, of which 114 (22%) were women, were randomly assigned to receive amiodarone. All patients had advanced chronic HF and reduced left ventricular EF (≤35%). Amiodarone use was associated with a significant reduction in the primary end point of all-cause mortality and hospital admission rates. No significant difference in the primary end point was observed between sexes (relative risk reduction, 26% for men and 48% for women).

A subsequent meta-analysis of amiodarone randomized clinical trials included 6,553 patients. This analysis, which comprised the 4 trials discussed earlier and an additional 9 studies of amiodarone therapy in patients who had experienced an MI or in patients who had HF, showed a significant reduction in total mortality ($P=.03$) and SCD mortality ($P<.001$) without an effect on nonarrhythmic death. Altogether, 17% of enrollees in this meta-analysis were women. A significant difference by sex was not observed for either total mortality or SCD mortality.

More recent clinical trials have raised concern about the safety of amiodarone in higher-risk patients. The SCD-HeFT was a 3-arm, double-blind, placebo-controlled trial with patients who were in New York Heart Association (NYHA) HF functional class II or III and who had ischemic or nonischemic dilated cardiomyopathy and EF of 35% or less. Patients were randomly assigned in equivalent proportions to receive an ICD or amiodarone. Of the 1,692 enrolled patients who received amiodarone or placebo, 24% (398) were women. Amiodarone was not associated with a reduction in all-cause mortality, and there was no difference in this outcome according to sex (men: hazard ratio [HR], 1.04; 95% CI, 0.72–1.90) (women: HR, 1.17; 95% CI, 0.83–1.30). However, among the 497 patients in NYHA class III, amiodarone was associated with an increase in all-cause mortality compared with the placebo drug (HR, 1.44; 95% CI, 1.05–1.97), with an equivalent effect regardless of sex (men: HR, 1.42; 95% CI, 1.00–2.01) (women: HR, 1.46; 95% CI, 0.70–3.04).

Excess mortality associated with amiodarone therapy has been observed in 2 other large randomized clinical trials. In a substudy of the COMET, 155 NYHA class II patients (of 1,466 total) and 209 NYHA class III or IV patients (of 1,563 total) were taking amiodarone at baseline entry into the trial. The trial randomly assigned 3,029 patients to receive carvedilol or metoprolol over a 58-month median follow-up. On multivariable analysis, a significant mortality difference was observed between patients who received amiodarone and those who did not ($P<.001$); the difference did not vary according to NYHA class. The excess mortality was entirely due to increased HF deaths (HR, 2.4; 95% CI, 1.9–3.1; $P<.001$), and arrhythmic death was not different between those who took amiodarone and those who did not. Women represented 20% of all patients enrolled in COMET; an effect of sex on outcomes with amiodarone was not reported.

Amiodarone was also assessed in a substudy of the VALIANT trial. VALIANT enrolled 14,700 patients (31% women) who had experienced an acute MI and who had left ventricular systolic dysfunction or HF. Patients were randomly assigned to receive valsartan or captopril or both. The primary outcome of VALIANT showed no difference in the randomized therapies on the outcome of all-cause mortality. In the substudy of amiodarone use, the outcomes for 14,700 patients were analyzed. At baseline, 825 patients (29% women) were treated with amiodarone and 13,875 patients (31% women) were not. Amiodarone was associated with an increase in early and late all-cause mortality and an increase in cardiovascular mortality. Among the female patients, amiodarone was associated only with decreased late mortality.

Two newer AADs have been studied in randomized clinical trials to test their benefit for atrial fibrillation. Dofetilide is a class III AAD approved by the US Food and Drug Administration for use in atrial fibrillation management. The SAFIRE-D trial was a placebo-controlled efficacy study that randomly assigned patients to receive dofetilide. Women represented 14% of the 273 patients enrolled in the SAFIRE-D trial; specific sex effects were not reported in this study.

The safety of dofetilide was assessed in 1,518 high-risk HF patients in the DIAMOND-CHF study. A significant difference between dofetilide and placebo was not observed in the primary end point of all-cause mortality. Women represented 27% of the patients enrolled in DIAMOND-CHF. No significant differences in mortality were observed between the sexes.

Dronedarone, an AAD indicated for atrial fibrillation, has electrophysiologic properties similar to those of amiodarone, but it lacks the iodine molecule. The safety of dronedarone was challenged after the results of the ANDROMEDA study were available. The study was terminated early after only 7 months of enrollment for excess deaths associated with dronedarone. A total of 627 patients were enrolled, of which 25% were women. The primary end point was all-cause mortality or hospitalization for HF. The excess deaths were associated with worsening HF and not with arrhythmic deaths or SCDs. Among covariates analyzed, the most significant predictor of death was treatment with dronedarone (HR, 2.13; 95% CI, 1.07–4.25; P=.03). Subanalysis by sex was not reported.

The concerns identified in ANDROMEDA were further supported by findings from the PALLAS trial, which evaluated the efficacy of dronedarone in patients with permanent atrial fibrillation. In this placebo-controlled study, 3,236 patients (35% women) who had permanent atrial fibrillation and major cardiovascular risk factors were randomly assigned to receive dronedarone. The study was terminated early because of excess risk associated with the use of dronedarone. Sex-specific differences were not reported.

RANDOMIZED CLINICAL TRIALS OF ICD THERAPY

As in the randomized clinical trials examining the role of AADs for primary prevention of SCD, women have been underrepresented in the randomized trials of ICD therapy in high-risk patients. The AVID trial was a large, multicenter US trial that enrolled patients who had survived cardiac arrest due to ventricular fibrillation, syncopal VT, or symptomatic VT (if EF ≤40%). Women represented 21% of the 1,016 patients enrolled in the trial. AVID showed that the use of an ICD was associated with improved survival compared with treatment with an AAD (primarily amiodarone). In a subsequent substudy, no difference in 1-year mortality was noted between women and men. Women were younger, more women had nonischemic heart disease, and more women had ventricular fibrillation rather than VT as the index arrhythmia.

The CIDS was a similar trial with 659 patients who had a history of cardiac arrest, syncopal VT, or symptomatic VT if the patient's EF was 35% or less and who were randomly assigned to receive an ICD or amiodarone therapy. Women represented 16% of the trial participants. The trial did not reach statistical significance for the primary end point of all-cause mortality despite a relative risk reduction of 19.7% in favor of ICD therapy.

The results of MADIT II and SCD-HeFT established the ICD securely as a primary prevention strategy for SCD in patients with moderate HF. In MADIT II, women and men experienced a similar benefit with ICD therapy (HR, 0.57 vs 0.66). Similarly, in SCD-HeFT, there was no significant difference in ICD benefit by sex, although the benefit for women was less than that observed for men (women: HR, 0.96; 95% CI, 0.58–1.61) (men: HR, 0.73; 95% CI, 0.57–0.93). In a subsequent substudy, women in SCD-HeFT were more likely to have nonischemic dilated cardiomyopathy compared with men (66% vs 43%) and were more likely to have NYHA class III HF compared with men (36% vs 26%). One additional explanation for the findings in SCD-HeFT was an observed lower mortality rate in the placebo arm for women compared with men; thus, the benefit of the ICD would be more difficult to demonstrate in women randomly assigned to receive ICD therapy. DEFINITE was a randomized trial of ICD therapy (compared with conventional medical therapy) for patients who had only nonischemic dilated cardiomyopathy. Although a statistically significant end point was not reached, ICD therapy was associated with a relative risk reduction of 35% in favor of ICD therapy. No difference in outcome by sex was observed.

Two trials have examined the role of ICD therapy in patients who have had a recent MI: the DINAMIT and the IRIS trial. Neither study demonstrated a benefit of ICD therapy on the end point of all-cause mortality, and neither study demonstrated a sex-specific difference in all-cause mortality. In each study, 24% of the enrolled patients were women.

Enrollment of women has been higher in the trials of CRT. The COMPANION study enrolled 1,520 patients, of which 33% were women, and the CARE-HF study enrolled 813 patients, of which 27% were women. Both trials enrolled patients with NYHA class III or IV HF, reduced EF, and a prolonged QRS interval. In each study, an interaction by sex was not observed for the primary outcome.

CRT-ICD therapy has been evaluated further in several large randomized clinical trials enrolling HF patients who are less ill according to the NYHA classification (REVERSE, RAFT, and MADIT-CRT). REVERSE was a crossover design trial evaluating 610 patients (21% women) who received a CRT-ICD. Patients were randomly assigned to CRT functionality (active CRT or control). Active CRT was associated with a nonsignificant ($P=.10$) improvement in the primary end point of HF clinical composite response, with no difference noted according to sex.

The RAFT enrolled 1,798 patients (17% were women) who had NYHA class II or III HF symptoms, EF of 30% or less, and a QRS duration of 120 ms or more (or a paced QRS duration ≥200 ms). Patients were randomly assigned to receive an ICD alone or an ICD in combination with CRT. The combination of an ICD with CRT was associated with an improvement in the primary outcome of all-cause death or hospitalization for HF (HR, 0.75; $P<.001$).

The MADIT-CRT enrolled patients with ischemic or nonischemic cardiomyopathy, NYHA class I or II HF, and EF of 30% or less. Patients who received an ICD in combination with CRT had a significant benefit in end-point events (all-cause mortality or nonfatal HF events) compared with those who received only an ICD. Female sex (26% of enrollees), compared with male sex, was associated with a significantly improved benefit from ICD-CRT therapy independently of QRS width (women: HR, 0.37; 95% CI, 0.22–0.61) (men: HR, 0.76; 95% CI, 0.59–0.97) ($P=.01$ for the interaction).

SUMMARY

Women have been underrepresented in all clinical trials examining the role of AADs, ICDs, and CRT. Few studies identified a significant sex-specific interaction since the trials were not powered to examine subgroup effects on the primary outcomes. The appropriate method to interpret any trial, in the absence of adequately powered trials, is to apply the results of the parent trial to the subgroups included in the trial. Trends of benefit within subgroups, including subgroups of sexes, are at best hypothesis generating. Given the recognized differences in cardiac disease prevalence and type between women and men, the question remains as to whether women would benefit from the studied therapy to the same extent as men. The ideal trial would be powered to detect differences in benefit or risk by sex.

To achieve adequate enrollment of women in randomized clinical trials, considerable effort needs to be directed toward a better understanding of the obstacles to enrollment. Barriers to enrollment may involve the physician or the patient. The benefits and risks of a trial may need to be presented to women in language that is different from that used with men. Addressing obstacles of transportation and frequency of study visits may be important to allow women, who are often the family caregivers, to dedicate their time to a clinical trial.

Initiatives must be undertaken to identify real solutions to the problem of enrollment of women into clinical trials. At a minimum, the reporting of sex-specific results should be included in all publications. Partnering of major stakeholders (eg, the NIH and the US Food and Drug Administration) with organizations interested in this issue (eg, WomenHeart, the American Heart Association Go Red for Women campaign, the American College of Cardiology, and the Heart Rhythm Society) is critical for identifying enrollment barriers and providing practical solutions. Without such efforts, we may never understand the relative benefits and risks of commonly used arrhythmia management strategies in women.

SUGGESTED READING

Bardy GH, Lee KL, Mark DB, Poole JE, Packer DL, Boineau R, et al; Sudden Cardiac Death in Heart Failure Trial (SCD-HeFT) Investigators. Amiodarone or an implantable cardioverter-defibrillator for congestive heart failure. N Engl J Med. 2005 Jan 20;352(3):225–37. Erratum in: N Engl J Med. 2005 May 19;352(20):2146.

Geller SE, Adams MG, Carnes M. Adherence to federal guidelines for reporting of sex and race/ethnicity in clinical trials. J Womens Health (Larchmt). 2006 Dec;15(10):1123–31.

Hayes SN, Redberg RF. Dispelling the myths: calling for sex-specific reporting of trial results. Mayo Clin Proc. 2008 May;83(5):523–5.

Inclusion of women and minorities in clinical research. [Website on the Internet]. [cited 2013 Mar 6]. Bethesda (MD): National Institutes of Health. Available from: http://orwh.od.nih.gov/research/inclusion/index.asp.

Moss AJ, Hall WJ, Cannom DS, Klein H, Brown MW, Daubert JP, et al; MADIT-CRT Trial Investigators. Cardiac-resynchronization therapy for the prevention of heart-failure events. N Engl J Med. 2009 Oct 1;361(14):1329–38. Epub 2009 Sep 1.

Moss AJ, Zareba W, Hall WJ, Klein H, Wilber DJ, Cannom DS, et al; Multicenter Automatic Defibrillator Implantation Trial II Investigators. Prophylactic implantation of a defibrillator in patients with myocardial infarction and reduced ejection fraction. N Engl J Med. 2002 Mar 21;346(12):877–83. Epub 2002 Mar 19.

Office of Research on Women's Health [Website on the Internet]. [cited 2013 Mar 6]. Bethesda (MD): National Institutes of Health. Available from: http://orwh.od.nih.gov/.

CHAPTER THREE

Genetic and Hereditary Considerations for Arrhythmias in Women

OHAD ZIV, MD, AND
ELIZABETH S. KAUFMAN, MD

INTRODUCTION

As the molecular basis for cardiac electrophysiology has become more clearly understood, the importance of heritable factors in the clinical manifestation of cardiac arrhythmias has become more apparent. The role of heritable factors may be subtle, as in atrial fibrillation (AF), or obvious, as in short QT syndrome (SQTS) and long QT syndrome (LQTS). It is also apparent that sex hormones exert an influence on cardiac electrophysiology. Cardiac myocytes have been found to express receptors to estrogen, progesterone, and testosterone. This chapter focuses on the intersection of the influence of heritable effects and sex effects on cardiac arrhythmias.

THE EFFECTS OF HORMONES ON THE QT INTERVAL

One of the most important differences between men and women in cardiac electrophysiology is the QT interval. As early as 1920, Bazett noted that the QT interval was longer in women. Subsequent electrocardiographic population studies supported the finding that when corrected for the heart rate, QT intervals in women were longer than in men. Furthermore, there is evidence that this difference in QT interval is directly related to differences in sex hormones. Receptors to estrogen, androgens, and progesterone have all been found in cardiac ventricular myocytes in several animal studies. Numerous studies have contributed to understanding more of the complex effects of sex hormones on the QT interval. However, the important aspects of these complex interactions can be distilled into a few key, clinically relevant points.

First, estrogen prolongs the QT interval. The initial observation that supported this finding was from human data. Women have a longer corrected QT interval (QTc) during the follicular phase, which is marked by an increased level of estrogen alone, than during the luteal phase, which is associated with an increased level of progesterone and a more modest increase in the estrogen level. A more recent population study echoed this finding, showing that QT intervals of postmenopausal women treated with estrogen-only hormone replacement therapy were significantly longer than those of women treated with estrogen in combination with progesterone. In the basic laboratory, estrogen exposure has reduced the rapid component of the delayed rectifier potassium current (I_{Kr}). The slow component of the delayed rectifier potassium current (I_{Ks}) is not affected by estrogen.

Second, estrogen appears to reduce repolarization reserve. *Repolarization reserve* is defined as a natural redundancy in the repolarization currents in ventricular myocytes. With this redundancy, a reduction in any single current has little effect on the overall change in repolarization and therefore little change in the QT interval. Thus, exposure to estrogen (with concomitant reduction in I_{Kr}) appears to make cardiac cells and, similarly, individuals, more susceptible to QT prolongation when exposed to a QT-prolonging drug. This notion is supported by Rodriguez and colleagues, who showed that the QT response to ibutilide infusion varied depending on the phase of women's menstrual cycles. In women in the follicular phase, with unopposed estrogen, the QT prolongation was more pronounced.

Third, both animal and human data suggest that testosterone and progesterone have the opposite effect of estrogen on the QT interval and ventricular repolarization. During infancy and childhood, there appears to be no sex difference in the QTc duration. At puberty, the QTc shortens in male adolescents by 20 ms. In animal laboratory studies, testosterone appears to increase repolarization reserve and thus reduce the QT-prolonging effects of I_{Kr}-blocking drugs such as dofetilide. Progesterone also shortens the action potential duration of cardiac myocytes,

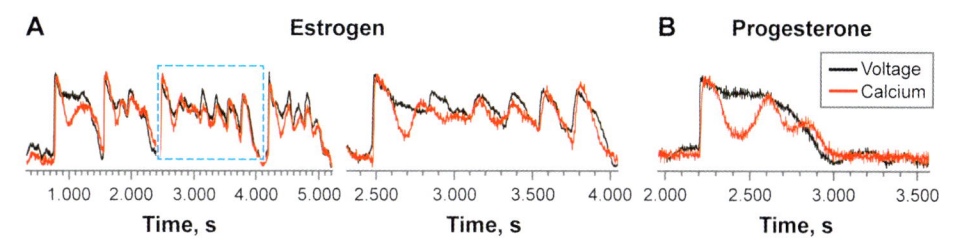

FIGURE 3.1. Hormonal Effects in a Long QT Syndrome Type 2 (LQT2) Rabbit Model. Tracings show voltage (black) and calcium (red) fluorescence signals from perfused whole hearts of transgenic LQT2 rabbits. Rabbits were exposed long-term to either estrogen (panel A) or progesterone (panel B). During short-term experiments, hearts were exposed to isoproterenol (both panel A and panel B). A, Left tracings show the first beat with a long action potential duration, a following beat with an early afterdepolarization, and 2 subsequent episodes of torsades de pointes. The section outlined by dashed lines is enlarged in the right tracing in panel A. Thus, under estrogen exposure, isoproterenol induces torsades de pointes readily in LQT2 hearts. B, An example of progesterone treatment is shown under the same isoproterenol condition. Despite calcium oscillations, no early afterdepolarization is seen and torsades de pointes is prevented. (From Odening KE, Choi BR, Liu GX, Hartmann K, Ziv O, Chaves L, et al. Estradiol promotes sudden cardiac death in transgenic long QT type 2 rabbits while progesterone is protective. Heart Rhythm. 2012 May;9[5]:823–32. Epub 2012 Jan 11. Used with permission.)

increases repolarization reserve, and, in both animal and computer modeling studies, reduces the likelihood of early afterdepolarizations. Odening and colleagues at the Cardiovascular Research Center at Brown University (Providence, Rhode Island) showed that treating LQTS rabbit hearts with progesterone reduced the onset of ventricular arrhythmias and the rate of sudden death. In this rabbit model, progesterone shortened the QT interval and reduced early afterdepolarizations (Figure 3.1). This model has led to the notion that progesterone and progesterone-type substances may be useful as antiarrhythmic medications in the future. In the basic laboratory, progesterone appears to increase I_{Ks}, while testosterone appears to increase I_{Kr}.

CONGENITAL AND ACQUIRED LQTS

Congenital LQTS

Given our understanding of the effects of hormones on QT, it is not surprising that there are marked sex differences in the manifestations of congenital and acquired LQTS. Among children with congenital LQTS, the risk of cardiac events (syncope and sudden cardiac death) is higher for boys than for girls. Boys with congenital LQTS type 1 (*KCNQ1* mutations causing loss of function in I_{Ks}) are at especially high risk. During adolescence, however, the sex and risk relationship changes, with the risk of cardiac events being higher for women than for men. This is especially true for women with congenital LQTS type 2 (*KCNH2* mutations causing loss of function in I_{Kr}), who, compared with men, have a markedly higher risk of both syncope and sudden death. This risk is increased during the postpartum period and persists during menopause. In LQTS type 3 (*SCN5A* mutations causing gain of function in the cardiac inward sodium channel [I_{Na}]), there does not appear to be a sex predisposition to syncope and sudden death, either in childhood or in adulthood. The other genetic subtypes of LQTS are relatively rare, and little is known about the sex effect on their clinical manifestations.

The interaction of sex and genotype appears to be quite complex. For example, a recent study compared event rates for men and women with respect to the type of LQTS type 2 mutation they carried. Men had a 2-fold higher risk of an event if they had a mutation in the pore region, compared with a mutation elsewhere. In contrast, the event rate for women was independent of the location of the mutation. One interpretation of these results is that pore mutations, which generally cause a greater reduction in I_{Kr} than nonpore mutations, are sufficient to cause events in men or women. Nonpore mutations are more likely to cause events in women, whose repolarization reserve is already compromised by the effect of estrogen on I_{Kr}.

LQTS and Shifts in Sex Hormones

Changes in hormone levels over a woman's lifetime also influence the risk of cardiac events in LQTS. Large changes in hormone levels occur during pregnancy and the postpartum period. In the first 9 months postpartum, the risk of cardiac events increases dramatically, especially for women with LQTS type 2. Figure 3.2 shows the steep increase in the event rate after childbirth.

At menopause, another large shift in hormone exposure occurs. A study from the International LQTS Registry showed that for women with LQTS type 1, the event rate may decrease after menopause. In contrast, women with LQTS type 2 have a dramatic increase in the risk of syncope after menopause. Estrogen replacement therapy did not appear to change the event rate for

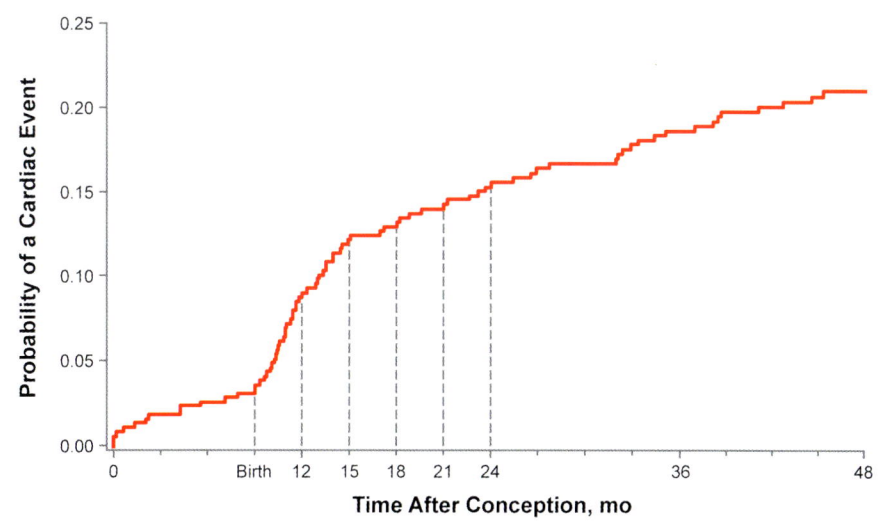

FIGURE 3.2. Probability of a Cardiac Event in Postpartum Women With Long QT Syndrome. The curve shows the increased probability of a cardiac event occurring within 48 months after conception. (From Seth R, Moss AJ, McNitt S, Zareba W, Andrews ML, Qi M, et al. Long QT syndrome and pregnancy. J Am CollCardiol. 2007 Mar 13;49[10]:1092–8. Epub 2007 Feb 27. Used with permission.)

women with LQTS type 1 or 2. As suggested by the study's authors, multiple factors may account for the different effects of menopause in LQTS types 1 and 2. Loss of testosterone in the presence of continued low-level extragonadal estrogen may reduce I_{Kr} without changing I_{Ks}, leading to a more profound effect on women with LQTS type 2. In addition, older adults tend to be less vigorously active than young adults (exercise is a trigger for arrhythmic events in LQTS type 1). Bradycardia, a trigger for arrhythmia in LQTS type 2, is more prevalent in the elderly.

Acquired LQTS

While congenital LQTS commonly results from disease-causing mutations in any of several genes, acquired LQTS is only rarely associated with subclinical mutations in the known congenital LQTS genes. More frequently, acquired LQTS occurs in individuals with more prevalent polymorphisms that usually do not cause disease in the absence of environmental provocation, such as drug exposure or electrolyte disorders. These individuals have a decreased repolarization reserve. In the presence of potentially QT-prolonging drugs (nearly all of which block I_{Kr}),

QT prolongation and torsades de pointes are more likely to develop in women than in men. In fact, up to two-thirds of drug-related torsades de pointes cases occur in women. Female sex remains a risk predictor for torsades de pointes even after adjusting for weight, renal function, and QTc. The steeper QT–RR interval relationship in women may explain this finding. In women, who have lower levels of I_{Kr} compared with men and thus depend more on I_{Ks} for repolarization, QT prolongation is most marked during bradycardia, causing particular vulnerability to torsades de pointes.

GENETIC BASES AND SEX DIFFERENCES IN OTHER INHERITED ARRHYTHMOGENIC DISEASES

Sex differences and differences in exposure to sex hormones are important in other inherited arrhythmogenic diseases. Like LQTS, Brugada syndrome, SQTS, and catecholaminergic polymorphic ventricular tachycardia (CPVT) are diseases caused by inherited mutations in genes coding for ion channels in the heart.

Brugada Syndrome

Brugada syndrome is most often caused by loss-of-function mutations in the *SCN5A* gene, which codes for the cardiac I_{Na} channel. These mutations lead to shorter repolarization in the right ventricle than in the left ventricle. This change shows up as a typical ST-segment elevation pattern in the early precordial leads on electrocardiography. Clinically apparent Brugada syndrome has been reported to be 8 to 10 times more prevalent in men than in women. In this case, the shortening of the QT interval by testosterone may worsen the shortening of the right ventricular repolarization and in turn contribute to the arrhythmogenic phenotype. Indeed, men with clinically evident Brugada syndrome have higher testosterone levels than age-matched controls. Conversely, one may speculate that QT prolongation associated with estrogen exposure may be clinically protective in women when associated with a loss-of-function *SCN5A* mutation. This protection may partly explain the male predominance of Brugada syndrome.

Short QT Syndrome

Like Brugada syndrome, SQTS manifests more often in men than in women. SQTS has been associated with several inherited mutations. In general, a mutation resulting in loss of inward current or gain of outward current may result in SQTS. Clinical manifestations of this syndrome include aborted cardiac arrest, syncope, AF, and family history of cardiac arrest. SQTS patients are 3 times more likely to be men than women. Women are slightly more likely than men to be asymptomatic carriers of the mutation, which is inherited as an autosomal dominant trait. The male predominance of the disease is explained by the hormonal effects on cardiac repolarization; in women, QT interval prolongation from estrogen may be protective.

Catecholaminergic Polymorphic Ventricular Tachycardia

CPVT is an inherited arrhythmogenic disease most often caused by a mutation in the ryanodine receptor that leads to diastolic calcium leak in cardiac myocytes. This leak results in pleomorphic ventricular tachycardia and ventricular fibrillation. From several studies, this disease appears to be equally prevalent in men and women. However, women tend to present at an older mean age and are less likely to present with aborted cardiac arrest. The cause of this difference in presentation is likely multifactorial. However, it is worth noting that testosterone increases the L-type calcium current while progesterone decreases it. From this simplified viewpoint, cardiomyocytes in men may be more susceptible to calcium overload. Further research is needed to decipher the full underlying cause of the clinical sex difference in CPVT and the interactions of genotypes and sex in Brugada syndrome and SQTS.

AF AND OTHER SUPRAVENTRICULAR TACHYCARDIAS

Atrial Fibrillation

By far, the most common narrow complex tachycardia is AF. AF affects an estimated 0.4% of the population. However, over half of these patients may have only a single episode. The prevalence of AF is higher for men than women across all age groups. In addition, in postcardiothoracic surgery series, AF was more likely to develop in men than in women. This finding suggests that the higher propensity for the arrhythmia in men may persist when accounting for comorbidities associated with AF. In 1 population study, AF patients had a shorter QTc than their age-matched controls. Given that women have a longer QTc than men in general, it is tempting to consider the longer QTc in women as a protective factor. While AF appears to occur less often in women, the prognosis for women with AF appears to be worse than for men. Thromboembolic events are more likely to occur in women than in men. Furthermore, in the Framingham cohort, women who had AF had a higher risk of death compared with men who had AF. The use of antiarrhythmic medications, especially class III agents, and the higher proarrhythmic potential in women may confound this finding.

While the sex difference in AF prevalence is suggestive of a hereditary electrophysiologic difference, the genetics of AF are extremely complex, and the interaction of sex, genetics, and AF is poorly understood. Monogenetic mutations have been found in families with AF, but these are rare cases. These single mutations have been found in genes encoding sodium channels (*SCN5A*, *SCN1B*, and *SCN2B*), potassium channels (*KCNQ1*, *KCNE2*, *KCNJ2*, *KCNE5*, and *KCNA5*), and connexin 40. More recently, genome-wide association studies have suggested the correlation of certain polymorphisms with AF. Examples of these findings are a locus near the transcription factor *PITX2* gene, which is important for left atrial differentiation, and a locus within the *KCNN3* gene, encoding for a calcium-dependent potassium channel. Further work is required to delineate the interaction of genetics, sex, and AF.

Regular Narrow Complex Tachycardia

Among regular supraventricular tachycardias (SVTs), atrioventricular (AV) nodal reentrant tachycardia (AVNRT) is the most common, accounting for an estimated two-thirds of these arrhythmias in adults. AVNRT is caused by reentry within the AV node, with the slow and fast pathways of the AV node constituting the reentrant circuit limbs. AVNRT has a 2:1 female predominance. AV reciprocating tachycardia is the second most common regular SVT. It results from reentry through the AV node as the antegrade limb and through a bypass tract as the retrograde limb. Bypass tracts may be concealed or manifest on the electrocardiogram. Manifest bypass tracts, as seen in Wolff-Parkinson-White syndrome, are twice as likely to be present in men than in women. Generally, sex is a poor predictor of SVT mechanism; furthermore, prognosis and treatment of these arrhythmias are identical in men and women. In both sexes, these arrhythmias are treatable and usually curable.

THE ROLE OF GENETIC TESTING

Genetic testing can be extremely helpful when it is performed and interpreted in a proper clinical context. If performed apart from this context, genetic testing can be confusing and misleading. The 2 primary reasons to perform genetic testing are to refine a clinical diagnosis and to screen family members when a family's pathogenic mutation is known.

As an example, consider an asymptomatic 20-year-old woman with a QTc of 510 ms and a family history of LQTS. For this patient, genetic testing will not be used to confirm or fail to confirm the diagnosis of LQTS—the diagnosis is clear. However, knowledge of the genetic subtype will be beneficial for risk stratification. If the subtype is LQTS type 1, β-blocker therapy alone will likely be highly protective. If the subtype is LQTS type 2, this young woman's risk is higher, and therapies beyond β-blocker medication should be considered. The mutation reported should be considered pathogenic or likely pathogenic for the results to be meaningful. A genetic polymorphism that is also found in many healthy individuals should not be assumed to be pathogenic.

After the mutation has been identified, the woman's first-degree relatives, especially those without convincing evidence of LQTS, can undergo testing for the pathogenic mutation. A negative genetic result in a phenotypically normal relative can reassure that individual that further evaluation, lifestyle restriction, and medication are not needed. A positive genetic result should lead to individualized advice for the affected individual and to screening of that individual's other first-degree relatives.

Genetic testing is not useful if good clinical evidence does not exist for the disease being tested and if the family's mutation is not known. The sensitivity and specificity of genetic testing are not high enough to support this kind of use and can result in confusion and misdirection. As an example, consider a 45-year-old woman with syncope, significant nonsustained ventricular tachycardia, and inducible polymorphic ventricular tachycardia who was treated by her local electrophysiologist with an implantable cardioverter-defibrillator. Because she had borderline QT prolongation on a single electrocardiogram, she underwent genetic testing and was found to have a mutation of uncertain significance on the gene responsible for LQTS type 12. Her 3 children were referred for consideration of genetic testing. On further evaluation, neither she nor the children had clinical evidence of LQTS. However, the patient and her oldest son did have right ventricular enlargement. It is unlikely that LQTS is the correct diagnosis for this patient. Testing of the children for her "mutation of uncertain significance" would be fruitless; a positive result would not confirm presence of disease, while a negative result might offer false reassurance, since the test would not be probing for the right disease.

While genetic testing has facilitated diagnosis for many patients, the interpretation and explanation of genetic results remain complex. It is advisable for genetic testing to be performed by a knowledgeable physician who can address the ambiguities that may arise. A genetic counselor can be an extremely helpful member of the team.

SUGGESTED READING

Benito B, Sarkozy A, Mont L, Henkens S, Berruezo A, Tamborero D, et al. Gender differences in clinical manifestations of Brugada syndrome. J Am Coll Cardiol. 2008 Nov 4;52(19):1567–73.

Buber J, Mathew J, Moss AJ, Hall WJ, Barsheshet A, McNitt S, et al. Risk of recurrent cardiac events after onset of menopause in women with congenital long-QT syndrome types 1 and 2. Circulation. 2011 Jun 21;123(24):2784–91. Epub 2011 May 31.

Burke JH, Ehlert FA, Kruse JT, Parker MA, Goldberger JJ, Kadish AH. Gender-specific differences in the QT interval and the effect of autonomic tone and menstrual cycle in healthy adults. Am J Cardiol. 1997 Jan 15;79(2):178–81.

Goldenberg I, Moss AJ, Peterson DR, McNitt S, Zareba W, Andrews ML, et al. Risk factors for aborted cardiac arrest and sudden cardiac death in children with the congenital long-QT syndrome. Circulation. 2008 Apr 29;117(17):2184–91. Epub 2008 Apr 21.

Napolitano C, Bloise R, Monteforte N, Priori SG. Sudden cardiac death and genetic ion channelopathies: long QT, Brugada, short QT, catecholaminergic polymorphic ventricular tachycardia, and idiopathic ventricular fibrillation. Circulation. 2012 Apr 24;125(16):2027–34.

Odening KE, Hyder O, Chaves L, Schofield L, Brunner M, Kirk M, et al. Pharmacogenomics of anesthetic drugs in transgenic LQT1 and LQT2 rabbits reveal genotype-specific differential effects on cardiac repolarization. Am J Physiol Heart Circ Physiol. 2008 Dec;295(6):H2264–72. Epub 2008 Oct 3.

Probst V, Veltmann C, Eckardt L, Meregalli PG, Gaita F, Tan HL, et al. Long-term prognosis of patients diagnosed with Brugada syndrome: Results from the FINGER Brugada Syndrome Registry. Circulation. 2010 Feb 9;121(5):635–43. Epub 2010 Jan 25.

Rautaharju PM, Zhou SH, Wong S, Calhoun HP, Berenson GS, Prineas R, et al. Sex differences in the evolution of the electrocardiographic QT interval with age. Can J Cardiol. 1992 Sep;8(7):690–5.

Rodriguez I, Kilborn MJ, Liu XK, Pezzullo JC, Woosley RL. Drug-induced QT prolongation in women during the menstrual cycle. JAMA. 2001 Mar 14;285(10):1322–6.

Sauer AJ, Moss AJ, McNitt S, Peterson DR, Zareba W, Robinson JL, et al. Long QT syndrome in adults. J Am Coll Cardiol. 2007 Jan 23;49(3):329–37. Epub 2007 Jan 4.

Seth R, Moss AJ, McNitt S, Zareba W, Andrews ML, Qi M, et al. Long QT syndrome and pregnancy. J Am Coll Cardiol. 2007 Mar 13;49(10):1092–8. Epub 2007 Feb 27.

Tsai CT, Lai LP, Hwang JJ, Lin JL, Chiang FT. Molecular genetics of atrial fibrillation. J Am Coll Cardiol. 2008 Jul 22;52(4):241–50.

Zareba W, Moss AJ, Locati EH, Lehmann MH, Peterson DR, Hall WJ, et al; International Long QT Syndrome Registry. Modulating effects of age and gender on the clinical course of long QT syndrome by genotype. J Am Coll Cardiol. 2003 Jul 2;42(1):103–9.

CHAPTER FOUR

Sex-Specific Electrophysiologic Properties

CHRISTINE TANAKA-ESPOSITO, MD, AND MINA K. CHUNG, MD

INTRODUCTION

Clinical and experimental observations suggest that myocardial tissue has sex-specific electrophysiologic properties. These differences, listed in Table 4.1, have important clinical implications and raise special therapeutic considerations in the management of arrhythmias in women.

ELECTROPHYSIOLOGIC PROPERTIES

Heart Rate

Sex-related differences apparent on the surface electrocardiogram have been recognized since 1920. Bazett observed that women have higher average resting heart rates than men, a finding corroborated by multiple subsequent studies. This difference in heart rate is apparent in the pediatric population as young as 5 years and persists into adulthood.

Burke and colleagues studied heart rate before and after pharmacologic-induced autonomic blockade at rest and during exercise in healthy young

TABLE 4.1. Sex-Related Electrophysiologic Differences

Electrophysiologic Property	Sex Difference
Resting heart rate	Female > Male
Corrected QT interval	Female > Male
P-wave duration	Male > Female
Atrial-His interval	Male > Female
His-ventricular interval	Male > Female

adults. Intrinsic heart rate remained higher in women, suggesting perhaps an inherent difference in sinus node automaticity determined by factors independent of the autonomic nervous system. These investigators also studied the relationship between phases of the menstrual cycle and heart rate trends in this same cohort of women. Heart rates were significantly lower during menses, when estrogen and progesterone levels are at a nadir, than during the luteal and follicular phases.

Ventricular Repolarization

Since the initial description by Bazett, numerous studies have reported that women have a longer corrected QT interval (QTc) than men despite having higher resting heart rates. Burke and colleagues reported that the sex difference in the QTc persists even after autonomic blockade, suggesting an intrinsic sex difference in ventricular repolarization (Table 4.2).

Using a validated computer algorithm, Merri and colleagues identified and quantified several electrocardiographic features of ventricular repolarization in a cohort of healthy adults. Prolongation of the early portion of repolarization, measured from the end of the S wave to the peak of the T wave, seemed to account for the longer QT intervals in women. Moreover, lengthening of this segment accounted for the disproportionate increase in ventricular repolarization at slower heart rates. Stramba-Badiale and colleagues subsequently quantified QT intervals in healthy participants under ambulatory conditions. They likewise showed that differences in the QT interval between the sexes were most marked during bradycardia.

TABLE 4.2. Corrected QT Intervals[a] by Sex, Autonomic State, and Menstrual Phase[b] or Visit Number[c]

Autonomic State and Sex	Menses or Visit 1	Follicular Phase or Visit 2	Luteal Phase or Visit 3	Mean (SD)
Baseline				
Women	421 (10)	423 (18)	420 (18)	421 (16)
Men	410 (15)	415 (18)	415 (13)	414 (15)
After autonomic blockade				
Women	446 (15)	444 (13)	438 (16)	443 (15)
Men	436 (12)	438 (12)	435 (13)	437 (12)

[a] Values are mean (SD) expressed in milliseconds.

[b] For women.

[c] For men.

Adapted from Burke JH, Ehlert FA, Kruse JT, Parker MA, Goldberger JJ, Kadish AH. Gender-specific differences in the QT interval and the effect of autonomic tone and menstrual cycle in healthy adults. Am J Cardiol. 1997 Jan 15;79(2):178–81. Used with permission.

Significant sex-related differences in the pattern of ventricular repolarization both globally and regionally have been shown in a cohort of healthy young adults. Using vectoral transformation, Smetana and colleagues characterized repolarization heterogeneity patterns. In striking contrast to men, women showed an inverse sequence pattern of global repolarization heterogeneity: Ventricular myocytes that were the last to depolarize were the first to repolarize. Moreover, even on a localized scale, the repolarization patterns of women showed greater heterogeneity.

Age-associated sex differences in the QTc suggest an influence of gonadal sex hormones. Rautaharju and colleagues studied 14,379 children and adults, ranging in age from birth through 75 years, and found a sex-related divergence in the QTc, which occurred from adolescence to age 50 years. At puberty, the

QTc shortened in male participants. It then increased linearly until midlife (Figure 4.1).

Data derived from castrated men and from women with virilization syndromes suggest a relationship between androgens and ventricular repolarization. Men with hypogonadism had longer corrected JT intervals than other men, and, consistent with this observation, women with hyperandrogenism had shorter corrected JT intervals than other women.

Moreover, in a cohort of hypogonadic men, Charbit and colleagues showed that exogenous testosterone administration shortened the QTc. With each man serving as an internal control, a significant inverse relationship was found between the QTc duration and the plasma free testosterone index.

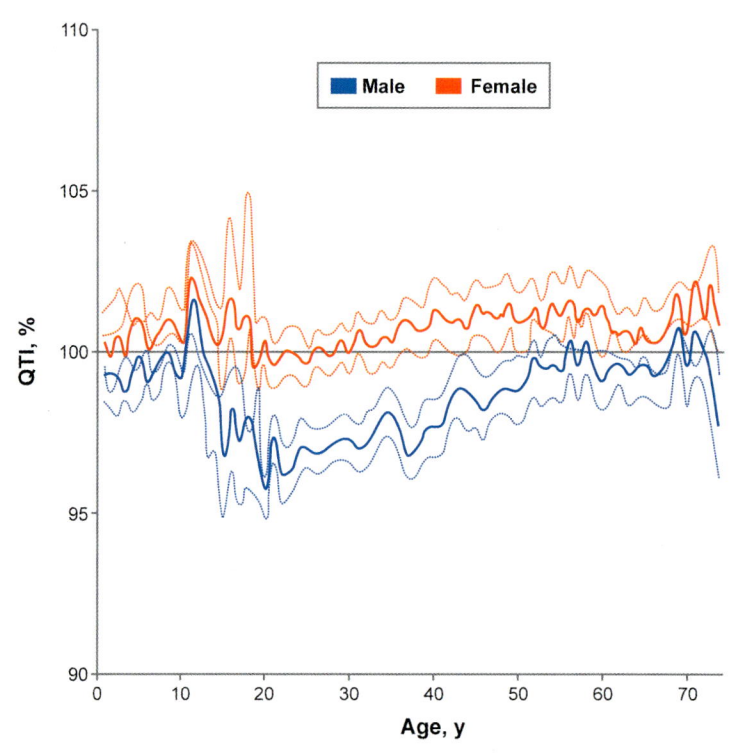

FIGURE 4.1. Mean QT Index (QTI) Values for Female and Male Participants. QTI = (QT/QTp) × 100, where QTp is the QT interval predicted from the formula QTp=656/(1+0.01 × heart rate). The 95% CIs (dotted lines) were calculated for each age subinterval of 1 year for male and female participants. The rate-corrected QT values for male participants distinctly decreased after puberty and then increased linearly through much of adult life.

(Adapted from Rautaharju PM, Zhou SH, Wong S, Calhoun HP, Berenson GS, Prineas R, et al. Sex differences in the evolution of the electrocardiographic QT interval with age. Can J Cardiol. 1992 Sep;8[7]:690–5. Used with permission.)

Conduction and Refractoriness

Sex-related differences in the atrial, atrioventricular nodal, and infranodal conduction system have been reported. However, these observations were primarily descriptions from cohorts of patients with clinical arrhythmias presenting for electrophysiologic study. Thus, it is not clear whether these findings represent true differences between the sexes or distinctions within a selected subpopulation.

Dhala and colleagues described longer P-wave duration among men. Differences in atrial effective refractory period have also been reported, with premenopausal women having significantly shorter atrial refractory periods than both their age-matched male and postmenopausal female counterparts. Taneja and colleagues reported that His-ventricular intervals and QRS duration were significantly longer in men. However, cardiac mass was not independently assessed in this study. S. Liu and colleagues similarly showed increased conduction times in men, who had longer atrial-His and His-ventricular intervals. These investigators found clear differences between the sexes in left ventricular mass normalized for body surface area, suggesting that the differences in conduction time could reflect greater distances of propagation.

POTENTIAL MECHANISMS

Electrophysiologic differences between the sexes likely have an important role in the recognized sex-related differences in the incidence of clinical arrhythmias. Although the exact mechanisms are yet to be fully elucidated, experimental studies with animal models have provided insight into possible mechanisms that underlie these sex-related differences (Table 4.3). The gonadal hormones have been at the forefront of these investigations. Differences in sex hormone levels exist throughout the human lifespan and are detectable even in utero. Yet, one cannot exclude the possibility of intrinsic genetic-based differences between the sexes that act independently of the sex hormones or confer a distinct response to the sex hormones.

TABLE 4.3. Potential Mechanisms Underlying Sex-Related Electrophysiologic Differences

Possible Mechanisms	Sex Difference
Autonomic responsiveness	Female > Male
Estrogen: ↑ muscarinic receptor density and affinity	
Estrogen: ↑ production of acetylcholine	
Estrogen: ↓ production of norepinephrine and epinephrine	
Ventricular myocyte (outward I_K)	Male > Female
Testosterone: ↑ I_K density	
Estrogen: ↓ I_K density	
Ventricular myocyte (↑ $I_{Ca,L}$, transmural gradient)	Female > Male
Ventricular myocyte (↑ $I_{Ca,L}$, base-apex gradient)	Female > Male
Testosterone: ↓ $I_{Ca,L}$	
Increased cardiac mass	Male > Female

Abbreviations: $I_{Ca,L}$, L-type calcium current; I_K, potassium current.

Autonomic Nervous System

The autonomic nervous system exerts a constant modulatory effect on the cardiac conduction system. Sex differences in the functioning of the autonomic nervous system have been described. In general, parasympathetic responsiveness is greater in females, while sympathetic responsiveness is greater in males. Accumulating evidence suggests that sex hormones have significant effects on the regions of the brain involved in cardiovascular regulation and the peripheral neurons of the autonomic nervous system.

Neurons containing estrogen, progesterone, and testosterone receptors have been described in brain centers that regulate cardiovascular function. In ovariectomized female and male rats, Rainbow and colleagues showed that intracerebral administration of estrogen increased vagal tone and suppressed sympathetic efferent activity by increasing the density and affinity of muscarinic receptors. This effect was blunted in the presence of a selective estrogen receptor antagonist.

Moreover, sex hormones regulate the synthesis and clearance of neurotransmitters in the central nervous system and in the peripheral nervous system. While testosterone promotes synthesis of catecholamines through a stimulatory effect on tyrosine hydroxylase, estrogen exerts an inhibitory effect. Additionally, estrogen enhances the production of acetylcholine.

Other mechanisms leading to sex differences in tissue responsiveness to neurotransmitters may exist. For example, differences in regulatory presynaptic receptors or neuronal transporters that uptake or degrade released neurotransmitters could account for differing responsiveness of the sympathetic and parasympathetic nervous systems between the sexes. And certainly, there may be inherent sex differences in how the myocardium and specialized conducting tissue respond to autonomic input.

Ionic Basis for Sex-Related Differences

The ionic basis for apparent sex-based differences in the atria and specialized conducting tissue is not well understood. Much of the focus has been on mechanisms that underlie the differences in ventricular repolarization. Sex differences in ventricular repolarization have been striking in nearly all species studied to date. Data from animal and human models support the premise that differences exist in cardiac cellular action potential electrogenesis. Voltage clamp data from several species consistently show sex-related differences in the major repolarizing potassium and calcium currents.

Like human hearts, rabbit hearts show sex-specific differences in the QTc. Using patch clamp techniques, X. K. Liu and colleagues recorded membrane currents of individual ventricular myocytes isolated from these hearts. Ventricular myocytes from females, compared with those from males, showed significantly smaller outward potassium currents. Given that outward potassium channels are major determinants of repolarization, this finding could explain at least in part the difference in QT interval observed between the sexes.

Using similar techniques, Pham and colleagues found sex differences in the transmural distribution of the L-type calcium current ($I_{Ca,L}$). They described higher $I_{Ca,L}$ density in myocytes isolated from the epicardium of hearts from adult female rabbits compared with those from adult male rabbits. In contrast, there was no sex difference in the density of $I_{Ca,L}$ in cells from the endocardium. Sims and colleagues further characterized sex-related differences in the regional dispersion of $I_{Ca,L}$. While $I_{Ca,L}$ density was significantly higher in myocytes isolated from the base of the left ventricle of females compared with males, there was no apparent sex-specific difference in cells taken from the apex. This base-apex gradient in $I_{Ca,L}$, seen only in cardiomyocytes from adult females, correlated with different levels of expression of calcium channel protein CaV 1.2α in these regions.

Androgens

Accumulating data support a key role for androgens. X. K. Liu and colleagues, studying orchiectomized male rabbits, found that administration of exogenous dihydrotestosterone attenuated rate-induced QT lengthening and increased the density of repolarizing potassium currents.

Classically, testosterone is thought to act as a transcription factor through binding to the androgen receptor. A novel nontranscriptional mode of regulation by testosterone has been elegantly described. Using an isolated ventricular myocyte model, Bai and colleagues showed that testosterone, administered at doses consistent with men's physiologic levels, shortened the action potential duration. This effect was due to augmentation of slowly activating potassium current (I_{Ks}) and suppression of $I_{Ca,L}$. These effects of testosterone were reversed by either an inhibitor of nitric oxide synthase or a scavenger of nitric oxide. The findings support the premise that testosterone, through cytosolic nitric oxide–dependent pathways, shortens repolarization by modulating I_{Ks} and $I_{Ca,L}$.

Estrogens

Although less clear, some data do suggest that ovarian hormones may also be important. Limitations of studies that reported the effects of the estrogen on prolonging the action potential and altering the ionic currents included the administration of estrogen at doses higher than physiologic concentrations. Other results are conflicting and difficult to reconcile partly because of the use of animal models, which have various estrous cycles and levels of ovarian hormones.

A study by Saito and colleagues, which accounted for these variables, supports a potentially important role for estrogen in modulating ventricular repolarization. They used a mouse model and compared male mice with female mice during 2 phases: proestrus, when the estrogen level is highest, and diestrus, when the estrogen level is lowest. Plasma estrogen concentrations were quantified. Action potential duration and QTc directly correlated with estrogen levels. They were longest in female mice in proestrus and shortest in male mice; female mice in diestrus had intermediate values. Repolarizing outward potassium currents were inversely related to plasma estrogen levels. Lower potassium current densities under conditions of higher estrogen levels were attributed to lower densities of I_{Ks} and fast transient outward current ($I_{to,f}$). This in turn was associated with lower levels of channel protein transcripts. These findings suggest a mechanistic role of estrogen in the transcriptional downregulation of potassium channel proteins.

Furthermore, studies have shown that right ventricular outflow tract tachycardia occurs in women more often than in men. In 1 study, 11 pregnant women experienced new-onset ventricular arrhythmias or premature ventricular contractions that originated from the right ventricular outflow tract. The frequency of premature ventricular contractions decreased by more than 95% in 83% of the patients during pregnancy; couplets and ventricular tachycardia disappeared completely in all patients during the postpartum period. The QTc did not change through the pregnancy. High levels of estrogen and progesterone during pregnancy may be the factors predisposing pregnant women to ventricular arrhythmia. In contrast, lower levels of estrogen may facilitate ventricular arrhythmias in postmenopausal women. Hu and colleagues found that the mean (±SD) concentration of estradiol was significantly lower in postmenopausal patients with outflow tract tachyarrhythmia than in control postmenopausal women (8.4±3.4 vs 36.9±12.8 pg/mL, $P<.001$). The burden of ventricular arrhythmias was significantly higher in postmenopausal patients than in controls (10,171±6,091 vs 209 ±468 per 24 hours, $P<.001$). After 3 months of estrogen replacement therapy, the ventricular arrhythmia count was significantly reduced.

CONCLUSION

Although data so far suggest that the gonadal sex hormones are key in the mechanisms that underlie the sex differences in human electrophysiology, other mechanisms that are independent of the sex hormones probably exist. For instance, hearts in men and women might differ in their responses to stimuli such as the gonadal steroids or in their basic electrophysiologic nature. A unique population of cells in the midmyocardium, M cells, have been shown to contribute to the heterogeneity of repolarization in the human ventricle. Sex-specific characterization of this cell type has not been done. While data particularly from animal models have provided insight into the sex differences, further work is needed to fully elucidate the underlying mechanisms.

SUGGESTED READING

Bai CX, Kurokawa J, Tamagawa M, Nakaya H, Furukawa T. Nontranscriptional regulation of cardiac repolarization currents by testosterone. Circulation. 2005 Sep 20;112(12):1701–10. Epub 2005 Sep 12.

Bidoggia H, Maciel JP, Capalozza N, Mosca S, Blaksley EJ, Valverde E, et al. Sex differences on the electrocardiographic pattern of cardiac repolarization: possible role of testosterone. Am Heart J. 2000 Oct;140(4):678–83.

Charbit B, Christin-Maitre S, Demolis JL, Soustre E, Young J, Funck-Brentano C. Effects of testosterone on ventricular repolarization in hypogonadic men. Am J Cardiol. 2009 Mar 15;103(6):887–90. Epub 2009 Jan 24.

Courant F, Aksglaede L, Antignac JP, Monteau F, Sorensen K, Andersson AM, et al. Assessment of circulating sex steroid levels in prepubertal and pubertal boys and girls by a novel ultrasensitive gas chromatography-tandem mass spectrometry method. J Clin Endocrinol Metab. 2010 Jan;95(1):82–92. Epub 2009 Nov 20.

Dhala A, Underwood D, Leman R, Madu E, Baugh D, Ozawa Y, et al; Multicenter PHi-Res Study. Signal-averaged P-wave analysis of normal controls and patients with paroxysmal atrial fibrillation: a study in gender differences, age dependence, and reproducibility. Clin Cardiol. 2002 Nov;25(11):525–31.

Hu X, Wang J, Xu C, He B, Lu Z, Jiang H. Effect of oestrogen replacement therapy on idiopathic outflow tract ventricular arrhythmias in postmenopausal women. Arch Cardiovasc Dis. 2011 Feb;104(2):84–8. Epub 2011 Feb 17.

Liu S, Yuan S, Kongstad O, Olsson SB. Gender differences in the electrophysiological characteristics of atrioventricular conduction system and their clinical implications. Scand Cardiovasc J. 2001 Oct;35(5):313–7.

Liu XK, Katchman A, Whitfield BH, Wan G, Janowski EM, Woosley RL, et al. In vivo androgen treatment shortens the QT interval and increases the densities of inward and delayed rectifier potassium currents in orchiectomized male rabbits. Cardiovasc Res. 2003 Jan;57(1):28–36.

Merri M, Benhorin J, Alberti M, Locati E, Moss AJ. Electrocardiographic quantitation of ventricular repolarization. Circulation. 1989 Nov;80(5):1301–8.

Pham TV, Robinson RB, Danilo P Jr, Rosen MR. Effects of gonadal steroids on gender-related differences in transmural dispersion of L-type calcium current. Cardiovasc Res. 2002 Feb 15;53(3):752–62.

Rainbow TC, Degroff V, Luine VN, McEwen BS. Estradiol 17 beta increases the number of muscarinic receptors in hypothalamic nuclei. Brain Res. 1980 Sep 29;198(1):239–43.

Saito T, Ciobotaru A, Bopassa JC, Toro L, Stefani E, Eghbali M. Estrogen contributes to gender differences in mouse ventricular repolarization. Circ Res. 2009 Aug 14;105(4):343–52. Epub 2009 Jul 16.

Sims C, Reisenweber S, Viswanathan PC, Choi BR, Walker WH, Salama G. Sex, age, and regional differences in L-type calcium current are important determinants of arrhythmia phenotype in rabbit hearts with drug-induced long QT type 2. Circ Res. 2008 May 9;102(9):e86–100. Epub 2008 Apr 24.

Smetana P, Batchvarov VN, Hnatkova K, Camm AJ, Malik M. Sex differences in repolarization homogeneity and its circadian pattern. Am J Physiol Heart Circ Physiol. 2002 May;282(5):H1889–97.

Stramba-Badiale M, Locati EH, Martinelli A, Courville J, Schwartz PJ. Gender and the relationship between ventricular repolarization and cardiac cycle length during 24-h Holter recordings. Eur Heart J. 1997 Jun;18(6):1000–6.

Taneja T, Mahnert BW, Passman R, Goldberger J, Kadish A. Effects of sex and age on electrocardiographic and cardiac electrophysiological properties in adults. Pacing Clin Electrophysiol. 2001 Jan;24(1):16–21.

Tse HF, Oral H, Pelosi F, Knight BP, Strickberger SA, Morady F. Effect of gender on atrial electrophysiologic changes induced by rapid atrial pacing and elevation of atrial pressure. J Cardiovasc Electrophysiol. 2001 Sep;12(9):986–9.

CHAPTER FIVE

Supraventricular Arrhythmias

CEVHER OZCAN, MD, AND ANNE B. CURTIS, MD

INTRODUCTION

Supraventricular tachyarrhythmias (SVTs) include atrioventricular (AV) nodal reentrant tachycardia (AVNRT), AV reciprocating tachycardia (AVRT), atrial tachycardia (AT), atrial fibrillation (AF), atrial flutter (AFL), and sinus tachyarrhythmias. They are common clinical problems in men and women, but there are significant sex-based differences in the incidence and prevalence of the various SVTs. In the general population, the relative risk of paroxysmal SVT is higher for women than for men. Paroxysmal SVT without underlying cardiovascular disease is particularly more common among women. In this population, the prevalence of paroxysmal SVT is 2.25 per 1,000 person-years, and the incidence is 35 per 100,000 person-years. The distribution of the types of paroxysmal SVT is different between men and women among patients with symptomatic SVT who undergo an electrophysiology study (EPS) and

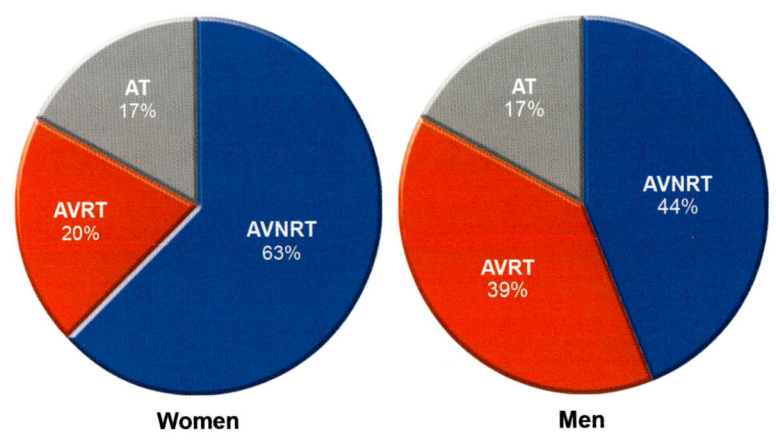

FIGURE 5.1. **Distribution of Supraventricular Tachycardias in Women and Men Undergoing Electrophysiology Study.** AT indicates atrial tachycardia; AVNRT, atrioventricular nodal reentrant tachycardia; AVRT, atrioventricular reciprocating tachycardia.

catheter ablation (Figure 5.1). While the most common diagnosis for both women and men is AVNRT, the incidence of AVRT is much higher among men than among women.

Morbidity and mortality are higher among women with SVT. The majority of hospital admissions for heart rhythm diseases or outpatient cardiac electrophysiology clinic visits are due to SVT, although AF dominates over other forms of SVT. Women have more frequent symptomatic episodes of SVT than men. Although there is only a modest increase in mortality among patients with SVT, morbidity increases considerably. In particular, quality of life is significantly impaired among women with SVT.

The effects of hormones on triggering SVT episodes are well known. Premenopausal women may have more episodes of symptomatic SVT during the luteal phase of the menstrual cycle. Accordingly, an EPS is more likely to induce SVT during the perimenstrual phase. It is worthwhile to ask premenopausal women whether they have noticed a pattern of SVT episodes possibly related to the menstrual cycle. If they have, the EPS should be scheduled during the perimenstrual phase of the cycle, increasing the diagnostic and therapeutic yield of the procedure with a higher probability of successful induction of SVT and ablation.

Sex-specific differences in the management of SVT have also been reported. For example, compared with men, women are referred for catheter ablation or cardioversion later, with more symptoms, and after more antiarrhythmic drugs have failed. Catheter ablation is equally effective and is a safe procedure in both sexes for the treatment of SVT.

Thus, it is important to acknowledge that there are sex-based differences in SVT. This chapter presents a comprehensive overview of the incidence, clinical presentation, general evaluation, management, and outcomes of SVT in women by focusing on AVNRT, AVRT, AT, AFL, and sinus tachyarrhythmias. Junctional tachycardia is also briefly summarized. AF is discussed in Chapter 6 ("Atrial Fibrillation in Women").

ATRIOVENTRICULAR NODAL REENTRANT TACHYCARDIA

AVNRT is a narrow complex tachycardia at a rate of 150 to 250 beats per minute. In its typical form, a reentrant circuit involves slow and fast AV nodal pathways (ie, dual AV nodal physiology). The fast pathway, which has a longer refractory period, includes the compact AV node and the anterior septum. The slow pathway involves atrial myocardium at the septal part of the tricuspid annulus near the coronary sinus ostium. The typical form of AVNRT uses the slow pathway in the anterograde direction and the fast pathway in the retrograde direction. Atypical AVNRT is much less common and is associated with conduction in the anterograde fast and retrograde slow pathways. The P wave is buried in the QRS complex and is not visible on the electrocardiogram (ECG) during tachycardia because of the nearly simultaneous activation of the atria and ventricles in typical AVNRT. The ECG may be helpful if it is obtained at the initiation and termination of tachycardia. An EPS with programmed stimulation is diagnostic.

Incidence

The prevalence of AVNRT in the general population is approximately 1 to 2 per 1,000 persons. AVNRT is the most common paroxysmal SVT in women, and both typical and atypical AVNRT occur more often in women than in men. The reason for the increased incidence of AVNRT among women is not clear, but it is likely associated with hormonal effects and AV conduction properties. Although dual AV nodal pathways are present equally in both sexes (and shown to occur in about 85% of all patients with AVNRT), AV conduction properties are significantly different (Figure 5.2). In patients with AVNRT, EPS shows that the following are shorter in women than in men: PR intervals, atrial-His (AH) intervals, His-ventricular (HV) intervals, and atrial effective refractory periods (ERPs). The ventricular ERP is longer in women than in men (Figure 5.2 and Table 5.1). During decremental atrial pacing, the AV block cycle length is shorter in women. Women have better ventriculoatrial conduction, while men have ventriculoatrial dissociation more often during ventricular pacing. The prevalence of AVNRT in patients with implantable cardioverter-defibrillators has been shown to be higher (3.5%) than in the general population. That study indicated the potentially increased risk of AVNRT with electroanatomical changes in the AV node in patients with underlying cardiac disease.

Management

Initial diagnostic evaluation of clinically suspected AVNRT includes a 12-lead ECG with Holter monitoring or event monitoring. An exercise stress test is usually not helpful. During an episode of tachycardia, termination of the tachycardia with an AV nodal blocking agent or vagal maneuver favors a diagnosis of AVNRT. However, an EPS is required for definitive diagnosis. Symptomatic and recurrent AVNRT requires effective short-term and long-term management. Overall, the therapeutic approach to AVNRT is similar for both sexes, although women may need closer monitoring and management because of more frequent episodes of symptomatic tachycardia. An acute episode of AVNRT is managed like any other narrow complex tachycardia. A Valsalva maneuver, carotid sinus massage, or AV blocking agents (adenosine, calcium channel blockers, β-blockers, or digoxin) successfully terminate AVNRT in almost all cases. Rarely, direct current cardioversion or overdrive pacing is required.

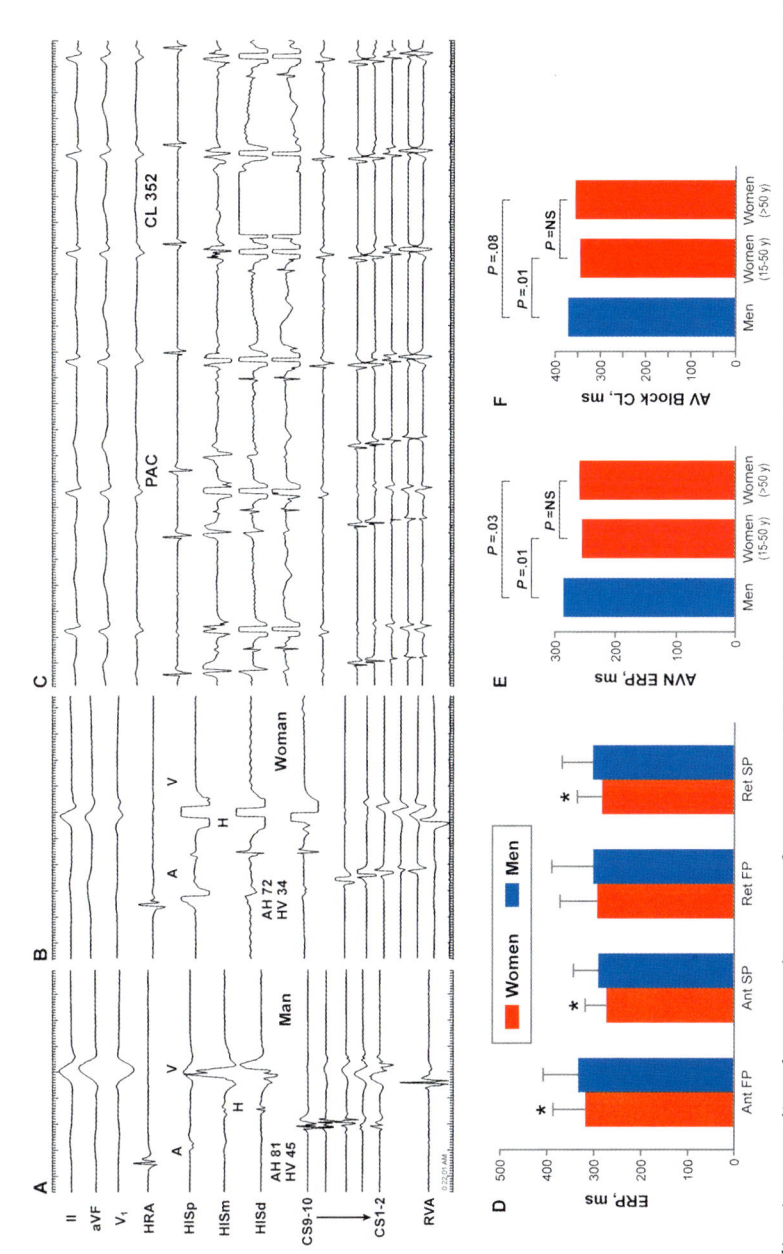

FIGURE 5.2. Baseline intracardiac electrocardiograms from a man (A) and a woman (B) with atrioventricular (AV) nodal reentrant tachycardia (AVNRT). Atrial-His (AH) and His-ventricular (HV) intervals are typically shorter in women; a premature atrial contraction induces AVNRT (cycle length [CL], 352 ms) in a woman (C). The mean CL of AVNRT in women is typically shorter than in men. D, Differences in slow and fast pathway (anterograde [Ant] and retrograde [Ret]) conduction are shown for men and women with AVNRT. Asterisks indicate statistically significant differences (P<.05); error bars, standard deviations of the means. E, Sex-based differences are shown for AV nodal (AVN) effective refractory periods (ERPs). F, AV block CL is shown for younger (15–50 years) and older (>50 years) women and for men. All intervals are in milliseconds. A indicates atrium; CS, coronary sinus; FP, fast pathway; H, His; HISd, distal area of His bundle region; HISm, middle area of His bundle region; HISp, proximal area of His bundle region; HRA, high right atrium; NS, not significant; PAC, premature atrial contraction; RVA, right ventricular apex; SP, slow pathway; V, ventricle. (Panel D, adapted from Suenari K, Hu YF, Tsao HM, Tai CT, Chiang CE, Lin YJ, et al. Gender differences in the clinical characteristics and atrioventricular nodal conduction properties in patients with atrioventricular nodal reentrant tachycardia. J Cardiovasc Electrophysiol. 2010 Oct;21(10):1114–9. Used with permission. Panels E and F, adapted from Liuba I, Jonsson A, Safstrom K, Walfridsson H. Gender-related differences in patients with atrioventricular nodal reentry tachycardia. Am J Cardiol. 2006 Feb 1;97(3):384–8. Epub 2005 Dec 1. Used with permission.)

TABLE 5.1. Electrophysiologic Characteristics of Patients With Atrioventricular Nodal Reentrant Tachycardia

Characteristic	Women[a]	Men[a]
Incidence of AVNRT	+++	++
Sinus cycle length	780 (140)	830 (161)
AH interval	75 (19)	82 (15)
HV interval	38 (6)	42 (6)
Atrial ERP	208 (33)	215 (36)
Ventricular ERP	222 (25)	216 (23)
Anterograde slow pathway ERP	265 (45)	287 (62)
Retrograde slow pathway ERP	283 (51)	302 (65)
Fast pathway ERP	322 (58)	333 (55)
AV block cycle length	348 (53)	371 (75)
Retrograde VA conduction	349 (78)	357 (78)
AVNRT cycle length	354 (58)	383 (60)
Incidence of multiple jumps	10%	7%
Baseline VA dissociation	8.6%	12%
Induction with stimulation	+++	++

Abbreviations: AH, atrial-His; AV, atrioventricular; AVNRT, atrioventricular nodal reentrant tachycardia; ERP, effective refractory period; HV, His-ventricular; VA, ventriculoatrial.

[a] *Durations are presented as mean (standard deviation) in milliseconds.*

The long-term management of AVNRT includes pharmacologic and catheter ablation treatment. The choice is dependent on the frequency of the tachycardia episodes, the hemodynamic tolerance of the patient, and the patient's preference. If AVNRT episodes occur occasionally and are well tolerated hemodynamically, the wide spectrum of management options ranges from no therapy to treatment with the Valsalva maneuver, "pill-in-the-pocket" (β-blocker or diltiazem), verapamil, diltiazem, β-blocker, or catheter ablation. However, if AVNRT causes hemodynamic intolerance or occurs frequently (or both), catheter ablation or medical management should be considered. In addition to AV nodal blockers, long-term pharmacologic therapy may include flecainide, propafenone, or sotalol. In rare cases, amiodarone may be used if the patient declines catheter ablation.

Catheter ablation is a class I indication with level B evidence for the treatment of recurrent symptomatic AVNRT in both sexes. At EPS, the characteristics of AVNRT are different for women than for men (Table 5.1). The anterograde and retrograde slow pathway ERPs are shorter. The anterograde fast pathway ERP is also shorter in women. Multiple jumps are often documented during EPS in women with AVNRT, particularly in younger patients (50 years or younger). Also, younger women have been noted to have shorter anterograde and retrograde slow pathway ERPs than women older than 50. In general, the tachycardia cycle length is shorter in women. AVNRT is usually induced with electrical stimulation. Pharmacologic intervention is less often required to induce tachycardia in women during EPS.

SVT may become more frequent during pregnancy. A calcium channel blocker, such as diltiazem (pregnancy category C), can be chosen to control the rhythm. Sotalol (pregnancy category B) is the alternative drug selection if the corrected QT interval and renal function allow its use. On occasion, with drug-refractory SVT or severe drug side effects, ablation may be undertaken during the second or third trimester. The arrhythmia management plan should be shared with the patient's obstetrician. Chapter 14 ("Pregnancy and Arrhythmias") discusses the topic in more detail.

Outcomes

Heart rate is the primary determinant of AVNRT symptoms, which include palpitations, fatigue, dyspnea, light-headedness, chest discomfort, and presyncope (but rarely syncope). In about half of the patients, symptoms may be successfully suppressed by slowing the heart rate or preventing the episodes with pharmacologic agents. However, catheter ablation is preferred for the majority of patients with recurrent symptomatic AVNRT because of potential side effects from the medications and the need to take them lifelong. There is no sex difference in outcomes with pharmacologic or nonpharmacologic treatment of AVNRT. Overall, slow pathway modification by catheter ablation in AVNRT is equally successful and is a safe procedure in men and women. Several studies have shown no significant sex differences in procedure times, radiation exposure, complication rates, or immediate success rates. Overall, the rate of recurrence is reported to be 3% to 7%. However, a study has shown that the highest rate of immediate procedural failure (5.5%) is among women younger than 20 years. Independent predictors of recurrence of AVNRT after ablation are age younger than 20 years and female sex. The risk of iatrogenic high-grade AV block and the need for a pacemaker after slow pathway modification is 1% in both sexes.

ATRIOVENTRICULAR RECIPROCATING TACHYCARDIA

AVRT is an AV accessory pathway (AP)-mediated macroreentrant tachycardia. The circuit includes the native AV nodal conduction system in addition to anterograde or retrograde AP conduction. Ventricular preexcitation, or a *manifest* AP, is associated with a short PR interval (<120 ms) and a delta wave (slurred upstroke of the QRS complex). If an AP is *concealed* (retrograde conduction only), the QRS complex will be normal in sinus rhythm with no evidence of preexcitation. The Wolff-Parkinson-White (WPW) syndrome is defined as recurrent symptomatic tachycardia in the presence of preexcitation on the ECG. The most common tachycardia in patients with APs is AVRT (orthodromic reciprocating tachycardia). AVRT usually has a narrow QRS complex, although bundle branch block aberration may be seen. Wide complex (antidromic reciprocating) tachycardia is less common. AF with preexcitation can be associated with very rapid heart rates. The ventricular insertion of the AP is usually located along the mitral or tricuspid valve.

Incidence

AVRT is a relatively common SVT in younger adults. Preexcitation on the ECG is found in 0.15% to 0.25% of the general population. Half of the community patients with preexcitation on the ECG report no symptoms at diagnosis. During follow-up, symptoms related to arrhythmia subsequently develop in only one-third of them. Also, preexcitation on the ECG may be intermittent. In fact, 22% of the patients with WPW syndrome may not show preexcitation on the ECG on initial evaluation, but a delta wave may develop after an average follow-up of 7 years. Most patients with AVRT are young and have no significant structural heart disease. The highest incidence of new cases of WPW syndrome in both sexes is in the first year of life, although approximately 50% of those spontaneously resolve within the first year.

The second peak for a new diagnosis of WPW syndrome occurs in the fourth decade of life for women and in the third decade for men. The incidence of AVRT among men is twice that among women (Box 5.1). Manifest WPW syndrome is more common in adult men, but concealed AVRT is almost equally distributed in both sexes. Also, boys and girls show a similar frequency of preexcitation on the ECG. The cause of these differences is not known, but shorter PR intervals in women compared with age-matched

---

BOX 5.1.
DIFFERENCES IN CHARACTERISTICS OF SUPRAVENTRICULAR TACHYCARDIAS IN WOMEN COMPARED WITH MEN

AVRT
- Less common (ratio of men to women, 2:1)
- Longer anterograde accessory pathway ERP
- Less antidromic AVRT
- More often have multiple accessory pathways
- Lower incidence of atrial fibrillation
- Lower incidence of ventricular fibrillation

Focal AT
- Paroxysmal focal AT more common
- Incessant AT less common
- Less tachycardia-mediated cardiomyopathy
- Develops at a younger age
- Fewer cardiac comorbidities
- Higher incidence of AVNRT

Atrial flutter
- Lower incidence (ratio of men to women, 2.5:1)
- Less frequent use of cardioversion
- Higher incidence of atrial fibrillation after ablation
- Similar long-term outcome

Abbreviations: AT, atrial tachycardia; AVNRT, atrioventricular nodal reentrant tachycardia; AVRT, atrioventricular reciprocating tachycardia; ERP, effective refractory period.

men are thought to contribute to a lower incidence of AVRT among women. While orthodromic AVRT occurs in the majority of patients with WPW syndrome, antidromic tachycardia, which is documented in about 5% of patients, is more prominent among men. AF develops in about 30% of patients with WPW syndrome.

Management

WPW syndrome is associated with a slight risk of sudden cardiac death (SCD) due to rapid tachycardia, in particular preexcited AF that degenerates into ventricular fibrillation. Therefore, risk stratification for possible SCD is essential for tailoring therapy for patients with preexcitation on the ECG. Risk stratification methods are similar for both sexes and include noninvasive testing such as exercise stress testing or procainamide challenge. Loss of preexcitation during exercise or procainamide infusion is associated with a lower risk of SCD, because either indicates a longer AP ERP and, hence, a smaller risk of rapid ventricular rates during AF. However, EPS provides the optimal risk stratification by determining the AP ERP and the shortest preexcited R-R interval in AF. There is no indication for a routine EPS for every person with asymptomatic preexcitation on the ECG. These patients should be followed clinically for the development of symptoms consistent with sustained tachycardia. An EPS is considered for asymptomatic people with preexcitation only if they are in a special circumstance such as being an athlete, pilot, or bus driver.

AVRT may manifest with a narrow or wide QRS complex tachycardia. Initial management of a narrow complex tachycardia is similar to that for AVNRT as outlined previously. Pharmacologic intervention is the first step in hemodynamically stable patients; if it fails, direct current cardioversion is required. However, if a patient presents with a hemodynamically unstable wide complex tachycardia, immediate direct current cardioversion is the treatment of choice. If a patient has a wide complex tachycardia and is hemodynamically stable, pharmacologic intervention should be provided with procainamide, sotalol, or amiodarone before overdrive pacing or mechanical cardioversion is considered. Administration of adenosine is also an option if antidromic tachycardia or AVRT with aberration is suspected since transient AV nodal block will terminate the tachycardia.

The long-term management of AVRT consists of pharmacologic treatment or catheter ablation of the AP (or both). Catheter ablation is a class I indication with level B evidence for the treatment of WPW syndrome and recurrent symptomatic AVRT. Antiarrhythmics (selected class I and III agents) are class IIa indications in these patients. Asymptomatic patients with preexcitation or infrequent AVRT without preexcitation should be followed without treatment (class I indication). In these patients, catheter ablation treatment is a class IIa indication and antiarrhythmics are a class IIb indication. In the presence of preexcitation, class I (flecainide and propafenone) and class III (sotalol and amiodarone) antiarrhythmics may be used to depress anterograde AP conduction.

Electrophysiologic characteristics of the AP are important in the management of AVRT. The anterograde AP ERP is usually longer in women (>250 ms). Men have more antidromic AVRTs. Women more often have multiple APs compared with men. Anatomic locations of the AP based on the preexcitation pattern on the ECG in the general population are shown in Figure 5.3. Women have a higher incidence of right free wall pathways and posteroseptal pathways than men, while men have a higher incidence of left free wall and anteroseptal pathways. AP location has been studied in a large cohort of patients (mean age, 34 years) who underwent EPS and ablation. This patient population had a male dominance (64%). The majority of APs were located at the left free wall in both sexes (58% in men and 57% in women). However, there was a significant

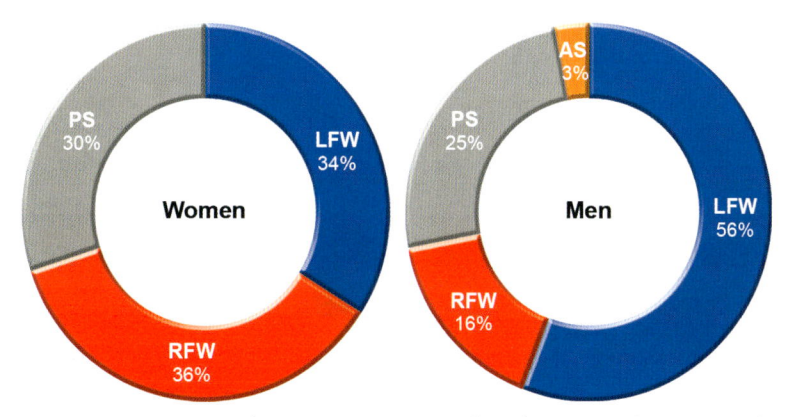

FIGURE 5.3. Accessory Pathway Location on the Electrocardiograms of Patients With Wolff-Parkinson-White Syndrome. AS indicates anteroseptal; LFW, left free wall; PS, posteroseptal; RFW, right free wall.

sex-based difference in AP location. Women more often had a right free wall location (13% in women and 7% in men), while men had twice the incidence of a right anteroseptal location compared with women. The frequency of a posteroseptal location was comparable in both sexes (23% in men and 22% in women) in this cohort.

Outcomes

Pharmacologic and nonpharmacologic treatments of AVRT are equally effective in men and women. The success rates with catheter ablation, the complication rates, and the rates of recurrence of AP conduction after ablation are similar for both sexes. Results from many studies show that the initial success rate of ablation for eliminating the AP is about 95%. The location of the AP is important for successful catheter ablation. Left free wall AP ablation is more successful than other locations. If catheter ablation fails, surgical intervention may be needed. Data are inadequate to determine the long-term efficacy of pharmacologic treatment of AVRT. Drug side effects and the efficacy of long-term pharmacologic treatment are significant concerns.

The incidence of SCD was 0.15% to 0.39% in a 10-year follow-up period for patients with WPW syndrome. Known risk factors for SCD in WPW syndrome include symptomatic tachycardia, multiple APs, a short preexcited R-R interval (<250 ms) during AF, Ebstein anomaly, and familial WPW syndrome. Men with WPW syndrome have a higher risk of atrial and ventricular fibrillation than women.

ATRIAL TACHYCARDIA

AT is a regular atrial tachyarrhythmia at rates of 100 to 250 beats per minute. The mechanism may be abnormal automaticity, triggered activity, or reentry. In most cases, the mechanism can be determined during EPS by initiation or termination of AT with programmed stimulation or overdrive pacing, entrainment, or responsiveness to isoproterenol, β-blockers, or adenosine. The majority of patients with focal AT do not have significant structural heart disease, and the arrhythmia originates from the right atrium (>70% of patients).

Incidence

Although nonsustained focal AT is commonly seen in the general population, sustained focal AT is less common (10%-15%) among patients who undergo EPS. The prevalence of AT is reported to be 0.3% to 0.4% in symptomatic and asymptomatic patients. The reported sex-based difference in the incidence and prevalence of AT varies with the population studied, but overall, AT develops at a similar frequency in men and women. However, paroxysmal AT is more common in women than in men, while the incidence of incessant AT is relatively higher in men (Box 5.1). Focal AT develops at a younger age in women than in men. Women with focal AT have fewer cardiac comorbidities than men. However, the incidence of associated SVTs (eg, AVNRT) is higher among women with focal AT than among men. Incessant AT causes tachycardia-induced cardiomyopathy. The mechanism of AT is commonly automaticity in premenopausal women.

Radiofrequency ablation for AF has become one of the most common catheter ablation procedures performed worldwide. The ablation involves circumferential pulmonary vein isolation; in persistent AF, multiple left atrial linear ablations may be required for modifying the left atrial substrate. Macroreentrant AT associated with ablation lesion gaps and new focal AT is a proarrhythmic complication of extensive atrial ablation in both men and women, with an incidence of 2.6% to 31%. These ATs are often resistant to antiarrhythmic medication and require subsequent ablation.

Management

Patients with nonsustained AT are rarely symptomatic and do not require therapeutic intervention. However, patients with sustained focal AT may be highly symptomatic and in a hemodynamically significant state. These patients initially require treatment that is pharmacologic or nonpharmacologic (or both), as with other narrow QRS complex tachycardias. During AT, P-wave morphology on the 12-lead ECG may be helpful in determining the location of the focus, but ultimate localization requires intracardiac electroanatomic mapping in the electrophysiology laboratory. AT may originate from the right or left atrium. The crista terminalis in the right atrium is the most common site of origin for focal AT. Left-sided

AT usually triggers AF and is most often located at the pulmonary veins or in the interatrial septum.

The mechanism of AT—whether it be abnormal automaticity, reentry, or triggered activity—may influence the efficacy of treatment options. AV nodal blocking agents or vagal maneuvers may not be as effective in terminating acute episodes of paroxysmal focal AT due to abnormal automaticity or triggered activity. An adenosine-sensitive form of AT exists, and cases of AT termination with β-blockers or verapamil have been reported. Class IA and IC antiarrhythmic drugs may inhibit AT due to abnormal automaticity. Amiodarone infusion may be necessary in some cases. Rarely, cardioversion may be required to treat AT, but it would be expected to be effective only for arrhythmias due to reentry or triggered activity. β-Blockers and calcium channel blockers are routinely given initially to control the ventricular rate. The long-term management of AT includes all of these pharmacologic agents in addition to catheter ablation. If a patient is symptomatic with recurrent episodes of AT, catheter ablation is a class I indication for treatment. β-Blockers and calcium channel blockers are a class I indication for suppression of recurrent episodes, while disopyramide, flecainide, propafenone, amiodarone, and sotalol are class IIA choices for symptomatic recurrent AT. The goal of long-term management is to prevent recurrence of episodes. During EPS, no significant sex differences in electrophysiologic characteristics of AT have been found. The number of foci, left atrial involvement, and tachycardia cycle length have all been found to be comparable in both sexes.

Outcomes

In general, AT is a benign condition and rarely causes serious conditions. Tachycardia-mediated cardiomyopathy secondary to incessant AT may occur in both sexes, but it is less common in women than in men. The outcome with pharmacologic treatment is similar in men and women. Catheter ablation is effective in both sexes, with an 80% to 85% immediate success rate and an approximately 10% rate of recurrence of AT during follow-up. No therapeutic intervention is recommended for asymptomatic patients or nonsustained AT. Catheter ablation is a class III indication in this group of patients.

ATRIAL FLUTTER

AFL is a regular, rapid atrial tachyarrhythmia at a rate of 240 to 350 beats per minute. It is an intra-atrial reentrant dysrhythmia with an excitable gap that can be entrained. *Typical AFL*, the most common type, is characterized by a reentrant circuit involving the isthmus between the tricuspid annulus and the inferior vena cava–eustachian ridge–coronary sinus ostium. The circuit travels counterclockwise up the atrial septum and down the right atrial free wall. If the same circuit is used in a clockwise direction, the arrhythmia is *reverse typical AFL*. Isthmus-dependent AFL comprises 90% of cases. Atypical AFL has a similar rate and macroreentrant mechanism, but the circuit is located in other parts of the atrium and around scar tissue. The ECG is diagnostic in most cases of AFL, but determining the type of AFL requires EPS and mapping.

Incidence

In MESA, the overall incidence of AFL was 88 per 100,000 person-years. The incidence of AFL is significantly lower among women than among men (Box 5.1). After adjustment for age in both sexes, AFL is 2.5 times more common in men. However, the incidence and prevalence of AFL increase with age and comorbidities. While the incidence is 5 in 100,000 among those younger than 50 years, it increases to 587 in 100,000 among octogenarians. AFL is commonly associated with underlying heart failure or chronic obstructive lung disease. In addition, the coexistence of AFL and AF is well documented. An estimated 70,000 people in the US population have a diagnosis of AFL only, but 190,000 have both AFL and AF. The prevalence of AFL is projected to increase considerably over time with the aging of the population.

Management

In general, the clinical presentation of cava-tricuspid, isthmus-dependent, or isthmus–independent macroreentrant AFL is similar for men and women. The ECG is useful to determine the location of the reentrant circuit. AFL is commonly associated with an acute systemic disease process, and treatment of the underlying disease is an important step in the management of AFL. If the patient is hemodynamically unstable with rapid ventricular conduction of

AFL, direct current cardioversion is indicated. If the patient is hemodynamically stable, pharmacologic cardioversion with ibutilide or other drugs can be used. Intravenous β-blockers, diltiazem, digoxin, flecainide, propafenone, procainamide, amiodarone, sotalol, and dofetilide have been studied for cardioversion and rate control. Among these agents, ibutilide and dofetilide have been found to be more effective than the other drugs for cardioversion. Atrial overdrive pacing is an option for successful termination of AFL. For the long-term management of AFL, rate control can be achieved with β-blockers, verapamil, diltiazem, digoxin, or amiodarone. However, catheter ablation is the treatment of choice in current practice for patients with recurrent symptomatic AFL, particularly isthmus-dependent AFL. Ablation is also an option for non–isthmus-dependent AFL. Anticoagulation is indicated according to the CHADS2 score (which is based on 5 risk factors for stroke: congestive heart failure, hypertension, age 75 years or older, diabetes mellitus, and history of stroke or transient ischemic attack).

Outcomes

Patients with AFL usually have underlying diseases that trigger the episodes and may affect the efficacy of treatment strategies. Like AF, AFL is associated with significant morbidity. Direct current cardioversion with low energy successfully restores sinus rhythm in 95% to 100% of patients with AFL. While the efficacy of cardioversion is similar for men and women, there is a sex-based difference in the use of cardioversion for hospitalized patients with AFL—cardioversion is used less frequently in women.

Catheter ablation is effective (success rate >90%) for isthmus-dependent AFL. The success rate is slightly less for non–isthmus-dependent AFL. If bidirectional conduction block is achieved during the procedure, the long-term success rate may increase to 100%. There are no sex differences in the outcome of catheter ablation for AFL with respect to initial or long-term success rates or complication rates. However, women have a higher incidence of AF after successful catheter ablation. Antiarrhythmics are inferior to ablation in maintaining sinus rhythm in patients with AFL. Since AF commonly coexists with AFL, AF significantly affects the outcome and management of AFL.

SINUS TACHYARRHYTHMIAS

Sinus tachyarrhythmias include inappropriate sinus tachycardia, postural orthostatic tachycardia syndrome, and sinus node reentry tachycardia. Women have sinus tachyarrhythmias more often than men. Generally, patients with paroxysmal tachycardia episodes may be highly symptomatic, but there is no significant increase in mortality that can be attributed to sinus tachyarrhythmias.

Although physiologic sinus tachycardia is also a type of SVT, it occurs as a response to underlying pathologic conditions and resolves with correction of the trigger. Sinus tachycardia is common in women. If it is triggered by emotional stress or an anxiety disorder, β-blockers can be effective for prevention or treatment. As discussed in Chapter 11 ("Syncope and POTS"), postural orthostatic tachycardia syndrome is an exaggerated sinus node response to upright posture. It is an autonomic disorder that is present more often in women. Catheter ablation for sinus node modification should not be considered, but β-blockers and nonpharmacologic treatments, particularly exercise, may control symptoms.

Inappropriate sinus tachycardia is associated with a high resting heart rate that is out of proportion to a person's physical or emotional condition. It may result from abnormal autonomic regulation or enhanced automaticity of the sinus node. Inappropriate sinus tachycardia occurs predominantly in women (90%). In symptomatic patients, β-blockers may be effective. Sinus node modification with catheter ablation is reserved for highly symptomatic patients with inappropriate sinus tachycardia that is refractory to pharmacologic treatment. Immediate and long-term success rates with ablation are reported to be around 60% to 70%.

Sinus node reentry tachycardia is a paroxysmal sustained tachycardia with a heart rate up to 180 beats per minute. It is relatively uncommon in the general population and has been documented from a small percentage of patients with SVT who present for EPS. Catheter ablation should be considered only in highly symptomatic patients who have frequent episodes. Tachycardia episodes can be terminated with vagal maneuvers, adenosine, β-blockers, calcium channel blockers, or amiodarone.

JUNCTIONAL TACHYCARDIA

Focal junctional tachycardia is a rare arrhythmia that usually has a narrow QRS complex but can manifest as intermittent bundle branch block with a wide QRS complex. It originates from the AV junction at the AV node or His bundle area and leads to AV dissociation. Abnormal automaticity or triggered activity is likely the mechanism of this tachycardia. This condition is mainly found in children or young adults. Recurrent symptomatic junctional tachycardia that requires EPS is more common among adult and elderly women than men. It may cause heart failure if it becomes incessant. Patients can be significantly symptomatic with this arrhythmia, which is somewhat responsive to β-blockers or flecainide. Catheter ablation is reserved for highly symptomatic patients, but it is associated with a 5% to 10% risk of AV block and a permanent pacemaker requirement. If a patient has ventriculoatrial conduction, ablation should be performed at the site of the earliest retrograde atrial activation. If no ventriculoatrial conduction is present, slow pathway modification is recommended. The nonparoxysmal form of junctional tachycardia may be associated with underlying myocardial ischemia, inflammation, surgical scar, or digitalis toxicity. Underlying conditions must be treated. β-Blockers and calcium channel blockers can be used initially.

SUMMARY

Significant sex-based differences are present in the incidence, prevalence, and clinical characteristics of SVT. AVNRT, focal AT, and sinus tachyarrhythmias are more common in women, whereas AVRT, AFL, and incessant AT are more often diagnosed in men. Overall, symptomatic episodes of SVT occur more frequently in women. The outcome of pharmacologic or nonpharmacologic treatment of SVT is similar for women and men. However, advanced therapies such as catheter ablation are offered to women at a later stage in the course of their disease when they have had more symptoms and more antiarrhythmic drugs have failed. Thus, acknowledgment of sex differences in SVT is important for optimizing the management of these debilitating arrhythmias.

SUGGESTED READING

Birati EY, Eldar M, Belhassen B. Gender differences in accessory connections location: an Israeli study. J Interv Card Electrophysiol. 2012 Sep;34(3):227–9. Epub 2012 May 13.

Blomstrom-Lundqvist C, Scheinman MM, Aliot EM, Alpert JS, Calkins H, Camm AJ, et al; European Society of Cardiology Committee, NASPE-Heart Rhythm Society. ACC/AHA/ESC guidelines for the management of patients with supraventricular arrhythmias: executive summary: a report of the American College of Cardiology/American Heart Association task force on practice guidelines and the European Society of Cardiology Committee for practice guidelines (writing committee to develop guidelines for the management of patients with supraventricular arrhythmias) developed in collaboration with NASPE-Heart Rhythm Society. J Am Coll Cardiol. 2003 Oct 15;42(8):1493–531.

Granada J, Uribe W, Chyou PH, Maassen K, Vierkant R, Smith PN, et al. Incidence and predictors of atrial flutter in the general population. J Am Coll Cardiol. 2000 Dec;36(7):2242–6.

Hu YF, Huang JL, Wu TJ, Higa S, Shih CM, Tai CT, et al. Gender differences of electrophysiological characteristics in focal atrial tachycardia. Am J Cardiol. 2009 Jul 1;104(1):97–100. Epub 2009 May 3.

Huang SY, Hu YF, Chang SL, Lin YJ, Lo LW, Tuan TC, et al. Gender differences of electrophysiologic characteristics in patients with accessory atrioventricular pathways. Heart Rhythm. 2011 Apr;8(4):571–4. Epub 2010 Dec 13.

LaPointe NM, Sun JL, Kaplan S. In-hospital management of patients with atrial flutter. Am Heart J. 2010 Mar;159(3):370–6.

Liu S, Yuan S, Kongstad O, Olsson SB. Gender differences in the electrophysiological characteristics of atrioventricular conduction system and their clinical implications. Scand Cardiovasc J. 2001 Oct;35(5):313–7.

Liuba I, Jonsson A, Safstrom K, Walfridsson H. Gender-related differences in patients with atrioventricular nodal reentry tachycardia. Am J Cardiol. 2006 Feb 1;97(3):384–8. Epub 2005 Dec 1.

Porter MJ, Morton JB, Denman R, Lin AC, Tierney S, Santucci PA, et al. Influence of age and gender on the mechanism of supraventricular tachycardia. Heart Rhythm. 2004 Oct;1(4):393–6.

Suenari K, Hu YF, Tsao HM, Tai CT, Chiang CE, Lin YJ, et al. Gender differences in the clinical characteristics and atrioventricular nodal conduction properties in patients with atrioventricular nodal reentrant tachycardia. J Cardiovasc Electrophysiol. 2010 Oct;21(10):1114–9.

CHAPTER SIX

Atrial Fibrillation in Women

SUSAN J. EISENBERG, MD, AND
TAYA V. GLOTZER, MD

INTRODUCTION

Atrial fibrillation (AF) is the most common cardiac dysrhythmia and is responsible for approximately one-third of hospitalizations for rhythm disturbances. Population surveys have shown that paroxysmal or persistent AF is present in 2.2 million people in the United States and in 4.5 million people in Europe. Without proper medical treatment, AF patients have a 5 times greater risk of stroke than the general population.

Sex-based differences in the presentation, symptomatology, clinical course, and response to treatment of AF have been identified. The most worrisome is that women with AF have an increased risk of death, cardiovascular events, and stroke. Research since the early 2000s has yielded significant progress in the understanding, management, and treatment of AF. Identification of sex-specific differences related to AF allows for a more tailored approach to the management of this disorder in women (Table 6.1). This chapter reviews sex-based differences in the presentation, treatment, and outcome of patients with AF. With these differences in mind, clinicians can be alert to clinical issues unique to women and thereby improve therapies and, consequently, outcomes.

TABLE 6.1. Major Sex Differences That Characterize Atrial Fibrillation in Women

Factor	Feature More Common in Women
Electrophysiology	Increased corrected QT interval Decreased atrial refractoriness after menopause
Clinical presentation	Older patient More comorbidities Hypertension Diastolic congestive heart failure More symptoms Lower quality of life; possible underlying depression
Mortality	Increased
Stroke risk	Increased despite anticoagulation
Bleeding risk	Same for both sexes
Rhythm vs rate control	No survival advantage with rhythm control for either sex Rhythm control for women: more complications with abdominal aortic aneurysm (torsades de pointes, bradycardia, symptoms), increased congestive heart failure, increased stroke rate Increased recurrence of atrial fibrillation with direct current cardioversion
Antiarrhythmics	Increased bradycardia, increased torsades de pointes, increased side effects
Atrial fibrillation ablation	Referred less often and referred later during course of atrial fibrillation Similar success rates as men with great improvement in quality of life More procedural bleeding complications More nonpulmonary vein triggers

Adapted from Michelena HI, Powell BD, Brady PA, Friedman PA, Ezekowitz MD. Gender in atrial fibrillation: ten years later. Gend Med. 2010 Jun;7(3):206–17. Used with permission.

PREVALENCE

The prevalence of AF in all age groups is higher among men than among women. However, since women generally live longer than men, more women than men are older than 75 years in the general population. Accordingly, the absolute number of women with AF is equal to or greater than the number of men with AF. Overall, 50% to 55% of all patients with AF are women, and this increases to around 60% in those older than 75 years. Data from the Framingham Heart Study from 2004 showed that at age 40, the lifetime risk of AF for men was 26.0% (95% CI,

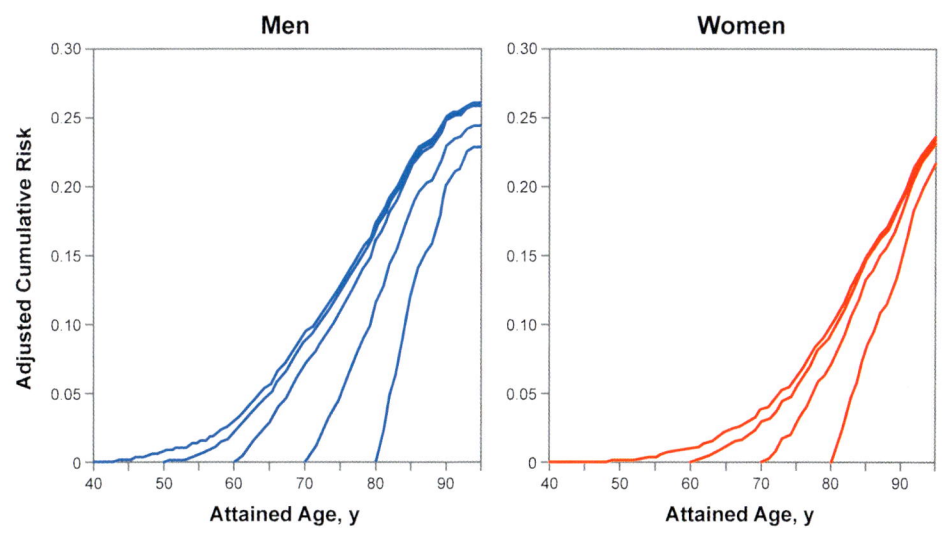

FIGURE 6.1. Risk of Atrial Fibrillation (AF). Cumulative risk of AF in men and women at selected index ages, with death free of AF considered a competing event. Lifetime risk at a given index age is cumulative risk through age 94 years. (Adapted from Lloyd-Jones DM, Wang TJ, Leip EP, Larson MG, Levy D, Vasan RS, et al. Lifetime risk for development of atrial fibrillation: the Framingham Heart Study. Circulation. 2004 Aug 31;110[9]:1042-6. Used with permission.)

24.0%-27.0%) and for women, 23.0% (95% CI, 21.0%-24.0%); prevalence was not significantly different (Figure 6.1). Lifetime risks did not vary substantially with advancing age because the incidence of AF increases rapidly with increasing age. In the Framingham Heart Study, at age 80 years, the lifetime risk of AF for men was 22.7% (95% CI, 20.1%-24.1%) and for women, 21.6% (95% CI, 19.3%-22.7%). Progression to permanent AF is the same for men and women over 3 years.

SYMPTOMS AND CLINICAL PRESENTATION

Compared with men, women who present with AF are older and more symptomatic and their heart rates during AF are significantly higher (Table 6.1). The Euro Heart Survey on AF enrolled 5,333 patients, of which 2,249 were female (42%). In that 2007 study, the women were older, had more symptoms and a lower quality of life, and were more likely to have concomitant diseases such as hypertension, valvular heart disease, diabetes mellitus, and hyperthyroidism. Men were more likely to have coronary artery disease (CAD) and idiopathic (ie, lone) AF. The univariate analysis of 1-year outcomes showed that women, compared with men, had significantly higher rates of stroke (2.2% vs 1.2%, P=.011) and major bleeding

(2.2% vs 1.3%, P=.028). The Euro Heart Survey also showed that women with AF were more likely to have heart failure (HF) with preserved left ventricular systolic function (18% vs 7%, P=.001) and to have less HF with systolic dysfunction (17% vs 26%, P=.001).

In a study of new-onset AF, the mean age at presentation was 5 years older for women than for men. Again, women were more likely to experience longer (>24 hours) episodes, more frequent recurrences, significantly higher ventricular rates, and more symptoms than men. A 2006 Canadian study of AF patients from tertiary care centers also found that, compared with men, women more frequently reported an impaired quality of life and that some of this impaired quality of life was caused by depression. Scores from the 36-Item Short Form Health Survey (SF-36) showed that the quality of life of female patients was consistently lower than that of male patients (Figure 6.2A). Compared with a healthy age-matched female control group without AF, the quality of life of female patients with persistent AF was significantly less on SF-36 subscales for measures of general health, physical role limitations, pain, and vitality (Figure 6.2B).

In summary, women with AF are more symptomatic than men, and subsequently, women with AF have a lower quality of life than men. These findings underscore the importance of open communication between patients and physicians and an awareness of the unique psychologic contributors to the well-being of the AF patient, particularly female patients.

ELECTROPHYSIOLOGY OF AF

The electrophysiologic properties of the atria have been studied to elucidate mechanisms of AF in both men and women. It is known that women have higher resting heart rates, shorter sinus node recovery times, and longer corrected QT intervals than men (Table 6.1). Some properties that may contribute to the development of AF include left atrial (LA) size, atrial effective refractory period (AERP), atrial conduction times, and response of these properties to rapid pacing. It is notable that baseline atrial refractoriness is shorter in premenopausal women than in postmenopausal women. Furthermore, the degree of AERP shortening that occurs during rapid atrial pacing (a surrogate for AF) and the elevation of atrial pressure due to rapid atrial pacing is smaller

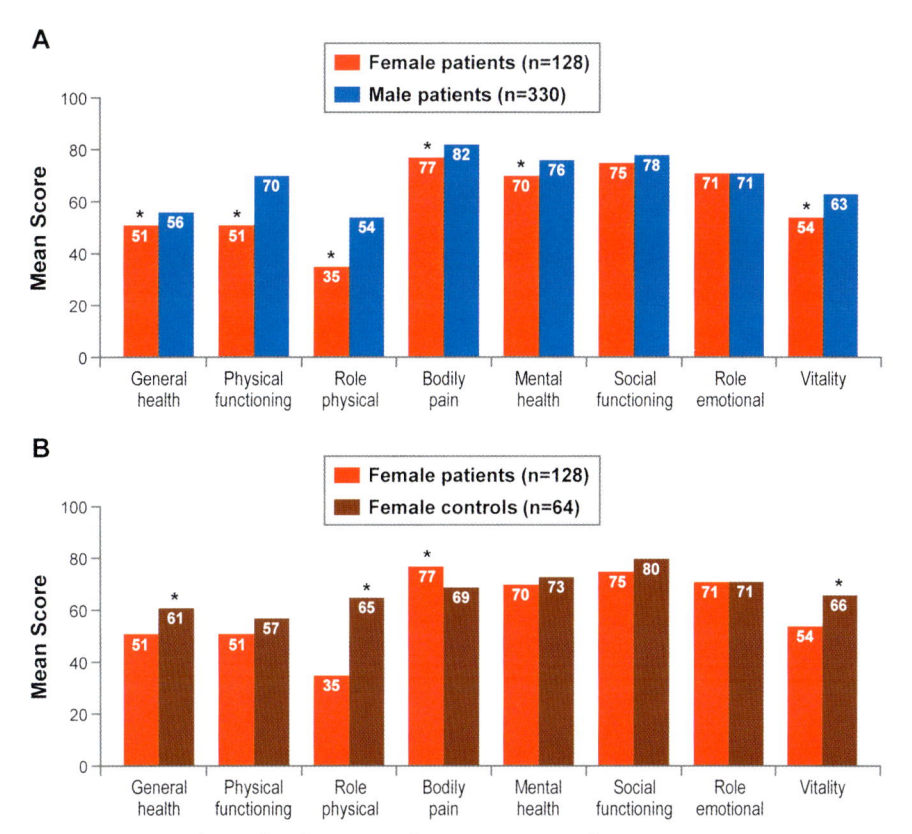

FIGURE 6.2. Quality of Life Scores for Patients With Recurrent Persistent Atrial Fibrillation. Scores are from the 36-Item Short Form Health Survey (SF-36). A, Female patients versus male patients. B, Female patients versus female controls (matched for age). Asterisks indicate $P<.05$. (Adapted from Rienstra M, Van Veldhuisen DJ, Hagens VE, Ranchor AV, Veeger NJ, Crijns HJ, et al; RACE Investigators. Gender-related differences in rhythm control treatment in persistent atrial fibrillation: data of the Rate Control Versus Electrical Cardioversion [RACE] study. J Am Coll Cardiol. 2005 Oct 4;46[7]:1298–306. Used with permission.)

in premenopausal women than in postmenopausal women. These changes are not due simply to aging because the same changes do not occur when assessed in men of different ages. AERP shortening in response to AF is directly correlated to age in women but not in men.

In a study from 2011 that analyzed P-wave dispersion (a marker for AF) in women at various stages of their menstrual cycle, P-wave dispersion was increased during the luteal phase of the menstrual cycle (higher sympathetic activity) compared to the follicular phase (highest estrogen). It may be that estrogen blunts AERP shortening; as a result, younger women have less AF (less AERP shortening due to more estrogen). Perhaps it is estrogen that protects young women from

AF, and perhaps estrogen withdrawal during menopause causes the increased incidence of AF in older women. Further study is needed in this area.

STROKE RISK

In multiple studies, female sex has been associated with an increased risk of stroke in AF, especially among women older than 75 years. In the SPAF I through III trials from the 1990s, female sex was 1 of the 5 independent predictors for stroke (along with age, hypertension, systolic blood pressure [BP] >160 mm Hg, and prior stroke or transient ischemic attack) in AF patients receiving aspirin therapy (relative risk [RR], 1.6; $P=.01$). AF did not seem to affect the stroke rate in younger women, but for women older than 75 who had at least 1 concomitant stroke risk factor, the stroke rate was significantly higher (9.7% per year) than for older men (3.2% per year) ($P<.001$). For older patients with AF and without other thromboembolic risk factors, the stroke rate for women was 7.8% per year compared to 1.2% per year for men ($P=.002$).

In the ATRIA study (published in 2005), 13,559 patients with AF were prospectively followed for 2.4 years. The annual rates of thromboembolism among patients not taking warfarin were higher for women (3.5%) than for men (1.8%). There was no sex difference in 30-day mortality after the thromboembolic event (23% for both sexes). Warfarin use correlated with significantly lower adjusted thromboembolism rates for both men (RR, 0.4; 95% CI, 0.3–0.5) and women (RR, 0.6; 95% CI, 0.5–0.8), with similar annual rates of major hemorrhage for men (1.0%) and women (1.1%). The ATRIA investigators proposed that female sex is an independent risk factor for thromboembolism and stated that sex should influence the decision to use anticoagulant therapy in patients with AF.

This finding was echoed in the Copenhagen City Heart Study (a population-based cohort of more than 16,000 adults) in 2004: the effect of AF on the risk of stroke was 4.6-fold greater for women (hazard ratio [HR], 7.8; 95% CI, 5.8–14.3) than for men (HR, 1.7; 95% CI, 1.0–3.0) after adjustment for age and comorbidities. A very large population-based cohort study (published in 2012) included 83,000 patients (women, 52.8%) 65 years or older who had been hospitalized with recently diagnosed AF in Quebec, Canada; in that study, the risk of stroke was also greater for women than for men, independently of warfarin use (Figure 6.3). On admission to the hospital with a diagnosis of AF, women were older and had higher

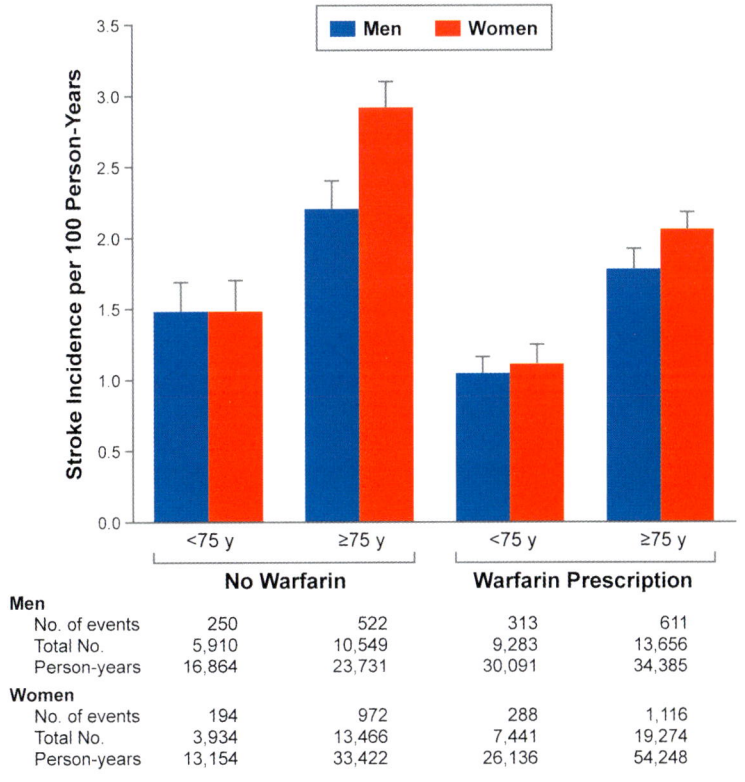

FIGURE 6.3. Incidence of Stroke in Patients With and Without Prescriptions Filled for Warfarin in the First 30 Days After Hospital Discharge, Stratified by Age Group and Sex. In the group that did not receive warfarin, $P=.96$ for comparison of patients younger than 75 years and $P<.001$ for comparison of patients 75 years or older. In the group that received warfarin, $P=.48$ for comparison of patients younger than 75 years and $P=.003$ for comparison of patients 75 years or older. Error bars indicate 95% confidence intervals. (Adapted from Avgil Tsadok M, Jackevicius CA, Rahme E, Humphries KH, Behlouli H, Pilote L. Sex differences in stroke risk among older patients with recently diagnosed atrial fibrillation. JAMA. 2012 May 9;307[18]:1952-8. Used with permission.)

CHADS2 (congestive heart failure, hypertension, age ≥75 years, diabetes mellitus, prior stroke or transient ischemic attack) scores than men. In the multivariable Cox regression analysis, women had a higher risk of stroke than men (adjusted HR, 1.14; 95% CI, 1.07–1.22; $P=.001$), even after adjusting for CHADS2 scores, warfarin use, and baseline comorbid conditions (Table 6.1).

Several hypotheses have been generated to explain the increased stroke rate in women compared to men. Women tend to have an elevated level of von Willebrand factor, which could cause a procoagulable state and might contribute to the higher stroke risk for women with AF. The WHI showed that among healthy postmenopausal women, estrogen replacement therapy increased the risk of stroke, leading to the hypothesis that hormone replacement therapy may cause a procoagulant effect. Data also suggest that diabetes mellitus and metabolic syndrome increase the risk of stroke in women to a greater degree than they do in men. It is also possible that women with AF have a higher stroke risk because of sex bias in the treatment of other concomitant stroke risk factors such as hypertension. Further study is required to determine whether the elevated risk of stroke in women with AF is due to their presentation with more clinical risk factors and possible undertreatment of these conditions due to sex bias, or whether female sex itself is associated with an inherent thromboembolic risk during AF.

MORTALITY AND MORBIDITY

Currently available data indicate that mortality for women with AF is higher than for men. In a study conducted in Sweden in 2001, women with AF had a 5-year mortality rate of 43% compared to an expected mortality rate of 23% ($P<.001$) for women without AF; for men with AF, the 5-year mortality rate was 30% compared to an expected mortality rate of 24% ($P<.05$). This is an excess mortality from AF of 49% for men and 88% for women. In the Copenhagen City Heart Study from 2004, the effect of AF on cardiovascular mortality among women was 2.5 times greater (HR, 4.4; 95% CI, 2.9–6.5) than among men (HR, 2.2; 95% CI, 1.6–3.1) (Table 6.1).

The WHS was a study of 34,715 women who were healthy at the time of enrollment. Published in 2005, the study included a comprehensive 12.4 years of follow-up, and it has provided much of the data presented in the present chapter. WHS data published in 2011 showed that new-onset AF was independently associated with all-cause, cardiovascular, and noncardiovascular mortality. Compared with women who were free of AF, women in whom AF developed represented a higher-risk subgroup and had a higher prevalence of hypertension, left ventricular hypertrophy, increased LA size, diabetes mellitus, hypercholesterolemia, smoking, and body mass index (BMI) (calculated as weight in kilograms divided by height in meters squared) greater than 25 at baseline.

Similar results were echoed in data from the Framingham Heart Study (1998), which showed that women with AF had an increased mortality after adjusting for known cardiovascular disease (men: HR, 1.5; women: HR, 1.9). It is impossible to definitively attribute the cause of increased mortality for women with AF to AF itself or to more severe comorbidities, but it is clear that AF in women is independently associated with increased mortality.

Hypertension has been shown to be a risk factor for the development of AF in both men and women. In the WHS, elevated BP was strongly associated with subsequent AF, and systolic BP was a better predictor of AF than diastolic BP. There was a continuous relationship between systolic BP and the incidence of AF in this study. Even systolic BP levels in the nonhypertensive range were independently associated with AF when BP changes over time were assessed. Left ventricular hypertrophy and increased LA size were also important concomitant findings linking BP and incident AF. Several potential mechanisms could underlie the relationship between elevated BP and AF. For example, elevated systolic BP may be associated with an increase in LA fibrosis, which in turn is related to the development of AF. Arterial stiffness may also contribute to the incidence of AF. Regardless of the mechanism, it is clear that careful control of BP may reduce the growing burden of AF in the community, especially among women.

The WHS also looked at AF and BMI in the study's population of apparently healthy women. The data showed an association of increased BMI with short- and long-term increases in AF risk that were responsible for a large proportion of the AF independently of traditional risk factors. During 12.9 years of follow-up, BMI was linearly associated with AF risk, with an increase in risk of 4.7% (95% CI, 3.4–6.1; $P<.001$) for each kilogram per square meter. The association was stronger for younger women. There was a 41% adjusted increase in risk for the development of AF ($P=.02$) in participants who became obese during the first 5 years of the study. Given that there are more obese women than obese men in the population, a strategy of weight control, especially for women, could reduce the increasing incidence of AF.

In the same study, data on birth weight and AF showed a significant, direct linear relationship between birth weight and incidence of AF ($P=.002$): Women in the highest birth weight category, compared with women in the lowest, had a significant 71% increased risk of AF. These data suggest that factors that affect the heart in childhood may be important in the pathogenesis of AF in adulthood.

ALCOHOL AND CAFFEINE INTAKE

An association between alcohol use and AF is well known, but little has been done to look at this association specifically in women. A 2010 meta-analysis and literature review of the association between alcohol intake and AF in women showed that alcohol consumption of 2 or fewer drinks per day was not significantly associated with the risk of AF. In fact, the risk with low-volume consumption was almost identical to the risk for nondrinkers (RR, 0.99; 95% CI, 0.91–1.07; P=.775). However, women who consumed more than 2 or 3 drinks daily had a 17% increased risk of AF, and those consuming more than 4 drinks daily had a 50% increased risk of AF.

Analysis of data from the Copenhagen City Heart Study in 2005 showed that alcohol consumption of 35 or more drinks per week was associated with an increased risk of AF among men. There were not enough women consuming this amount of alcohol in that study to draw any conclusions about the subgroup of women. The WHS (with 12.4 years of follow-up) showed a statistically significant 1.6-fold greater risk of AF for women who had 2 or more drinks per day.

Short- or long-term alcohol consumption has various effects on the electrical activity of the heart in men and women. These include direct alcohol cardiotoxicity, hyperadrenergic activity during drinking and withdrawal, and impairment of vagal tone, with a subsequent increase in intra-atrial conduction time leading to increased P-wave dispersion and susceptibility to AF. Another potential explanation for alcohol-related AF is LA remodeling due to the hypertension that typically occurs during alcohol intoxication.

Fewer studies have been published on the effects of caffeine on incident AF. The WHS, however, did show that caffeine consumption of up to 656 mg daily was not associated with an increased risk of AF. In addition, none of the specific caffeine-containing products (coffee, tea, cola, and chocolate) was associated with risk of AF. From the limited data available, elevated caffeine consumption does not appear to contribute to the increasing burden of AF in women.

AF IN PREGNANCY

The initial evaluation of a pregnant woman with AF should include an electrocardiogram, measurement of serum electrolytes, urine drug screen, serum thyroid studies, and an echocardiogram. The electrocardiogram will show the diagnosis of possible underlying conditions, such as Wolff-Parkinson-White syndrome. The echocardiogram will show other causes of previously undetected structural or congenital abnormalities. Most cases of AF in pregnancy do occur in women with underlying cardiac structural defects or underlying medical problems (eg, rheumatic heart disease or other valvular pathology, cardiac conduction or structural anomalies, hyperthyroidism, drug toxicity, electrolyte disturbances, or pulmonary embolus). When the primary problem is properly treated, the secondary AF will resolve. Even more rarely, however, lone AF may occur in pregnancy.

The initial treatment of pregnant women who present with AF should be to control the ventricular rate while the patient is being evaluated. Ultimately, the goal is restoration of normal sinus rhythm either chemically or electrically. Restoring normal rhythm will preserve adequate blood flow to the woman's vital organs and to the placenta and eliminate the need for long-term anticoagulation during pregnancy. Before cardioversion, transesophageal echocardiography should be performed if indicated (depending on the duration of the AF episode) to be certain that there is no LA thrombus. Procainamide, digoxin, propranolol, and flecainide have been used successfully in pregnancy. Theoretically, electrical cardioversion of the mother during pregnancy can induce fetal arrhythmias; however, reported cases of cardioversion in pregnancy have shown good fetal tolerance to this procedure. Fortunately, most of the time an underlying cause of AF that manifests during pregnancy can be determined and corrected, so that long-term antiarrhythmic therapy and anticoagulation are not required.

TREATMENT OF AF IN WOMEN

Stroke Prevention

Antithrombotic therapy with oral anticoagulation (OAC) is recommended for all patients, male and female, who have AF and more than 1 moderate stroke risk factor according to the CHADS2 stroke risk assessment score. The CHADS2 score assigns 1 point each for 4 comorbidities (congestive heart failure, hypertension, age ≥75 years, and diabetes mellitus) and 2 points for stroke or transient ischemic attack. Aspirin (81–325 mg) can be used as an alternative to OAC in low-risk patients who do not have associated comorbidities (ie, lone AF) or in those with contraindications to OAC. OAC traditionally only included the vitamin K antagonist warfarin, but now there are several newer anticoagulation agents. These include the factor Xa inhibitors rivaroxaban and apixaban, the direct thrombin inhibitor dabigatran, and others awaiting approval by the US Food and Drug Administration.

Warfarin has been the most extensively studied and widely used drug for stroke prevention in AF. Anticoagulation with adjusted-dose warfarin is highly efficacious in stroke prevention, with a risk reduction of more than 60% compared with placebo or antiplatelet therapy. For patients taking vitamin K antagonists, the target international normalized ratio (INR) for nonvalvular AF is 2 to 3 as assessed by a blood level determination at a minimum of monthly intervals. Unfortunately, the use of vitamin K antagonists can be confounded by food and drug interactions, which require frequent laboratory monitoring and dose adjustments in some patients.

Dabigatran, approved for use in the United States and Europe, was found to be noninferior to warfarin in the RE-LY study. Rivaroxaban was compared to warfarin in the ROCKET AF study and was also found to be noninferior. Apixaban was first shown to prevent stroke in the AVERROES trial and was shown to be noninferior to warfarin in the ARISTOTLE study. All studies of the new OAC agents showed a trend toward less intracranial and fatal bleeding when compared with the traditional vitamin K antagonist, warfarin, and therefore offer the promise of a superior safety profile.

Factors such as advanced age, uncontrolled hypertension, CAD, cerebrovascular disease, anemia, and concomitant antiplatelet agent use are associated with increased bleeding risk. Most bleeding complications occur at times of excessive anticoagulation with warfarin (INR >3.0), and thus, appropriate INR monitoring is of paramount importance for both men and women. In the CARAF, in 1998, women older than 75 years were 54% less likely to receive warfarin then men in the same age group and they were twice as likely to receive acetylsalicylic acid, a treatment for stroke prevention that is not as effective. Despite having similar

CHADS2 scores, older women received less OAC than older men with similar risk scores.

Because some studies have suggested that women have an increased risk of bleeding compared to men, physicians are occasionally less inclined to prescribe adequate OAC for women. However, current data have not proved a clear increased bleeding risk for women compared to men (Table 6.1). Given the significantly higher reported rates of stroke in women, awareness of treatment biases needs to be raised and therapies need to be more evidence-based. Women may benefit even more than their male counterparts with appropriate and adequate anticoagulation. Further study of the newer agents may show that they are superior in this regard.

Alternatives to OAC are currently under investigation (eg, LA appendage occlusion with either surgical ligation or occlusion devices). Whether these techniques will provide a permanent and effective treatment for stroke prevention in AF remains to be determined.

Drug Therapy

Drug therapy for AF may be divided into 2 broad categories: a rate control strategy, in which the ventricular response during AF is slowed but the patient remains in AF, or a rhythm control strategy, in which an attempt is made to restore and maintain normal sinus rhythm. Selection of appropriate drugs for either of these strategies is based on the type of underlying heart disease, the magnitude of symptoms, and the type of AF (ie, paroxysmal, persistent, or permanent).

Long-term rate control can be maintained by using AV nodal blocking agents, such as β-blockers, calcium channel blockers, and digoxin. Intravenous agents, such as digoxin and amiodarone, can be used for acute rate control when there is concomitant HF associated with rapidly conducted AF. Digoxin alone is no longer considered adequate as a single agent for rate control given its limited effect on resting heart rates and lack of efficacy on heart rates during exertion. If the ventricular rate cannot be adequately controlled with drug therapy, or the patient experiences intolerable side effects to medications, complete atrioventricular nodal ablation and pacemaker implantation can be performed as a permanent solution. Studies have shown that women are referred for this procedure more often than men.

For the rate control strategy, it is important to assess the effectiveness of the rate control medications in the resting state and during exertion. Resting heart rates should be between 60 and 80 beats per minute, and heart rates should be between 90 and 115 beats per minute during moderate exercise. Adequacy of rate control is best assessed by a combination of ambulatory monitoring and stress testing in appropriate patients. Data from the RACE II trial, published in 2010, showed that a more lenient range of heart rates, such as a resting heart rate less than 110 beats per minute, may be acceptable in some patients with preserved left ventricular systolic function without compromising long-term outcomes.

Selection of antiarrhythmic drugs for a rhythm control strategy must be carefully based on the type of underlying structural heart disease. For patients without structural heart disease, the European Society of Cardiology and the American Heart Association guidelines recommend flecainide, propafenone, sotalol, or dronedarone as first-line therapy and amiodarone or dofetilide as second-line therapy. For hypertensive patients and particularly those with left ventricular hypertrophy, amiodarone is considered to be the safest agent, with a lower incidence of torsades de pointes (TdP). Dofetilide, dronedarone, and sotalol are recommended for patients with CAD; only amiodarone and dofetilide have been proved safe for patients with concomitant AF and HF. The recommended algorithm for antiarrhythmic drug selection is shown in Figure 6.4.

It is well recognized that women, compared with men, have a significantly higher risk of proarrhythmia and other side effects when using antiarrhythmic drugs (Table 6.1). Women, compared with men, have longer QT intervals at baseline and have hypokalemia more frequently because of their greater use of diuretics. Longer baseline QT intervals increase the risk of TdP in women. In a study of D,L-sotalol, women had a 4.1% incidence of TdP, compared to 1% for men. Increased TdP due to sotalol was also seen in the SWORD trial, and the study was prematurely terminated because of excess mortality in the treatment group. The DIAMOND-CHF trial, designed to evaluate dofetilide, similarly showed that female sex was an independent risk factor for the occurrence of TdP. The incidence of drug-induced sick sinus syndrome due to flecainide, sotalol, and amiodarone

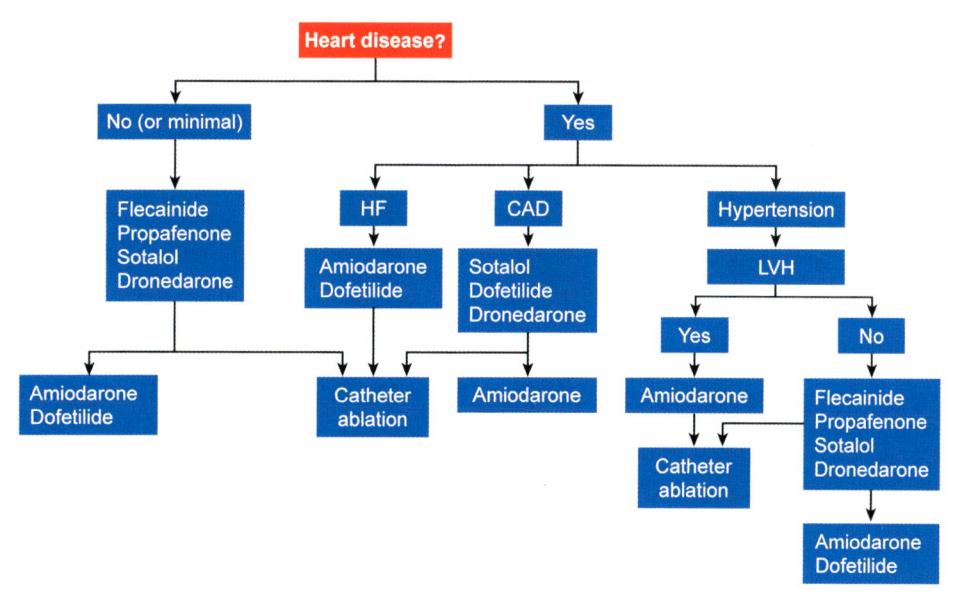

FIGURE 6.4. Antiarrhythmic Drug Therapy to Maintain Sinus Rhythm in Patients With Recurrent Paroxysmal or Persistent Atrial Fibrillation. CAD indicates coronary artery disease; HF, heart failure; LVH, left ventricular hypertrophy.

therapy is notably higher for women than for men, leading to a higher rate of pacemaker implantation for women than for men.

The risk of proarrhythmia also changes with hormonal fluctuations. The postpartum period is particularly arrhythmogenic because progesterone and estradiol levels abruptly decrease. Unopposed estrogen replacement hormonal therapy, rather than combination estrogen and progesterone therapy, also makes women more susceptible to arrhythmias. Women's higher risk of proarrhythmia from antiarrhythmic drugs must be considered when deciding on a rate or rhythm control strategy for each patient.

AFFIRM, published in 2002, was a randomized trial that included 4,060 patients with AF. The patients were divided into 2 treatment arms: rhythm control strategy and rate control strategy. After a mean of 3.5 years of follow-up, the investigators found no survival advantage with rhythm control for men or women. Sex did not predict any difference in response to the 2 treatment strategies.

The RACE trial, published in 2002, also investigated the outcome of AF patients randomly assigned to a rate control strategy or a rhythm control strategy. Again, there was no statistically significant difference in the cardiovascular end points of death from a cardiovascular cause, thromboembolic events, severe adverse drug

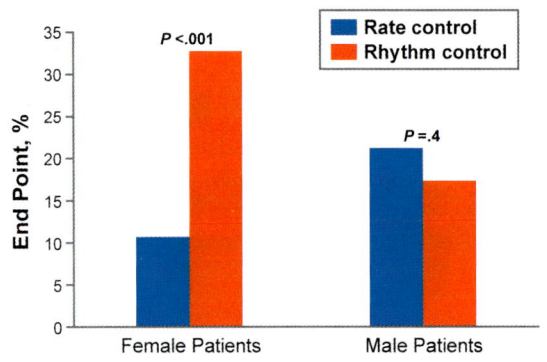

FIGURE 6.5. Occurrence of Primary End Point According to Sex and Randomized Strategy. Patients were randomly assigned to a rate control strategy (blue bars) or a rhythm control strategy (red bars). (Adapted from Rienstra M, Van Veldhuisen DJ, Hagens VE, Ranchor AV, Veeger NJ, Crijns HJ, et al; RACE Investigators. Gender-related differences in rhythm control treatment in persistent atrial fibrillation: data of the Rate Control Versus Electrical Cardioversion [RACE] study. J Am Coll Cardiol. 2005 Oct 4;46[7]:1298-306. Used with permission.)

reactions, implantation of a pacemaker, HF, or bleeding in all patients. However, in a substudy of the RACE trial published in 2005, adverse events (HF, thromboembolic complications, and adverse effects of antiarrhythmic drugs) were 3 times as likely to occur in women randomly assigned to the rhythm control arm compared to women assigned to the rate control arm (Table 6.1). This finding was absent for the 2 male treatment groups (Figure 6.5). Notably, there was a lower quality of life for women in both arms of the study.

Adjuvant Medical Therapy

Statins

In addition to standard antiarrhythmic drugs for treatment of AF, statins may help protect against AF, as suggested by some data. However, there is not a plethora of data on the effect of statin treatment on the incidence of AF specifically in women. In 2009, HERS authors reported the effect of statin treatment on the incidence and prevalence of AF in 2,673 postmenopausal women with stable CAD. First, the data showed that women with AF were significantly less likely to be taking a statin at study enrollment than those without AF (22% vs 37%, $P=.003$). Second, statin users had a 65% lower chance of having AF at baseline after controlling for age, race, history of myocardial infarction or revascularization, and history of HF (odds ratio, 0.35; 95% CI, 0.13–0.93; *P*=.04). Third, for women free of AF at baseline, the adjusted risk of AF developing during the study was 55% less for those receiving statin therapy (HR, 0.45; 95% CI, 0.26–0.78; *P*=.004).

Statins are thought to prevent AF through their anti-inflammatory and antioxidant effects. Other potential mechanisms of the effect of statins include improvement in endothelial function, reduction of neurohormonal activation, attenuating leukocyte infiltration, and beneficial effects on atrial cellular and electrophysiologic remodeling. Statins may also potentially protect the atrial myocardium during ischemia. Unfortunately, statins have not been shown to reduce recurrent AF after pulmonary vein isolation. In addition, women are less likely to be treated with statins than men, and this could be a factor in the increased prevalence of AF in women.

Angiotensin-Converting Enzyme Inhibitors

Limited data suggest that the use of angiotensin-blocking drugs lowers the rate of AF recurrences. Studies have shown that estrogen inhibits the renin-angiotensin system through elevation of plasma levels of angiotensin II and, by negative feedback, lowers angiotensin-converting enzyme levels and renin activity. Postmenopausal women therefore have increased activity of the renin-angiotensin system, which could lead to AF and can be reversed by using hormone replacement therapy. Galinier and colleagues reported in 2006 that irbesartan used along with amiodarone (compared with use of amiodarone alone) lowered AF recurrence after cardioversion. Whether this also holds true for AF after catheter ablation is not known.

Bisphosphonates

Since the WHI in 2003 showed an increased risk of cardiovascular events in women taking hormone replacement therapy, there has been interest in the effects of bisphosphonates on cardiovascular heart disease and AF. Several studies of postmenopausal women, including a 2010 meta-analysis of 4 randomized trials and 3 population-based clinical trials, have shown a significant increase in the incidence of AF in patients treated with bisphosphonates. A population-based case-control study showed that women who had taken alendronate at any time (compared with those who had never taken the drug) were more likely to have

AF after adjustment for age, hypertension, osteoporosis, and cardiovascular disease. The authors of that study estimated that 3% of incident AF in their population might be explained by alendronate use. In contrast, a Danish study (published in 2008) that used medical databases with over 80,000 patients and a case-control study from the United Kingdom (published in 2009) found no strong evidence of a long-term increased risk of AF or atrial flutter in connection with use of the oral bisphosphonates alendronic acid and risedronate sodium. The mechanisms by which bisphosphonates could contribute to AF have been hypothesized to be hypocalcemia, alterations in atrial conduction properties, and possibly hypoparathyroidism, but no study has proved these hypothetical mechanisms. The relationship between bisphosphonate use and AF is still controversial and speculative.

Thyroid Replacement

A study at the Karolinska Institute in Sweden (published in 2011) showed that thyroid replacement therapy in women with AF correlated with a lower total mortality after adjusting for other comorbidities. The study included 5,642 women older than 45 at the time of the AF diagnosis; 907 were already taking levothyroxine, and 4,735 were not receiving thyroid supplement therapy. The women receiving replacement therapy had a lower mortality than those not receiving replacement therapy. Levothyroxine is known to improve the dyslipidemia associated with hypothyroidism. The lipid-lowering effect of levothyroxine not only decreases arterial plaque formation, but it may also have effects on the cardiac ion channels that benefit patients with AF. Thus, the lower mortality among women with AF who take levothyroxine could reflect undiagnosed cases of clinical or subclinical hypothyroidism in the untreated women. A careful evaluation for hypothyroidism in women who present with AF may be warranted.

Cardioversion

Direct current cardioversion (DCCV) is a safe and effective means of restoring sinus rhythm. DCCV is indicated for patients who have uncontrolled rapid ventricular response, for patients who are hemodynamically unstable, and for patients who need an ultimate strategy for restoring sinus rhythm by other means, such as drug therapy or catheter ablation. The short-term success rate with a biphasic waveform is 94% to 97%. However, 50% of patients who undergo electrical cardioversion have a recurrence of AF within 1 year. Predictors of AF recurrence include older age, underlying structural heart disease, prolonged duration of AF, and increased LA size. A study by Gurevitz and colleagues (published in 2006) showed that female sex was a strong univariate and multivariate predictor of earlier and higher rates of AF recurrence after DCCV.

Catheter Ablation

Catheter ablation of AF offers a potential cure for patients who are resistant to pharmacologic therapy and remain symptomatic. The resumption of sinus rhythm after ablation has been shown to significantly improve quality of life, symptomatology, exercise tolerance, and left ventricular function. Catheter ablation with a strategy of pulmonary vein antrum isolation has a broad 2-year success rate, ranging from 60% to 85%, depending on the severity of the antecedent AF. The possibility of a cure is particularly attractive for women because women have worse outcomes in terms of stroke, mortality, and poorer quality of life.

Despite the potential advantages of catheter ablation for women, significant sex disparities exist in the referral patterns. Women ultimately referred for ablation are generally older and more symptomatic than their male counterparts. Women tend to have more longstanding AF, larger LA, and a history of not responding to more antiarrhythmic drugs than men (Table 6.1). In a study by Roten and colleagues (published in 2009), women were referred 3 times less often for AF ablation then men. This sex bias in referral patterns persisted even when a cardiologist was caring for the patient before referral. However, after patients were referred to a tertiary center or to an electrophysiologist, there appeared to be no sex-based differences in subsequent treatment decisions. It seems that the bias in referrals may be at the level of the primary care provider or the referring cardiologist. Women with AF report a poorer quality of life and have a higher risk of death than men. In addition, women have a higher stroke risk and a poorer overall prognosis than men. Therefore, with a curative strategy of catheter ablation therapy, women may benefit more than men. This background provides a valid argument for referring women for catheter ablation even sooner than men.

Studies have shown that ablation success and AF recurrence rates are similar between men and women, but women face referral delays and have higher-risk clinical profiles when they are ultimately referred for ablation. Even though they have smaller bodies, women tend to have larger LA because their disease is more advanced at ablation. In a study by Forleo and colleagues (published in 2007), catheter ablation of AF provided uniform benefit for both men and women (Figure 6.6). At a mean (SD) follow-up of 22.5 (11.8) months after the last ablation, the overall freedom from AF recurrence was similar for women (83.1%) and men (82.7%), and SF-36 quality of life scores improved for both sexes.

Success rates for catheter ablation of AF depend on the stage of AF at presentation and on the presence or absence of structural heart disease. In contrast to the findings of Forleo and colleagues, Patel and colleagues reported in 2010 that the success rate with catheter ablation was lower for female patients (68.5%) than for male patients (77.5%). This apparent discrepancy may be explained by the fact that the study by Forleo and colleagues included more patients with paroxysmal AF and structurally normal hearts than the study by Patel and

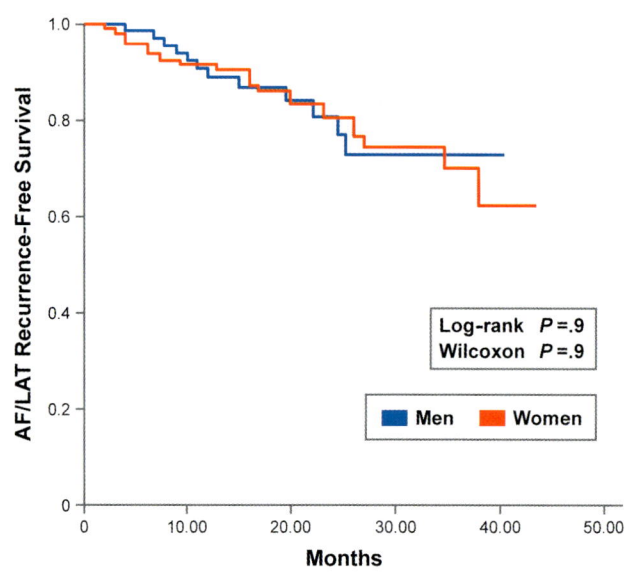

FIGURE 6.6. Kaplan-Meier Curve of Survival Free From Recurrence of Atrial Fibrillation (AF) and Left Atrial Tachycardia (LAT) After 1 Month of the Blanking Period. The time until first recurrence was not different between men and women. (Adapted from Forleo GB, Tondo C, De Luca L, Dello Russo A, Casella M, De Sanctis V, et al. Gender-related differences in catheter ablation of atrial fibrillation. Europace. 2007 Aug;9[8]:613–20. Used with permission.)

colleagues. Paroxysmal AF is known to be more amenable to successful catheter ablation. In a 2005 article, Lee and colleagues reported on their study of consecutive patients referred for catheter ablation of AF: women had a higher incidence of nonpulmonary vein sources, and women tended to have more firing from the superior vena cava than men. The authors postulated that this resulted from higher parasympathetic tone in women. Sauer and colleagues in 2003 also reported that female sex was associated with more nonpulmonary vein sources. Given the higher prevalence of more advanced AF in women referred for ablation, it is not surprising that they have more nonpulmonary vein firing and a potentially lower success rate with catheter ablation than men who were referred at earlier stages of their disease.

In several studies, the incidence of procedural complications has been higher for women than for men. Women have a higher incidence of femoral vascular complications, such as hematoma requiring evacuation, and pseudoaneurysms. Female sex is also an independent risk factor for pericardial tamponade.

There is an increasing awareness that women are underrepresented in studies of many invasive cardiac procedures, including catheter ablation for AF. It is notable that the proportion of women enrolled in single-center or multicenter AF ablation studies has been consistently less than 30%. This awareness should drive physicians to enroll more women in trials to discover which treatments are safest and most effective specifically in women.

CONCLUSIONS

Cardiovascular disease is the leading cause of death among women, and AF is the most common cardiac arrhythmia. Because of the greater longevity of women in older age groups, women with AF currently outnumber men. Sex-related differences in clinical presentation are clear, with more women than men complaining of intolerable symptoms and a worse quality of life with AF. Women are at increased risk of proarrhythmia and other adverse events associated with the use of antiarrhythmic drugs. OAC therapy should be prescribed equally to patients of either sex, although currently it is not. The advent of the novel oral anticoagulants may change this practice in the future. Women with AF have a worse prognosis than men, with higher death rates and more frequent cardioembolic strokes.

Women have received more conservative treatment of AF than men, and they have typically been offered fewer cardioversions and are more likely to receive atrioventricular nodal ablation and pacemaker implantations than men after antiarrhythmic drug therapy has failed. These facts present a strong case for more aggressive and earlier therapy for AF in women, including risk factor modification, treatment with OAC, and early referral for catheter ablation.

SUGGESTED READING

Avgil Tsadok M, Jackevicius CA, Rahme E, Humphries KH, Behlouli H, Pilote L. Sex differences in stroke risk among older patients with recently diagnosed atrial fibrillation. JAMA. 2012 May 9;307(18):1952–8.

Conen D, Chae CU, Glynn RJ, Tedrow UB, Everett BM, Buring JE, et al. Risk of death and cardiovascular events in initially healthy women with new-onset atrial fibrillation. JAMA. 2011 May 25;305(20):2080–7.

Cook NR, Lee IM, Gaziano JM, Gordon D, Ridker PM, Manson JE, et al. Low-dose aspirin in the primary prevention of cancer: the Women's Health Study: a randomized controlled trial. JAMA. 2005 Jul 6;294(1):47–55.

Dagres N, Nieuwlaat R, Vardas PE, Andresen D, Levy S, Cobbe S, et al. Gender-related differences in presentation, treatment, and outcome of patients with atrial fibrillation in Europe: a report from the Euro Heart Survey on Atrial Fibrillation. J Am Coll Cardiol. 2007 Feb 6;49(5):572–7. Epub 2007 Jan 22.

Fang MC, Singer DE, Chang Y, Hylek EM, Henault LE, Jensvold NG, et al. Gender differences in the risk of ischemic stroke and peripheral embolism in atrial fibrillation: the AnTicoagulation and Risk factors In Atrial fibrillation (ATRIA) study. Circulation. 2005 Sep 20;112(12):1687–91. Epub 2005 Sep 12.

Flaker G, Ezekowitz M, Yusuf S, Wallentin L, Noack H, Brueckmann M, et al. Efficacy and safety of dabigatran compared to warfarin in patients with paroxysmal, persistent, and permanent atrial fibrillation: results from the RE-LY (Randomized Evaluation of Long-Term Anticoagulation Therapy) study. J Am Coll Cardiol. 2012 Feb 28;59(9):854–5.

Friberg J, Scharling H, Gadsboll N, Truelsen T, Jensen GB; Copenhagen City Heart Study. Comparison of the impact of atrial fibrillation on the risk of stroke and cardiovascular death in women versus men (The Copenhagen City Heart Study). Am J Cardiol. 2004 Oct 1;94(7):889–94.

Lee IM, Cook NR, Gaziano JM, Gordon D, Ridker PM, Manson JE, et al. Vitamin E in the primary prevention of cardiovascular disease and cancer: the Women's Health Study: a randomized controlled trial. JAMA. 2005 Jul 6;294(1):56–65.

Lloyd-Jones DM, Wang TJ, Leip EP, Larson MG, Levy D, Vasan RS, et al. Lifetime risk for development of atrial fibrillation: the Framingham Heart Study. Circulation. 2004 Aug 31;110(9):1042–6. Epub 2004 Aug 16.

Miyasaka Y, Barnes ME, Bailey KR, Cha SS, Gersh BJ, Seward JB, et al. Mortality trends in patients diagnosed with first atrial fibrillation: a 21-year community-based study. J Am Coll Cardiol. 2007 Mar 6;49(9):986–92. Epub 2007 Feb 16.

Patel D, Mohanty P, Di Biase L, Sanchez JE, Shaheen MH, Burkhardt JD, et al. Outcomes and complications of catheter ablation for atrial fibrillation in females. Heart Rhythm. 2010;7(2):167–72. Epub 2009 Oct 23.

Patel MR, Mahaffey KW, Garg J, Pan G, Singer DE, Hacke W, et al; ROCKET AF Investigators. Rivaroxaban versus warfarin in nonvalvular atrial fibrillation. N Engl J Med. 2011 Sep 8;365(10):883–91. Epub 2011 Aug 10.

Ridker PM, Cook NR, Lee IM, Gordon D, Gaziano JM, Manson JE, et al. A randomized trial of low-dose aspirin in the primary prevention of cardiovascular disease in women. N Engl J Med. 2005 Mar 31;352(13):1293–304. Epub 2005 Mar 7.

Rienstra M, Van Veldhuisen DJ, Hagens VE, Ranchor AV, Veeger NJ, Crijns HJ, et al; RACE Investigators. Gender-related differences in rhythm control treatment in persistent atrial fibrillation: data of the Rate Control Versus Electrical Cardioversion (RACE) study. J Am Coll Cardiol. 2005 Oct 4;46(7):1298–306.

Roten L, Rimoldi SF, Schwick N, Sakata T, Heimgartner C, Fuhrer J, et al. Gender differences in patients referred for atrial fibrillation management to a tertiary center. Pacing Clin Electrophysiol. 2009 May;32(5):622–6.

Van Gelder IC, Hagens VE, Bosker HA, Kingma JH, Kamp O, Kingma T, et al; Rate Control versus Electrical Cardioversion for Persistent Atrial Fibrillation Study Group. A comparison of rate control and rhythm control in patients with recurrent persistent atrial fibrillation. N Engl J Med. 2002 Dec 5;347(23):1834–40.

CHAPTER SEVEN

Drug Treatment in Women

KATHERINE T. MURRAY, MD

INTRODUCTION

In the quest for a personalized approach to modern drug therapy, there is increasing evidence that sex matters. In cardiovascular therapeutics, sex-based considerations are particularly important with the use of antiarrhythmic drugs. In general, women have a greater incidence of adverse outcomes, especially drug-mediated proarrhythmia. Despite numerous studies, the mechanisms responsible for these sex-related differences are not fully understood. This chapter reviews the evidence for the disparate responses between men and women to electrophysiologically active agents and highlights potential drug interactions of unique clinical significance for women.

DRUG-INDUCED LONG QT SYNDROME

It is well recognized that adult women have longer QT intervals than men. Cardiac repolarization is similar in male and female children at birth, but after puberty, the QT interval shortens in men. Some studies suggest that the duration of the QT interval fluctuates during menses, but this remains controversial. In 1 investigation, ibutilide-related QT prolongation in women was greatest during menses compared with the ovulatory or luteal phases. For patients with congenital long QT syndrome (LQTS), registry data indicate that women have a greater risk for a first cardiac event between the ages of 15 and 40 years. In general, pregnancy does not increase the arrhythmic risk in patients with congenital LQTS, but arrhythmias can be increased in the postpartum period, especially for women with the LQTS type 2 genotype (mutations in *KCNH2*). Taken together, these data suggest a role for gonadal steroids to modulate cardiac repolarization.

Animal studies have also shown sex differences in ventricular repolarization, ion channel expression, and transmural ion channel gradients, although results are markedly species dependent. For example, isolated female rabbit hearts, compared with male rabbit hearts, have greater QT prolongation at slower heart rates and reduced repolarizing potassium currents. Sex hormones have been shown to have acute effects on ion channels that are nongenomic (ie, independent of hormone-mediated changes in transcription). In general, exposure to estradiol-17β prolongs ventricular repolarization, while progesterone and testosterone shorten it. Nonetheless, existing data implicate testosterone as the major factor responsible for sex-based differences in cardiac repolarization. Acute exposure to testosterone shortens the action potential duration (APD) in isolated guinea pig ventricular myocytes, with enhanced slow component of the delayed rectifier potassium current (I_{Ks}) and reduced L-type calcium current ($I_{Ca,L}$). Other studies indicate that testosterone exposure shortens repolarization by increasing the rapid component of the delayed rectifier potassium current (I_{Kr}). In the failing human heart, ventricular myocytes from women had longer APDs and greater susceptibility to early afterdepolarizations than cells from men's hearts. These differences were attributed to tendencies for decreased transient outward potassium current (I_{To}) and increased $I_{Ca,L}$ in myocytes from women.

Beginning in the 1980s, published case reports and small series suggested that women were more prone to drug-induced QT prolongation and torsades de pointes (Figure 7.1). In a comprehensive review of published data for QT-prolonging drugs, 332 cases of torsades de pointes were identified; 70% of the cases were in women. This study and others have established that female sex, independently of other clinical variables, is a risk factor for this proarrhythmic event. For both cardiac and noncardiac QT-prolonging drugs, studies have repeatedly shown that approximately two-thirds of affected patients were women.

Additional findings from randomized clinical trials have provided similar findings. The SWORD trial compared outcomes with the pure class III drug D-sotalol or placebo in a randomized, blinded design with patients who had left

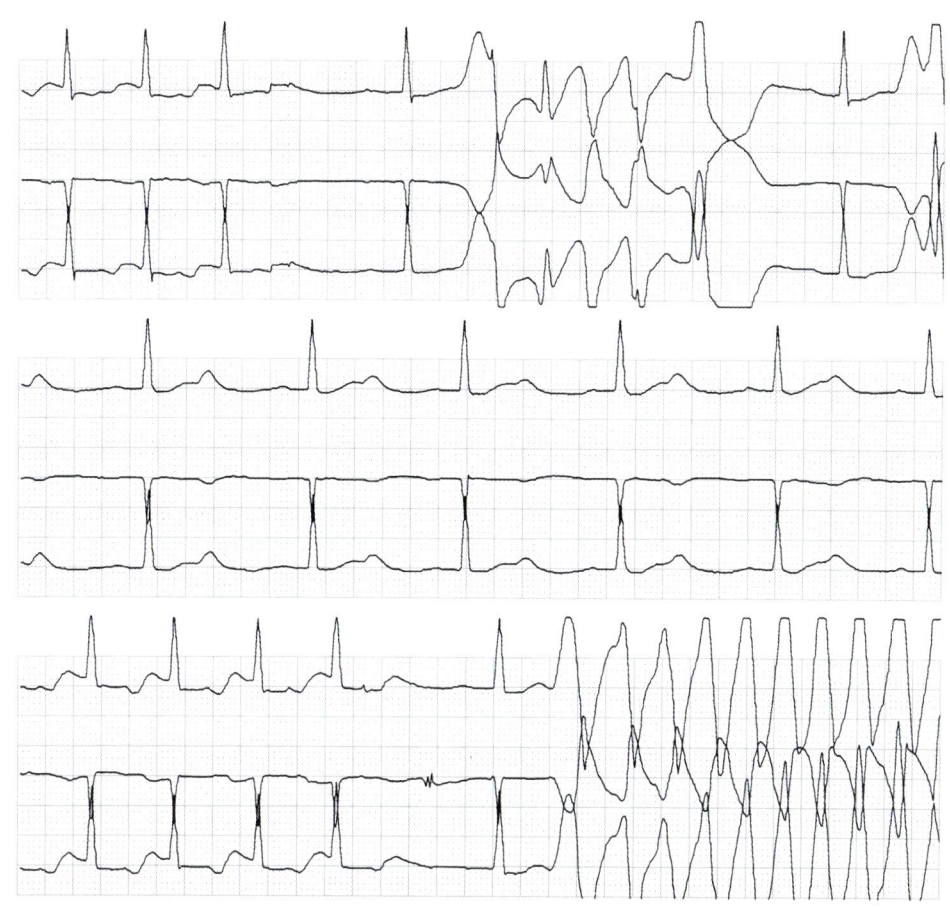

FIGURE 7.1. Electrocardiogram Showing Drug-Induced Long QT Syndrome and Torsades de Pointes. The patient was a 63-year-old woman taking sotalol for prevention of atrial fibrillation.

ventricular dysfunction after myocardial infarction. The trial was stopped early because of excessive mortality in the D-sotalol arm. Presumed arrhythmic death largely accounted for the increased mortality, with a rate for women (relative risk [RR], ~4) that exceeded that for men (RR, ~1.5). With the marketed racemic (D,L) preparation of sotalol, torsades de pointes occurs in a greater proportion of women (4.1%) than men (1.9%).

The DIAMOND-CHF trial randomly assigned patients with left ventricular dysfunction and congestive heart failure (CHF) to receive the class III drug dofetilide or placebo, with inpatient initiation of drug therapy and careful dose adjustment based on the creatinine value and QT response. Dofetilide had no effect on mortality, while torsades de pointes occurred only in the dofetilide arm. Logistic regression analysis showed that female sex (RR, 3.2) and New York Heart

Association class III or IV CHF (RR, 3.9) were significantly associated with the occurrence of torsades de pointes. Similarly, QT prolongation during ibutilide infusion was greater in women than men, with an increased incidence of torsades de pointes (5.6% for women vs 3% for men). Interestingly, the female preponderance of drug-induced LQTS does not change after menopause, arguing against an important role for estrogen.

With QT-prolonging drugs, animal studies have shown that androgens appear to have a protective effect, while estrogens may facilitate related arrhythmias. Ventricular tissue from oophorectomized female rabbits treated with testosterone had shorter APDs at baseline, less APD prolongation with the QT-prolonging drug E-4031, and fewer early afterdepolarizations compared with placebo- or estradiol-treated animals (Figure 7.2). Similar results have been obtained with female rabbits treated with dofetilide.

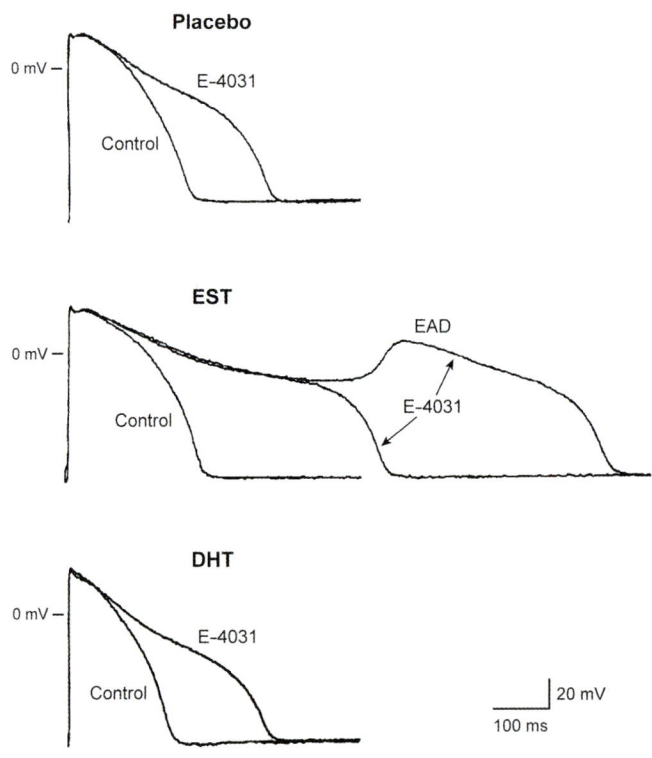

FIGURE 7.2. Effects of the QT-Prolonging Drug E-4031 on Ventricular Papillary Muscle From Oophorectomized Rabbits. The rabbits were treated with placebo, estradiol (EST), or dihydrotestosterone (DHT). Action potential prolongation was greatest in the animals treated with EST, which induced early afterdepolarization (EAD). (Adapted from Hara M, Danilo P Jr, Rosen MR. Effects of gonadal steroids on ventricular repolarization and on the response to E4031. J PharmacolExpTher. 1998 Jun;285[3]:1068–72. Used with permission.)

For drug-induced QT prolongation, the magnitude of hormone-mediated changes in experimental preparations is considerably smaller than the clinical effects observed in patients. Along with additional findings, these data suggest that other mechanisms besides gonadal steroids likely contribute to sex-related differences. Interestingly, available evidence shows sex-related differences in drug disposition. As a simple example, creatinine clearance is reduced in women compared with men because women have a smaller body mass. This factor could affect certain class III drugs that are renally excreted, such as sotalol and dofetilide. Cytochrome P450 3A isozyme (CYP3A) is the predominant cytochrome P450 subfamily in humans, and it accounts for the metabolism of more than 50% of marketed drugs (Figure 7.3). In addition, many drugs that are CYP3A substrates, including macrolide antibiotics, ketoconazole, and thioridazine, also bind to the human ether-à-go-go–related gene (*hERG*) channel, which forms the basis of I_{Kr}. Several studies have shown sex-based differences in CYP3A expression in the liver, with enhanced activity in women.

Many drugs are taken up into cells by membrane transporters, such as P-glycoprotein, and sex-based differences in transporter activity are also now recognized. An important substrate for P-glycoprotein is digoxin, and drugs such as

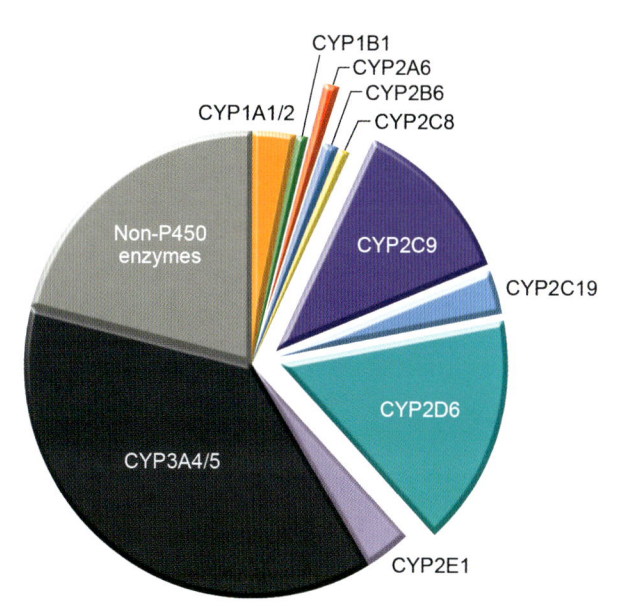

FIGURE 7.3. Contribution of Cytochrome P450 (CYP) Enzymes to the Phase I Metabolism of Marketed Drugs. The estimates are approximate and vary with time. Non–cytochrome P450 (Non-P450) enzymes include alcohol dehydrogenase and aldehyde dehydrogenase. (Adapted from Guengerich FP. Cytochromes P450, drugs, and diseases. MolInterv. 2003 Jun;3[4]:194–204.)

quinidine and amiodarone that inhibit P-glycoprotein cause elevated plasma concentrations of digoxin and digoxin toxicity. Expression of P-glycoprotein in the liver is 2-fold greater in men than in women, and this discrepancy may contribute to the increased mortality among women during digoxin therapy. Genetic-based activity of the organic anion-transporting polypeptide OATP1B1, which mediates hepatic uptake of various drugs, is now widely recognized to have a critical role in the risk of myopathic toxicity during simvastatin therapy. The role of sex-based variability in drug transport for compounds that block *hERG* is currently an area of active investigation.

CARDIOVASCULAR TOXICITY OF RHYTHM-CONTROL DRUGS

For both men and women, the AFFIRM trial showed that rhythm control with antiarrhythmic drugs did not afford a survival advantage compared with rate control for atrial fibrillation. These findings were confirmed in patients with persistent atrial fibrillation in the smaller European-based RACE study.

A substudy of RACE was conducted to determine whether sex affected overall outcomes in the trial's 2 treatment arms. A total of 522 patients were followed for a mean (SD) duration of 2.3 (0.6) years, with the primary end point being a composite of death from cardiovascular causes, heart failure, thromboembolic complications, bleeding, severe adverse antiarrhythmic drug effects, and need for pacemaker implantation. Cardiovascular morbidity and mortality were equally distributed between male and female patients. However, severe adverse effects of antiarrhythmic drugs and pacemaker implantation occurred primarily in the female patients (Table 7.1). Adverse effects included sick sinus syndrome (which required permanent pacing in some patients), torsades de pointes, and hemodynamically significant rapid atrial flutter. Female sex was associated with a significant risk of bradyarrhythmias (adjusted hazard ratio [HR], 4.8). Compared with patients assigned to rate control, patients treated with a rhythm control strategy experienced the primary end point more often (adjusted HR, 3.1). The primary end point was mainly heart failure, thromboembolic complications, or adverse effects of antiarrhythmic drugs. With no significant difference in quality of life between the 2 treatment arms, these data suggest that a rate control strategy is associated with more favorable outcomes for women with persistent fibrillation.

TABLE 7.1. Major Similarities and Differences Between Sexes in Antiarrhythmic Drug Therapy

Specific Factor	Similarities and Differences Between Sexes
Rhythm control vs rate control	Survival advantage with rhythm control: no advantage for either sex Rhythm control in women: ↑ cardioembolism, ↑ heart failure, ↑ antiarrhythmic complications After electrical cardioversion: women have higher atrial fibrillation recurrence rate Rhythm control in selected instances: both sexes may benefit
Antiarrhythmic drugs	Women: ↑ bradyarrhythmias in women Tolerance for antiarrhythmics: women less than men Risk of torsades de pointes with sotalol and dofetilide: 2-fold ↑ for women Amiodarone: low arrhythmia risk for both sexes

Adapted from Michelena HI, Powell BD, Brady PA, Friedman PA, Ezekowitz MD. Gender in atrial fibrillation: ten years later. Gend Med. 2010 Jun;7(3):206–17. Used with permission.

This is particularly true since women appear to have a higher recurrence rate of atrial fibrillation after electrical cardioversion.

Additional evidence for increased risk for women who take rhythm control drugs comes from the FRACTAL study. This study enrolled 973 patients with new-onset atrial fibrillation, leaving the patient treatment strategy to the discretion of the local physician. Patients were followed for a mean (SD) of 2.0 (0.9) years, until pacemaker implantation, death, or end of follow-up. The use of amiodarone was associated with an increased risk of pacemaker implantation in women (HR, 4.69) but not men. The interaction between sex and amiodarone remained significant after adjustment for the daily dose of amiodarone.

MORTALITY WITH DIGOXIN THERAPY

Despite the advent of newer agents, digoxin continues to be widely used for slowing atrioventricular nodal conduction during atrial tachyarrhythmias and for managing CHF. In the DIG trial, digoxin had no effect on overall mortality among patients with depressed left ventricular function and CHF, although fewer patients were hospitalized for worsening heart failure. After the trial, a post hoc subgroup analysis was conducted to determine whether there were sex-based differences in the effects of digoxin therapy. For all-cause mortality, women randomly assigned to receive digoxin had a higher rate of death than women in the placebo arm, while no difference was observed for men (Figure 7.4). The digoxin dose was standardized according to the body mass index (BMI) and was slightly higher in men (0.0093 ng/unit of BMI vs 0.0084 ng/unit of BMI). In groups of randomly selected patients, the median plasma digoxin concentration was slightly higher in women at 1 month (0.9 vs 0.8 ng/mL, $P=.007$) but essentially identical at 12 months (0.6 ng/mL in both groups). The proportion of patients with plasma concentrations exceeding 2.0 ng/mL was not different between men and women. Unfortunately, plasma concentrations were measured in less than one-third of patients, reducing the statistical power for examining the role of drug concentration in the increased mortality rate. Progesterone is known to inhibit P-glycoprotein, and a plausible mechanism is

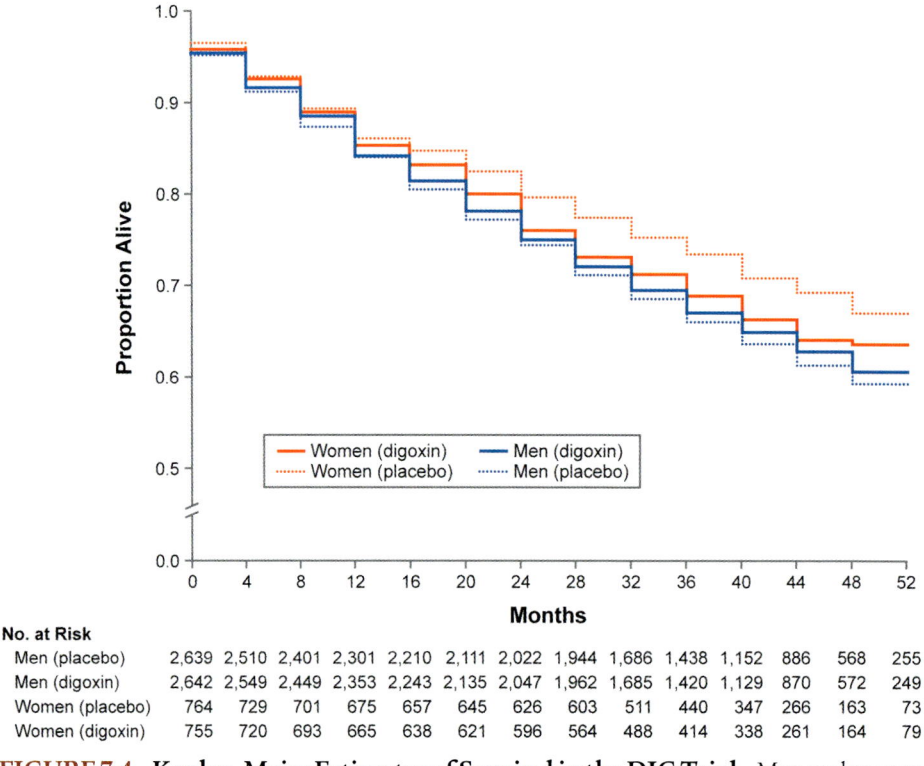

FIGURE 7.4. Kaplan-Meier Estimates of Survival in the DIG Trial. Men and women were randomly assigned to receive digoxin or placebo. (Adapted from Rathore SS, Wang Y, Krumholz HM. Sex-based differences in the effect of digoxin for the treatment of heart failure. N Engl J Med. 2002 Oct 31;347[18]:1403–11. Used with permission.)

an interaction between hormone replacement therapy and digoxin. However, data on hormone replacement therapy were not collected during the trial, so that hypothesis could not be tested.

ENDOCRINE THERAPY FOR BREAST CANCER

A selective estrogen receptor modulator, tamoxifen, is widely used in the treatment and prevention of breast cancer. Tamoxifen itself has weak affinity for the estrogen receptor and serves as a prodrug, while multiple cytochrome P450 enzymes convert tamoxifen into active metabolites. Available evidence indicates that the cytochrome P450 2D6 isozyme (CYP2D6) has a dominant role in generating 4-hydroxytamoxifen and endoxifen. Both of these products have at least a 10-fold higher affinity for estrogen receptors than tamoxifen and are considered the most potent metabolites. Variant alleles encoding CYP2D6 can also render it nonfunctional (ie, "poor metabolizers"). In addition, several drugs, including quinidine, dronedarone, fluoxetine, and several tricyclic antidepressants, are potent inhibitors of CYP2D6 and cause patients to become poor metabolizers. Multiple studies suggest that either a genetic-based or drug-induced reduction in CYP2D6 activity may be associated with inferior outcomes related to breast cancer treatment with tamoxifen. The present recommendation is that use of CYP2D6 inhibitors, including quinidine and dronedarone, should be avoided if possible in patients taking tamoxifen.

CONCLUSIONS

For optimal patient safety, practitioners must be aware of sex-based differences in outcomes related to antiarrhythmic drug therapy. Women are particularly prone to adverse electrophysiologic responses when exposed to QT-prolonging drugs, and other proarrhythmic risk factors (eg, hypokalemia, hypomagnesemia) should be avoided when these agents are used in female patients. Women are also especially susceptible to bradycardia and other adverse effects with other rhythm control agents, in particular amiodarone. Given the evidence that digoxin can increase mortality among women, the risk-benefit ratio for use of this drug in female patients should be carefully considered. Finally, use of the CYP2D6 inhibitors quinidine and dronedarone should be avoided in women taking tamoxifen for prophylaxis or treatment of breast cancer.

SUGGESTED READING

Higgins MJ, Stearns V. Pharmacogenetics of endocrine therapy for breast cancer. Annu Rev Med. 2011;62:281–93.

Hreiche R, Morissette P, Turgeon J. Drug-induced long QT syndrome in women: review of current evidence and remaining gaps. Gend Med. 2008 Jun;5(2):124–35.

Kannankeril P, Roden DM, Darbar D. Drug-induced long QT syndrome. Pharmacol Rev. 2010 Dec;62(4):760–81.

Michelena HI, Powell BD, Brady PA, Friedman PA, Ezekowitz MD. Gender in atrial fibrillation: Ten years later. Gend Med. 2010 Jun;7(3):206–17.

Sica DA, Wood M, Hess M. Gender and its effect in cardiovascular pharmacotherapeutics: recent considerations. Congest Heart Fail. 2005 May-Jun;11(3):163–6.

Yang PC, Clancy CE. Effects of sex hormones on cardiac repolarization. J Cardiovasc Pharmacol. 2010 Aug;56(2):123–9.

CHAPTER EIGHT

Sudden Cardiac Death in Women

LAURA M. GRAVELIN, MD, AND RACHEL J. LAMPERT, MD[*]

INTRODUCTION

The incidence of sudden cardiac death (SCD) in the United States is estimated to be 180,000 to 450,000 events annually. More than one-third (150,000) of the SCD cases occur in women; this number is more than twice the number of women who die of breast cancer annually. If death from coronary artery disease (CAD) is included with SCD, more women in the United States die of cardiovascular disease than of all cancers. Globally, cardiovascular disease is the leading killer of women.

A small segment of the population, both men and women, belong to a high-risk group for SCD and will experience an event. The majority of patients with SCD, however, are not in an identifiable high-risk group. In fact, a very small percentage of SCD occurs in patients who would meet guidelines for a primary prevention implantable cardioverter-defibrillator (ICD). SCD is a public health burden owing to its unexpected nature—there are no warning symptoms to identify a person who may experience SCD and, therefore, little opportunity to successfully intervene. Further, there are epidemiologic differences between men and women who experience SCD. These differences raise questions about possible variations

---

[*] Dr Lampert has received significant research funding from Boston Scientific, Medtronic, and St Jude Medical, for a study on safety of sports for patients with ICDs, and modest honoraria from Boston Scientific and Medtronic.

in arrhythmogenic substrates as well as in susceptibility to triggers, and they pose challenges to the development of risk stratification schema and risk reduction strategies.

SEX DIFFERENCES IN EPIDEMIOLOGY

For both sexes, the development of ventricular tachycardia (VT) and its degeneration to ventricular fibrillation (VF) have been reported in up to two-thirds of the SCD cases, with bradyarrhythmias accounting for the remainder, although these proportions may be changing over time. The overall incidence of SCD increases with age; in women, it doubles with each decade. There is also a difference in age at presentation, with women presenting at older ages. The Framingham Heart Study evaluated 5,209 men and women with SCD. For women, the incidence of SCD lagged behind that for men by more than a decade. Analysis of the MUSTT data showed a 20-year lag for SCD in women. These findings are likely a result of the complex relationship between sex hormones and the development of CAD.

In a study of the causative rhythm of SCD in a cohort of women, early data suggested that the majority were related to ventricular tachyarrhythmias. In a 2003 report from the NHS, which looked at both out-of-hospital cardiac arrests (OHCAs) and in-hospital cardiac arrests in patients with documented presenting rhythms, VT or VF was noted 76% of the time, pulseless electrical activity (PEA) or bradycardia accounted for 10% of SCDs, and asystole accounted for 14% (Figure 8.1). Not only have more contemporary studies shown a decrease in VT and VF as the rhythm mediating SCD, they have also identified differences between men and women in the rhythm at the time of SCD.

A study of OHCAs showed less VT in women than in men. Oregon SUDS looked at 1,568 cases of OHCA, of which 36% were in women, from 2002 to 2007. At presentation, the rhythm was VT or VF in 32.8% of the women and 47.7% of the men, and PEA or asystole in 63.8% of the women and 51% of the men. Since VT and VF may degenerate to asystole or PEA over several minutes, the difference may be related to the response time of emergency medical services; however, no sex difference was seen in response time in Oregon SUDS. Interestingly, while women were more likely to have PEA or asystole, they were also more likely to

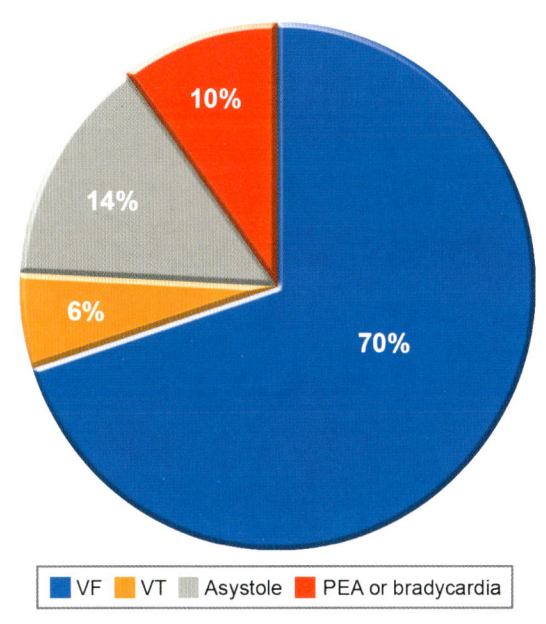

FIGURE 8.1. Cardiac Rhythm Underlying 109 Sudden Cardiac Deaths in the NHS. PEA indicates pulseless electrical activity; VF, ventricular fibrillation; VT, ventricular tachycardia. (Adapted from Albert CM, Chae CU, Grodstein F, Rose LM, Rexrode KM, Ruskin JN, et al. Prospective study of sudden cardiac death among women in the United States. Circulation. 2003 Apr 29;107[16]:2096–101. Epub 2003 Apr 14. Used with permission.)

have a return of spontaneous circulation (25% vs 21%); the reasons for this finding are not understood.

A decrease in ventricular arrhythmias as the underlying rhythm in SCD was documented in a report from King County, Washington, which retrospectively examined 6,713 cases of SCD treated by the emergency medical services in a 10-year period, in which 40% of the SCD cases occurred in women. SCD was attributed to VT or VF 36% of the time during the first 5 years (January 1, 2000, through December 31, 2004) compared with 31% during the following 5.25 years (January 1, 2005, through March 31, 2010).

ETIOLOGIES OF SCD: SEX DIFFERENCES IN ARRHYTHMIC SUBSTRATE

Overall, 80% of the SCD cases are attributed to CAD; however, among survivors of SCD, men and women have differences in the underlying cardiac structural abnormalities (Figure 8.2). In 1 study, 45% of women had underlying CAD, with dilated cardiomyopathy in another 19% and valvular heart disease in another 13%. For men, however, 80% had underlying CAD, 10% had dilated cardiomyopathy, and 5% had valvular heart disease (Figure 8.3).

CAD and SCD

The prevalence of CAD is less for women than for men across all age groups, except for patients aged 40 to 59 years, for whom the prevalence is equivalent (Figure 8.4). However, even among patients with a prior myocardial infarction, the risk of SCD is 2.5-fold higher for men than women. Among CAD patients older than 38, men are more than twice as likely as women to have SCD. Pathophysiologic differences between men and women with CAD may explain

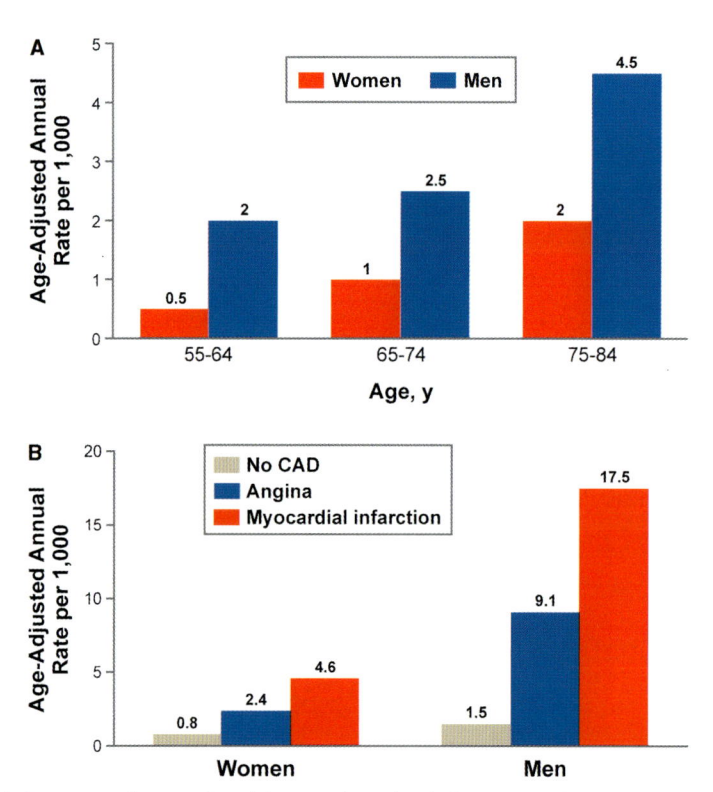

FIGURE 8.2. A. Incidence of sudden cardiac death by age and sex. B, Rates of sudden cardiac death attributed to coronary artery disease (CAD). (Adapted from Kannel WB, Wilson PW, D'Agostino RB, Cobb J. Sudden coronary death in women. Am Heart J. 1998 Aug;136[2]:205-12. Used with permission.)

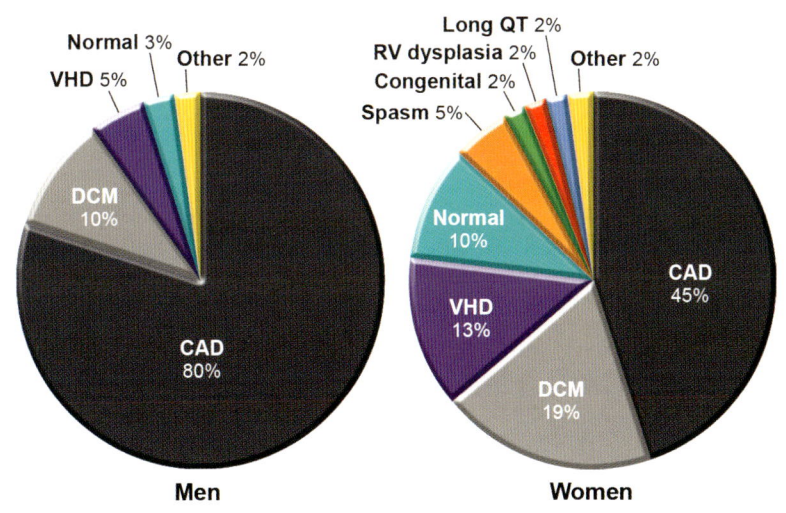

FIGURE 8.3. Cardiac Disease by Sex Among Survivors of Sudden Cardiac Death. CAD indicates coronary artery disease; DCM, dilated cardiomyopathy; RV, right ventricular; VHD, valvular heart disease. (Adapted from Deo R, Albert CM. Epidemiology and genetics of sudden cardiac death. Circulation. 2012 Jan 31;125[4]:620-37. Used with permission.)

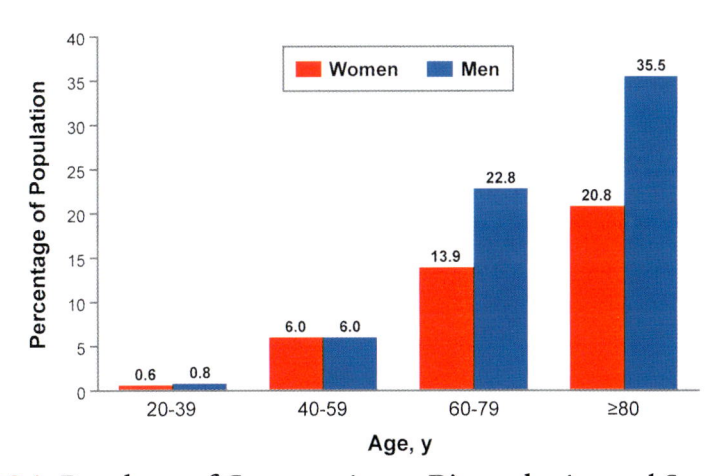

FIGURE 8.4. Prevalence of Coronary Artery Disease by Age and Sex. (Adapted from Roger VL, Go AS, Lloyd-Jones DM, Benjamin EJ, Berry JD, Borden WB, et al; American Heart Association Statistics Committee and Stroke Statistics Subcommittee. Heart disease and stroke statistics: 2012 update: a report from the American Heart Association. Circulation. 2012 Jan 3;125[1]:e2-e220. Epub 2011 Dec 15. Erratum in: Circulation. 2012 Jun 5;125[22]:e1002. Used with permission.)

the difference in propensity for the development of SCD. In CASS, women with angina were less likely to have obstructive CAD at angiography, although only a small fraction of the study population was women. These results suggested that ischemia was occurring without epicardial vessel occlusion. The WISE study showed that while men presented with classically described intraluminal plaque and rupture in the epicardial arteries, women were more likely to have microvasculature ischemia that can be identified with magnetic resonance imaging. Others have observed that CAD in women may be related to plaque erosion with less identifiable stenosis by the best diagnostic angiographic techniques. The methods by which CAD is assessed may not be adequate to quantify the disease burden in women nor to successfully risk stratify appropriately, which may contribute to women receiving less aggressive therapies for similar disease states. The development of other imaging methods, such as magnetic resonance imaging, to improve the diagnosis of CAD in women may be warranted. Whether these different mechanisms lead to variable substrates for arrhythmia has not been fully determined. Data from MUSTT showed that women meeting entry criteria were less likely to have an inducible arrhythmia at the electrophysiology study, suggesting that there was a different substrate for arrhythmia after myocardial infarction, but there was no sex difference in event-free survival or in all-cause mortality.

In acute coronary obstruction, unstable plaques lead to areas of ischemia and reperfusion alterations. These result in heterogeneous electrophysiologic properties with changes in local conduction velocity, alterations in anisotropy, and repolarization. It is also possible that in ischemia these dynamic cellular changes may differ between men and women.

The relationship between CAD and SCD may explain, in part, the decreasing incidence of VF among patients with SCD. It may reflect the decreasing prevalence of CAD or, in the era of reperfusion therapies, the prevention of scar formation from which monomorphic VT (and subsequent degeneration into VF) may occur. The use of β-blockers in the contemporary era of CAD management has also been postulated to contribute not only to the reduction in VT and VF but also to an increase in PEA and asystole. However, the use of therapies for CAD differs between men and women. A recent review of the GRACE and CANRACE trials reported that fewer women than men received heparin, glycoprotein IIb/IIIa inhibitors, and thienopyridines. Whether this disparity affects the risk of SCD has not been investigated.

Left Ventricular Dysfunction and SCD

The risk of SCD is greatly increased for patients with left ventricular (LV) dysfunction, especially if they have clinical heart failure. In these patients, progressive pump failure, ischemia, and a primary arrhythmia are all possible causal events for SCD. A survival benefit from use of ICDs in patients with LV dysfunction has been shown in data from several trials, including MUSTT, MADIT, MADIT II, and SCD-HeFT. However, since the majority of patients presenting with SCD do not have LV dysfunction, the ICD offers prevention to only a small percentage of these patients. Women are less likely than men to have LV dysfunction at the time of SCD. Compared with men, women were more likely to have normal LV function (48.9% vs 35.2%), underscoring the difficulty in predicting the risk of SCD for women.

Nonischemic Cardiomyopathies and SCD

Among the participants in SCD-HeFT, women were more likely than men to have nonischemic cardiomyopathy (NICM) and New York Heart Association class III symptoms. Researchers at Stanford University evaluated 140 consecutive patients undergoing ICD implantation for NICM and found no significant differences in age, LV dimensions or systolic function, electrocardiographic (ECG) parameters, or medical therapeutic regimens. They found no difference between men and women when evaluating the rate of appropriate discharges (36.4% vs 38.5%) and mortality (21.6% vs 11.5%, $P=.11$). These results suggest that men and women with NICM may be at similar risk for arrhythmic SCD.

Another structural abnormality associated with SCD is hypertrophic cardiomyopathy, which carries an overall SCD risk of 1% per year. Patients at high risk include those with massive hypertrophy, a family history of SCD, recurrent syncope, a history of prior SCD, or sustained VT. A cross-sectional analysis of a community-based cohort of 239 patients showed an inverse relationship between age and LV hypertrophy (ie, as age increased, LV wall thickness decreased). However, when these results were separated by sex, they were statistically significant for women only. This may reflect a higher rate of premature death among younger patients with more severe hypertrophy. No difference has been observed between men and women with hypertrophic cardiomyopathy and the risk of SCD.

Arrhythmogenic right ventricular dysplasia (ARVD), another rare cause of SCD, results from the fibrofatty replacement of normal tissue. The electrophysiologic dysfunction that occurs is implicated in the pathogenesis of SCD. ARVD is more prevalent in men. One study examined the features of 171 consecutive patients (29% were women) with ARVD; men had larger right ventricular dimensions and a greater frequency of LV involvement, and women had a milder form. This observation may explain why typical ECG features and late potentials were observed more commonly in men. Despite men having a more severe phenotype, the incidence of life-threatening ventricular arrhythmias was similar in both sexes.

Channelopathies and SCD

Although accounting for a much smaller fraction of overall mortality from SCD, channelopathies provide an intriguing avenue toward understanding sex differences in SCD. The Cardiovascular Research Center at Brown University (Providence, Rhode Island) has been investigating long QT syndrome (LQTS) in a rabbit model and the role of sex hormones. The investigators have reported that progesterone has a protective effect, while estrogen appears to be arrhythmogenic in the model for LQTS type 2. These data prompted a review of the LQTS Registry database, which showed that women who took oral contraceptives had a lower incidence of cardiac events than women who did not take oral contraceptives. The association with hormones in LQTS has been previously suggested because an increased incidence of SCD during the peripartum period has been noted for women with LQTS type 2. This increased risk has also been documented at the onset of menopause. In the absence of congenital LQTS, prolongation of the QT interval is dynamically associated with the menstrual cycle. These findings suggest that sex hormones may dynamically mediate the risk of SCD, particularly when repolarization reserve is taxed; specifically, estrogen may be proarrhythmic and progesterone may be protective. To what extent these differences may extend to patients without LQTS warrants further investigation. (The role of sex hormones in arrhythmogenesis is discussed in Chapters 3 and 4 in this book.)

In Brugada syndrome, which is caused by a mutation of the cardiac sodium channel encoded by the *SCN5A* gene, male sex portends a more malignant course. This gene was studied in 2 large, prospective cohorts of men and women (in the HPFS and the NHS) to evaluate the contribution of subclinical mutations in *SCN5A* to SCD risk. While not common, variants were present among women experiencing SCD. Further investigations with genome-wide association studies may provide further insights into SCD risks and point to opportunities for prevention.

POTENTIAL SEX DIFFERENCES IN THE TRIGGERING OF VENTRICULAR ARRHYTHMIAS

Arrhythmogenesis relies on the presence of a trigger to initiate an arrhythmia and a substrate to maintain it. Many studies have implicated fluctuations in autonomic tone triggered by psychologic stressors as contributing to SCD. For example, the incidence of SCD increases at times of natural disaster. A study evaluating the role of anger showed that anger-induced T-wave alternans predicted future ventricular arrhythmias in a population of ICD patients. Further, an increase in sympathetic tone increases the likelihood of VF during times of ischemia. Circadian patterns, another marker for autonomic tone, have been observed in SCD, with events occurring more frequently in the morning. This pattern is diminished by the use of β-blockers. Other studies have shown that the incidence peaks on Mondays and then decreases during the week.

Chronic psychologic stressors may also lead to autonomic changes, which may be arrhythmogenic. For example, depression was shown to be a risk factor for ventricular arrhythmias among men and women. In a group of 645 prospectively analyzed patients with ICDs, more severe symptoms of depression predicted shocks for VT or VF. Depressed patients were more often women. A strong association between depression and SCD was identified and was associated with the use of antidepressants. Whether the antidepressant medications are a marker of more severe depression or are directly related to increased SCD requires further investigation, particularly since many of the medications alter repolarization by modulating the rapid component of the delayed rectifier potassium current (I_{Kr}). The NHS prospectively looked at depression in women as a risk factor for SCD. Symptoms of depression were related to CAD events and were strongly associated with fatal CAD events.

Panic attacks have been associated with SCD in both men and women. These psychologic perturbations are associated with decreases in markers of autonomic function, such as heart rate variability, which are in turn associated with a higher risk of SCD. These data implicate an arrhythmogenic role for long-term changes in the autonomic nervous system. The WHI Observational Study prospectively studied 3,369 postmenopausal women and found that panic attacks were an independent risk factor for cardiovascular morbidity and mortality.

Data from HERS showed that postmenopausal women with CAD who exercised and engaged in regular physical activity (≥3 times weekly) had a decreased incidence of SCD. These findings further support the beneficial effect of modulating the autonomic nervous system by increasing vagal tone.

Autonomic nervous system function differs between men and women. The balance between sympathetic and parasympathetic activation has been studied by looking at heart rate variability (HRV), the amount of beat-to-beat variation in sinus rhythm over time. Reduced HRV has been associated with increased mortality after myocardial infarction. Resting vagal tone as assessed by HRV is higher in women, although this is not a consistent finding in all studies. Women are less likely to have exertion-related SCD.

Not only does resting autonomic tone differ between men and women, but differences in autonomic reactivity between men and women are well documented. These differences may further contribute to the differences in SCD among patients with similar substrate. Despite the popular stereotypes of sex and emotion, women have less adrenergic response to induced mental stress. These observations suggest that differences in autonomic modulation may temper susceptibility to SCD. One explanation may be related to the role of estrogen in modulating norepinephrine release (although the difference in vagal tone persists even in elderly women).

The concept that women may be less susceptible to triggers is supported by a study showing that men with CAD and ICDs were more likely to have ventricular arrhythmias at follow-up. In that study, there were no clinical differences between the sexes, and no differences in inducibility; the data implied that men and women had a similar arrhythmic substrate. The lower rate of ventricular arrhythmias among women with CAD, despite having a similar substrate as men, suggests a sex difference in the susceptibility to triggering events. Despite the presence of similar substrates in men and women (eg, scar after myocardial infarction), men with CAD are more susceptible to SCD. This may, in part, be explained by different susceptibilities to the triggers that initiate arrhythmia.

RISK STRATIFICATION

An area of intensive investigation has been to determine which patients have an SCD risk that is high enough that they will benefit from ICD therapy. Several parameters have been evaluated for risk stratification, including ECG markers, ejection fraction, electrophysiology testing, markers of autonomic tone (eg, HRV and baroreflex sensitivity), and inflammation. The ability to individualize risk remains a difficult task and is likely more so for women, who have been studied less well.

Over 2,760 postmenopausal women with CAD in the HERS study were evaluated for specific risk factors over a mean follow-up of 6.8 years. One observation was that SCD comprised the majority of cardiac deaths in this population. A second observation was that independent predictors of SCD included diabetes mellitus, atrial fibrillation, myocardial infarction, congestive heart failure, decreased glomerular filtration rate, and physical inactivity. These characteristics, when combined with LV ejection fraction, were a better predictor of risk than LV ejection fraction alone. Analysis of the NHS after 16 years of follow-up showed that an increased baseline level of the N-terminal fragment of the prohormone brain natriuretic peptide was independently associated with SCD. This same analysis showed no association with C-reactive protein levels. The complexity and heterogeneity of risk demands a broad range of investigation.

Current guideline-based models for primary prevention are predicated on ejection fraction, which accounts for only a small segment of the at-risk population; since women are less likely to have a reduced ejection fraction, efforts have been made to model risk more specifically for women. A 2010 report from the National Heart, Lung, and Blood Institute and the Heart Rhythm Society (Workshop for SCD Prediction and Prevention) identified the need for large population-based studies that would include women, address the knowledge gaps in the mechanisms of SCD, and define sex-specific risk factors. This need is especially important given that the inherent unexpected nature of SCD leaves little opportunity for prevention.

RISK REDUCTION

Early efforts at risk-reduction strategies focused on the use of antiarrhythmic drugs. However, patients in CAST had an increased mortality after myocardial infarction if they used antiarrhythmics, despite suppression of premature ventricular contractions. Among pharmacologic approaches, emphasis is now placed on the role of β-blockers and renin-angiotensin system blockers in the reduction of cardiovascular mortality and SCD. Data from the 1990s showed that women were less likely than men to receive an appropriate medical regimen for CAD. In a meta-analysis of primary prevention ICD trials, women were less likely to receive renin-angiotensin system blockers. This suggests that at the most basic level of health care—medical therapies—women do not receive the best possible care.

Current algorithms are based on many clinical trials that have shown the efficacy of the ICD in preventing SCD in patients with LV dysfunction (ejection fraction <30%-35%). These trials are the basis for practice guidelines that have led to an increase in ICD implantation. Despite this increase, event rates for SCD have not had a similar decrease. Less than 30% of SCDs occur in patients who meet the guidelines for a primary prevention ICD. Furthermore, the majority of patients in the clinical studies on which the guidelines are predicated were men. (Further discussion on women in clinical trials can be found in Chapter 2, "Women in Clinical Trials.") A meta-analysis of 5 major primary prevention studies (MADIT II, MUSTT, SCD-HeFT, DEFINITE, and COMPANION) examined 7,229 patients, of whom 1,630 (23%) were women. The findings of the analysis, while not statistically significant, suggested a smaller benefit for women and questioned the applicability of current practice-based risk reduction guidelines to women who may be not only underrepresented in clinical trials but may also have differences in arrhythmogenic triggers and substrate. (The use of ICDs in women is discussed in Chapter 9, "Implantable Cardioverter-Defibrillator Therapy in Women.")

SUMMARY

SCD continues to be an important public health burden. While women are less likely than men to die of SCD, cardiovascular disease (including SCD) is the number 1 killer of women. Differences between men and women in the presenting arrhythmia and age at presentation further add to the complexity of understanding the interactions of factors leading to SCD. Both a trigger and a substrate are required for SCD, and the variations between the sexes add to the challenges in determining the pathologic processes and interactions involved. Prediction and prevention of SCD is an area of active investigation, but current guidelines for preventive intervention are applicable to only a very small portion of the population at risk, and only small percentages of women were involved in the studies upon which the guidelines were constructed. Continued efforts to better understand not only SCD in women but also overall cardiovascular processes will improve understanding of arrhythmogenic substrate and susceptibility and will provide opportunities for improved risk stratification and decreased mortality from SCD.

SUGGESTED READING

Albert CM, Nam EG, Rimm EB, Jin HW, Hajjar RJ, Hunter DJ, et al. Cardiac sodium channel gene variants and sudden cardiac death in women. Circulation. 2008 Jan 1;117(1):16–23.

Chugh SS, Uy-Evanado A, Teodorescu C, Reinier K, Mariani R, Gunson K, et al. Women have a lower prevalence of structural heart disease as a precursor to sudden cardiac arrest: The Ore-SUDS (Oregon Sudden Unexpected Death Study). J Am Coll Cardiol. 2009 Nov 24;54(22):2006–11.

Deo R, Albert CM. Epidemiology and genetics of sudden cardiac death. Circulation. 2012 Jan 31;125(4):620–37.

Deo R, Vittinghoff E, Lin F, Tseng ZH, Hulley SB, Shlipak MG. Risk factor and prediction modeling for sudden cardiac death in women with coronary artery disease. Arch Intern Med. 2011 Oct 24;171(19):1703–9. Epub 2011 Jul 25.

Lampert R. Implantable cardioverter-defibrillator use and benefit in women. Cardiol Rev. 2007 Nov-Dec;15(6):298–303.

Lampert R, McPherson CA, Clancy JF, Caulin-Glaser TL, Rosenfeld LE, Batsford WP. Gender differences in ventricular arrhythmia recurrence in patients with coronary artery disease and implantable cardioverter-defibrillators. J Am Coll Cardiol. 2004 Jun 16;43(12):2293–9.

Lampert R, Shusterman V, Burg M, McPherson C, Batsford W, Goldberg A, et al. Anger-induced T-wave alternans predicts future ventricular arrhythmias in patients with implantable cardioverter-defibrillators. J Am Coll Cardiol. 2009 Mar 3;53(9):774–8.

Maron BJ, Casey SA, Hurrell DG, Aeppli DM. Relation of left ventricular thickness to age and gender in hypertrophic cardiomyopathy. Am J Cardiol. 2003 May 15;91(10):1195–8.

Moss AJ. Sex hormones and ventricular tachyarrhythmias in LQTS: new insights regarding antiarrhythmic therapy. Heart Rhythm. 2012 May;9(5):833–4. Epub 2012 Jan 20.

Olivotto I, Maron MS, Adabag AS, Casey SA, Vargiu D, Link MS, et al. Gender-related differences in the clinical presentation and outcome of hypertrophic cardiomyopathy. J Am Coll Cardiol. 2005 Aug 2;46(3):480–7.

Poon S, Goodman SG, Yan RT, Bugiardini R, Bierman AS, Eagle KA, et al. Bridging the gender gap: Insights from a contemporary analysis of sex-related differences in the treatment and outcomes of patients with acute coronary syndromes. Am Heart J. 2012 Jan;163(1):66–73.

Russo AM, Poole JE, Mark DB, Anderson J, Hellkamp AS, Lee KL, et al. Primary prevention with defibrillator therapy in women: results from the Sudden Cardiac Death in Heart Failure Trial. J Cardiovasc Electrophysiol. 2008 Jul;19(7):720–4. Epub 2008 Mar 26.

Russo AM, Stamato NJ, Lehmann MH, Hafley GE, Lee KL, Pieper K, et al; MUSTT Investigators. Influence of gender on arrhythmia characteristics and outcome in the Multicenter UnSustained Tachycardia Trial. J Cardiovasc Electrophysiol. 2004 Sep;15(9):993–8.

Santangeli P, Pelargonio G, Dello Russo A, Casella M, Bisceglia C, Bartoletti S, et al. Gender differences in clinical outcome and primary prevention defibrillator benefit in patients with severe left ventricular dysfunction: a systematic review and meta-analysis. Heart Rhythm. 2010 Jul;7(7):876–82. Epub 2010 Apr 7.

Whang W, Kubzansky LD, Kawachi I, Rexrode KM, Kroenke CH, Glynn RJ, et al. Depression and risk of sudden cardiac death and coronary heart disease in women: results from the Nurses' Health Study. J Am Coll Cardiol. 2009 Mar 17;53(11):950–8.

CHAPTER NINE

Implantable Cardioverter-Defibrillator Therapy in Women[*]

ANDREA M. RUSSO, MD

INTRODUCTION

Randomized clinical trials have clearly demonstrated the efficacy of the implantable cardioverter-defibrillator (ICD) for the primary and secondary prevention of sudden cardiac death (SCD). However, the benefit of prophylactic ICD therapy in certain subgroups of patients, particularly women, has been questioned. This chapter discusses sex differences in outcome, including mortality and arrhythmic events during follow-up, complications, and use of ICD therapy in clinical practice.

EPIDEMIOLOGY OF SCD

It is estimated that 300,000 SCDs occur each year in the United States. This number represents over 50% of all cardiovascular deaths. In the Framingham Heart Study, the absolute incidence of SCD in adults increased with age for both men and women; however, the incidence of SCD was less for women than for men in

---

[*] Portions previously published in Russo AM, Poole JE, Mark DB, Anderson J, Hellkamp AS, Lee KL, et al. Primary prevention with defibrillator therapy in women: results from the Sudden Cardiac Death in Heart Failure Trial. J Cardiovasc Electrophysiol. 2008 Jul;19(7):720-4. Epub 2008 Mar 26, and Russo AM, Day JD, Stolen K, Mullin CM, Doraiswamy V, Lerew DL, et al. Implantable cardioverter defibrillators: do women fare worse than men? Gender comparison in the INTRINSIC RV trial.J Cardiovasc Electrophysiol. 2009 Sep;20(9):973-8. Epub 2009 May 12. Used with permission.

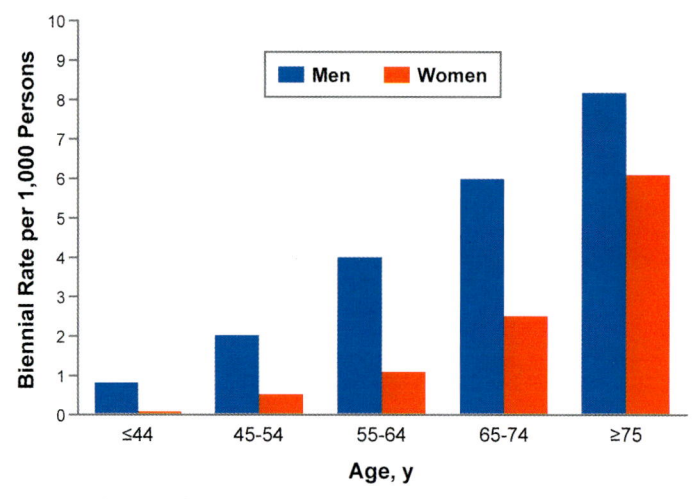

FIGURE 9.1. Incidence of Sudden Cardiac Death (SCD) by Age and Sex in People Free of Known Coronary Artery Disease. Data are from the Framingham Heart Study 26-year follow-up. A total of 5,128 men and women were enrolled, and SCD occurred in 147 men and 50 women. The absolute incidence of SCD increased with age for both men and women; the incidence was less for women than men in all age groups. (Adapted from Kannel WB, Schatzkin A. Sudden death: lessons from subsets in population studies. J Am CollCardiol. 1985 Jun;5[6 Suppl]:141B-9. Used with permission.)

all age groups, with a 10- to 20-year lag for women, which paralleled the incidence of ischemic heart disease (Figure 9.1). Men were more likely than women to have a history of known coronary artery disease (CAD) before the episode of SCD.

Arrhythmias at the time of presentation with SCD may differ in men and women. In studies of out-of-hospital cardiac arrests, women had a lower incidence of ventricular fibrillation (VF) compared with men. At the time of out-of-hospital cardiac arrest, VF and ventricular tachycardia (VT) were more common in men, while asystole and pulseless electrical activity were more common in women (Figure 9.2). The outcome from out-of-hospital cardiac arrest is typically better for patients presenting with VT or VF as the initially documented arrhythmia. However, despite these differences in clinical arrhythmias at presentation, resuscitation rates were better for women than for men (13.5% vs 10.7%, P=.005). With corrections for differences at baseline, women may have a slightly better survival advantage to hospital discharge (hazard ratio [HR], 1.66; 95% CI, 1.06–2.62; P=.03).

The type of underlying heart disease also differs between men and women who survive cardiac arrest: Men have a higher occurrence of CAD and women have a higher occurrence of dilated cardiomyopathy (Figure 9.3). Female survivors of out-of-hospital cardiac arrest have a higher mean left ventricular ejection fraction

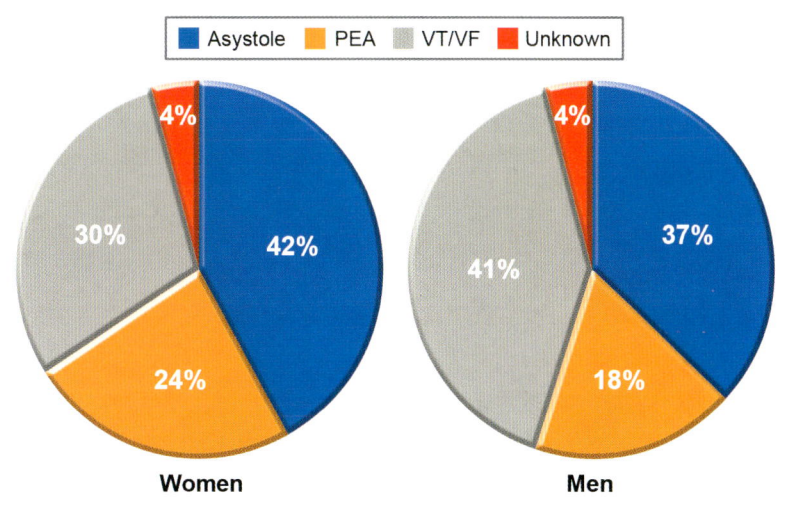

FIGURE 9.2. **Sex Differences in Presenting Rhythm for Out-of-Hospital Cardiac Arrest.** The presenting rhythm at the time of cardiac arrest is shown for men and women as a percentage of patients. Of the 4,147 total patients, 1,742 were women and 2,405 were men. In comparisons of the men and women who had asystole, pulseless electrical activity (PEA), or ventricular tachycardia (VT) or ventricular fibrillation (VF), $P<.05$. (Adapted from Wigginton JG, Pepe PE, Bedolla JP, DeTamble LA, Atkins JM. Sex-related differences in the presentation and outcome of out-of-hospital cardiopulmonary arrest: a multiyear, prospective, population-based study. Crit Care Med. 2002 Apr;30[4 Suppl]:S131-6. Used with permission.)

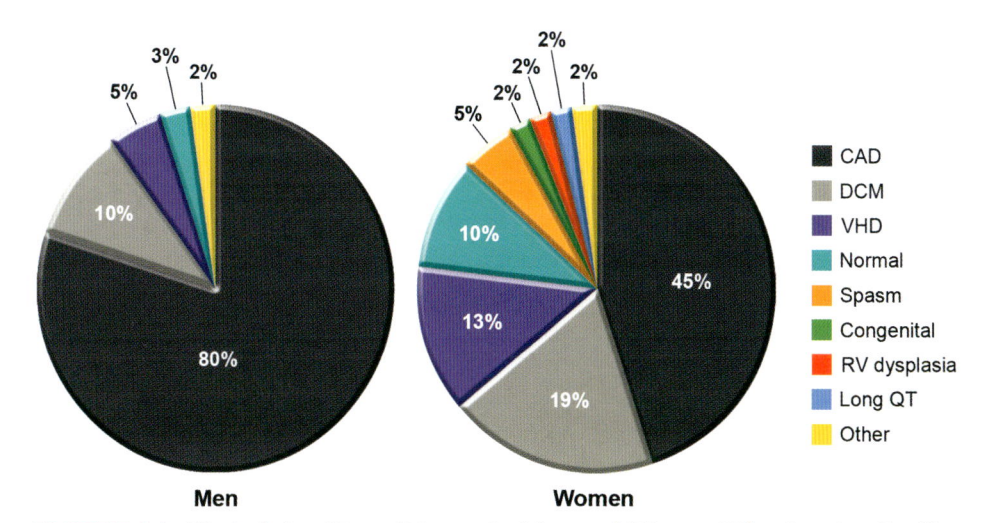

FIGURE 9.3. **Underlying Heart Disease in Men and Women Who Survive Cardiac Arrest.** Men are more likely to have coronary artery disease (CAD), and women are more likely to have nonischemic heart disease. DCM indicates dilated cardiomyopathy; RV, right ventricular; VHD, valvular heart disease. (Adapted from Albert CM, McGovern BA, Newell JB, Ruskin JN. Sex differences in cardiac arrest survivors. Circulation. 1996 Mar 15;93[6]:1170-6. Used with permission.)

(LVEF) than men. LVEF less than 40% was the strongest predictor of death for men, but LVEF did not have the same prognostic significance for women. These epidemiologic differences suggest the importance of including women in clinical trials evaluating ventricular arrhythmias and SCD, since trial results may not necessarily be extrapolated to women if women are not well represented.

CLINICAL CHARACTERISTICS AND OUTCOMES

Secondary Prevention ICD Trials

The benefit of ICD therapy in secondary prevention has been well established. Sex differences in baseline characteristics have been identified in studies of patients presenting with sustained ventricular arrhythmias. Women presenting with sustained VT or VF have a lower prevalence of CAD and a higher LVEF than men. Women are also more likely than men to have VF as a presenting arrhythmia.

In the AVID trial, ICD therapy, compared with class III antiarrhythmic drug therapy, improved survival after life-threatening ventricular arrhythmias. Compared with men enrolled in this trial, women were younger, had CAD less often, had a nonischemic cardiomyopathy more often, and had VF more often than VT as the index arrhythmia. Despite sex differences in baseline characteristics, there was no significant difference in ICD implantation rate, and the 1-year mortality rate was similar for women (14.4%) and men (15.5%). Findings were similar in other studies evaluating ICD therapy in patients presenting with life-threatening ventricular arrhythmias. After adjustment for baseline differences, overall survival was not different for men and women.

No significant difference in mortality between men and women was identified in CIDS, a secondary prevention ICD trial that randomly assigned ICD therapy or amiodarone therapy to 659 patients who had resuscitated VF or VT or unmonitored syncope. None of the tests for an interaction between baseline characteristics and treatment were significant, and no identifiable subgroup benefited significantly more or less from the ICD.

Primary Prevention ICD Trials

Randomized clinical trials have demonstrated the efficacy of prophylactic ICD therapy in reducing mortality or SCD risk. Table 9.1 shows the enrollment

TABLE 9.1. Implantable Cardioverter-Defibrillator (ICD) Studies

Study	Publication Year	Primary or Secondary Prevention	Patients, No.	Women Control, %	Women ICD, %	ICD, No.	Ischemic or Nonischemic	LVEF Cutoff, %	Follow-up, mo
AVID	1997	Secondary	1,016	19	22	112	Both	...	18
MADIT	1996	Primary	196	8	8	8	Ischemic	≤35	27
MUSTT	1999	Primary	704	10	10	18	Ischemic	≤40	39
MADIT II	2002	Primary	1,232	15	16	119	Ischemic	≤30	20
DEFINITE	2004	Primary	458	30	28	64	Nonischemic	≤35	29
SCD-HeFT	2005	Primary	2,521	23	23	185	Both	≤35	45
INTRINSIC RV	2007	Both	1,530	...	19	293	Both	...	11

criteria and characteristics of patients enrolled in several primary prevention trials.

Sex differences in baseline characteristics have been identified among patients undergoing ICD implantation for primary prevention. MUSTT evaluated the role of electrophysiologically guided therapy for men and women who had ischemic heart disease, prior infarction, and LVEF of 40% or less. In this primary prevention trial, women (compared with men) were older, were more likely to have had an infarction within 6 months, were more likely to have a history of heart failure, and were more likely to have recent angina before enrollment. In MADIT II, 1,232 patients with CAD and LVEF of 30% or less were enrolled, and 16% were women. Compared with men, women had an increased frequency of hypertension, diabetes mellitus, and left bundle branch block, and they underwent coronary artery bypass surgery less frequently.

SCD-HeFT included men and women with ischemic or nonischemic cardiomyopathy, LVEF of 35% or less, and New York Heart Association (NYHA) class II or III heart failure. In this trial, women were less likely to be white and were more likely to have NYHA class III heart failure or nonischemic heart disease. The DEFINITE study evaluated the role of primary prevention ICD in patients with nonischemic cardiomyopathy and LVEF of 35% or less. In contrast to sex differences in other primary prevention studies, men and women enrolled in DEFINITE had no significant differences in most baseline characteristics, including age, NYHA class, LVEF, heart failure duration, atrial fibrillation, QRS duration, presence of left bundle branch block or right bundle branch block, qualifying arrhythmia, and diabetes mellitus.

The benefit of ICDs implanted for primary prevention in women has been questioned. In subgroup analyses of MUSTT and MADIT II, both of which included only patients with underlying ischemic heart disease, there was no difference in outcome between men and women. However, these trials included only a small number of women, and small differences in overall survival or arrhythmia-free survival could have been missed.

In MUSTT, there were no significant sex influences on risk of arrhythmic death or cardiac arrest (the 2-year event rate was 9% for women and 12% for men; adjusted HR, 0.88) or overall mortality (the 2-year event rate was 32% for women and 21% for men; adjusted HR, 1.51). Figure 9.4 shows overall

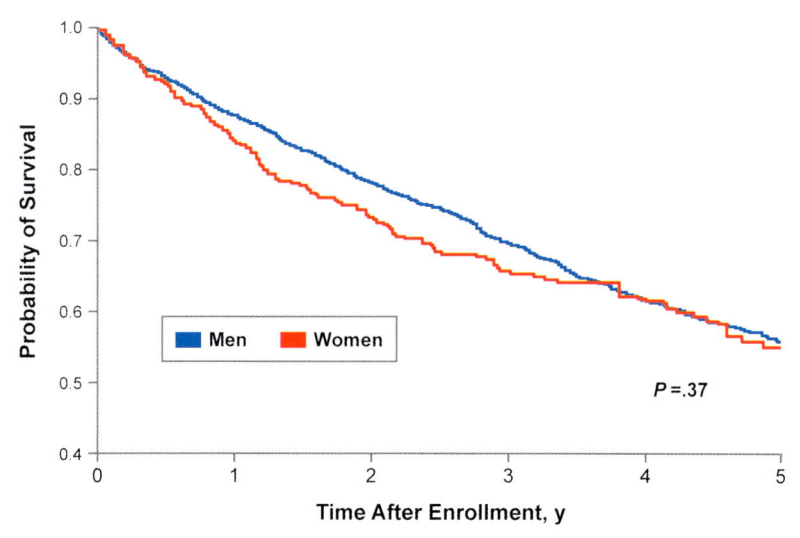

FIGURE 9.4. Overall Survival for All Patients in MUSTT. There was no sex difference in mortality.

survival by sex in MUSTT. However, there were only 68 women enrolled in the randomized group, and small differences in survival could have been missed.

In MADIT II, the 2-year mortality for patients randomly assigned to receive conventional therapy was not significantly different between men (20%) and women (30%) ($P=.19$) (Figure 9.5). After adjustment for relevant clinical

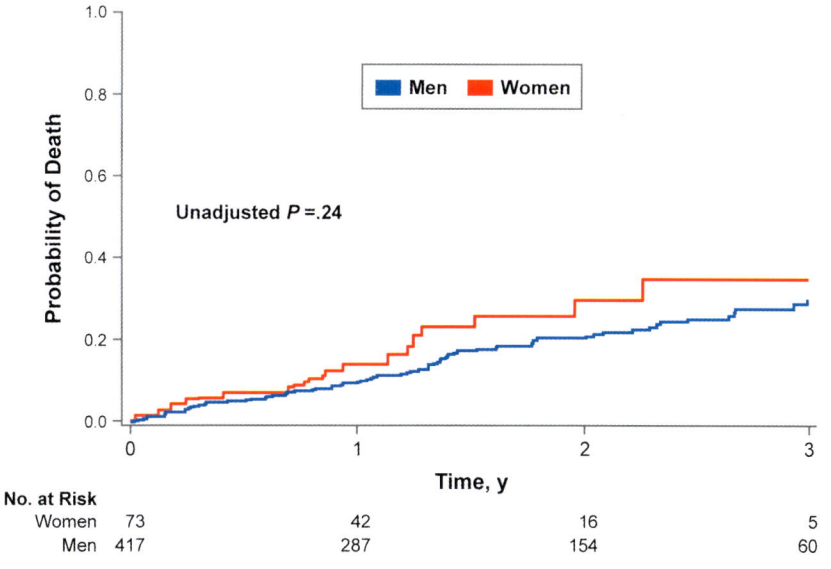

FIGURE 9.5. Mortality in MADIT II (Conventional Therapy Group). The 2-year cumulative total mortality in MADIT II for patients randomly assigned to receive conventional therapy was not significantly different between men and women. (Adapted from Zareba W, Moss AJ, Jackson Hall W, Wilber DJ, Ruskin JN, McNitt S, et al; MADIT II Investigators. Clinical course and implantable cardioverter defibrillator therapy in postinfarction women with severe left ventricular dysfunction. J CardiovascElectrophysiol. 2005 Dec;16[12]:1265–70. Used with permission.)

covariates, the HRs for ICD effectiveness were similar for women (HR, 0.57; 95% CI, 0.28–1.18; *P*=.13) and men (HR, 0.66; 95% CI, 0.48–0.91; *P*=.01). There was no significant interaction between sex, mortality, and ICD therapy (*P*=.72), indicating that ICD therapy was similarly effective for men and women.

Trials that included subjects with nonischemic heart disease, including SCD-HeFT and DEFINITE, suggest that women may derive less relative benefit from ICD therapy than men. In DEFINITE, for patients who received ICD therapy, all-cause mortality was decreased among men (*P*=.02) but not women (*P*=.75) (Figure 9.6). However, the test for an interaction between sex and ICD treatment on mortality was not significant in unadjusted analysis (*P*=.11) or multivariate adjusted analysis (*P*=.18). For cause-specific mortality, there was no sex difference in the incidence of arrhythmic death, but there was a relative excess of noncardiac deaths among women randomly assigned to ICD therapy (*P*=.02) compared with women randomly assigned to standard medical therapy. Although there was no conclusive evidence for a sex difference in the effectiveness of the ICD, the trial was not adequately powered to detect those interaction effects.

SCD-HeFT also showed that ICD therapy reduced overall mortality among patients with NYHA class II or III heart failure and LVEF of 35% or less, while amiodarone had no effect on survival. Women comprised 23% of

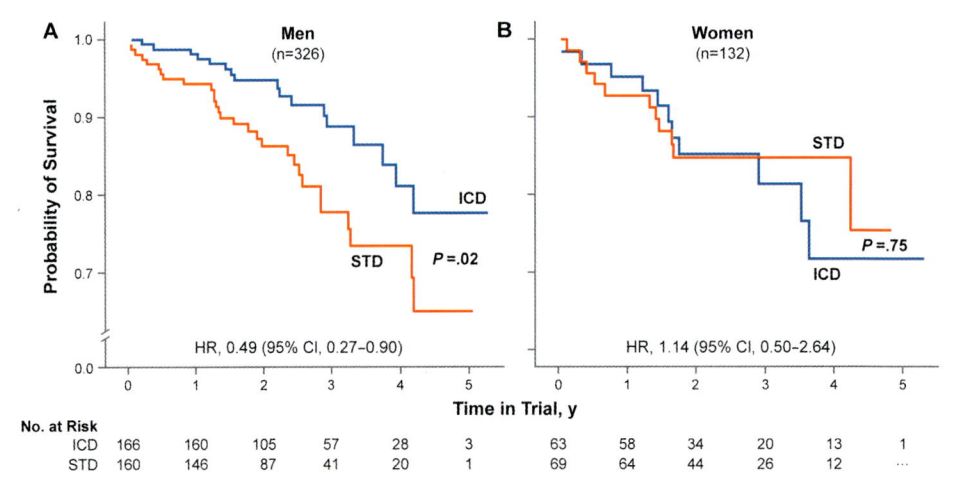

FIGURE 9.6. Survival in DEFINITE. A, Survival among men. B, Survival among women. For patients who received implantable cardioverter-defibrillator therapy (ICD) instead of standard therapy (STD), all-cause mortality was decreased among men (*P*=.02) but not women (*P*=.75). HR indicates hazard ratio. (Adapted from Albert CM, Quigg R, Saba S, Estes NA 3rd, Shaechter A, Subacius H, et al; DEFINITE Investigators. Sex differences in outcome after implantable cardioverter defibrillator implantation in nonischemic cardiomyopathy. Am Heart J. 2008 Aug;156[2]:367-72. Used with permission.)

the SCD-HeFT cohort. After adjustment for baseline differences between men and women, the overall mortality risk was lower for women than for men (Figure 9.7A). The sex difference in overall mortality was seen in the placebo group, but no sex difference in overall mortality was seen in the ICD group (Figure 9.7B). The absolute risk of death was significantly lower among the

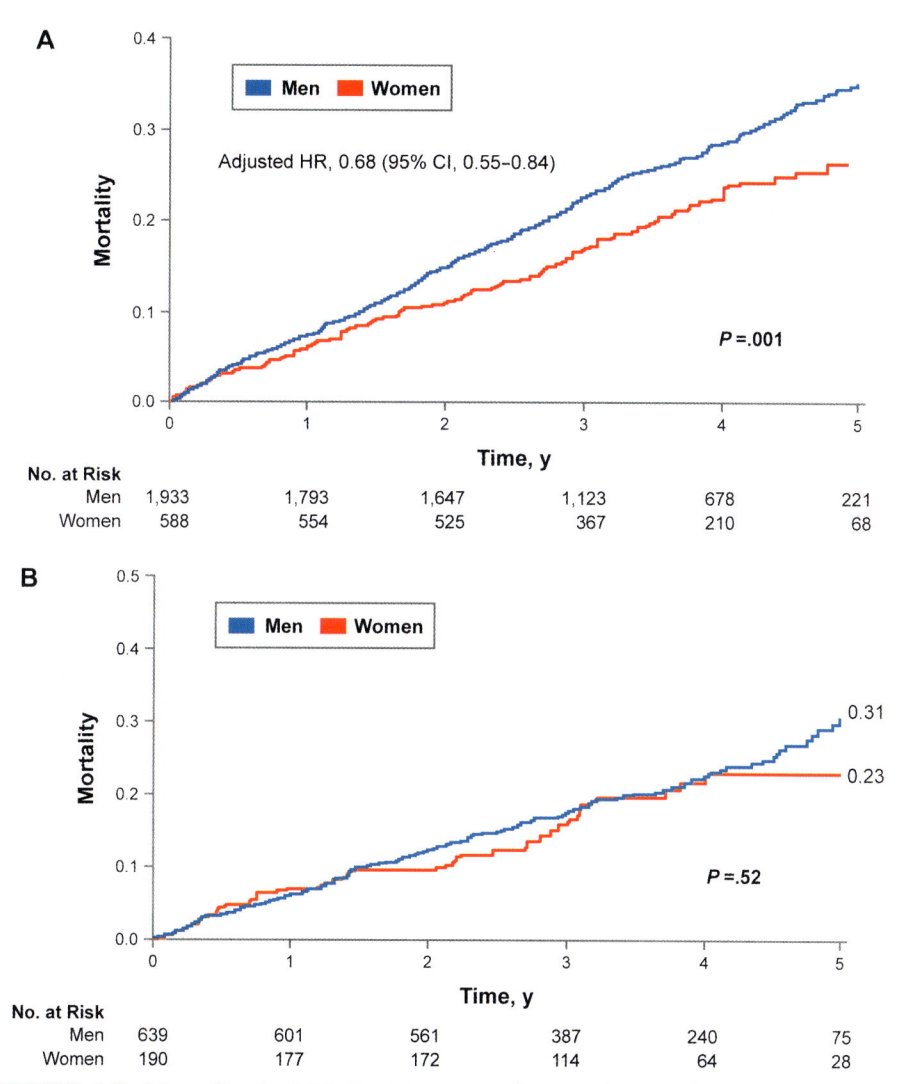

FIGURE 9.7. Mortality in SCD-HeFT. A, Overall mortality was lower among women than among men (*P*=.001). Mortality was lower among women in the placebo group; the difference was not statistically significant in the amiodarone group. B, In the ICD group, there was no difference in mortality between men and women. (A, Adapted from Russo AM, Poole JE, Mark DB, Anderson J, Hellkamp AS, Lee KL, et al. Primary prevention with defibrillator therapy in women: results from the Sudden Cardiac Death in Heart Failure Trial. J CardiovascElectrophysiol. 2008 Jul;19[7]:720–4. Epub 2008 Mar 26. Used with permission.)

women in the placebo group, compared with men in the placebo group (annual mortality rate, approximately 4% vs 6%). Although this suggests that women may have a smaller ICD benefit than men, the interaction between sex and therapy was not significant. The lower overall mortality risk for women in the placebo group and the smaller number of women enrolled may help to explain why treatment differences among women were much smaller and may have been more difficult to detect. Results from post hoc analyses must be interpreted with caution since small numbers of women were enrolled, and these trials may have been underpowered for showing any benefit of ICD therapy for women.

A meta-analysis of 5 primary prevention ICD trials (MADIT II, MUSTT, SCD-HeFT, DEFINITE, and COMPANION) evaluated the effect of prophylactic ICD therapy on the end points of total mortality, appropriate ICD therapies, and survival of women compared with men. This analysis included 7,229 patients with left ventricular dysfunction; in 74%, cardiomyopathy had an ischemic origin. Women represented 22% of the study group and presented with more comorbidities and more advanced heart failure. In addition, fewer women received renin-angiotensin blockers and underwent coronary revascularization procedures. After adjustment for baseline cofounders and covariates, there was no significant difference in overall mortality for women compared with men (HR, 0.96; 95% CI, 0.67–1.39; P=.84) (Figure 9.8). Prophylactic ICD implantation significantly reduced mortality for men (HR, 0.67; 95% CI, 0.58–0.78; P<.001), while there was no significant reduction in mortality for women (HR, 0.78; 95% CI, 0.57–1.05; P=.1) (Figure 9.9).

This meta-analysis included a cardiac resynchronization therapy (CRT) trial (COMPANION), which evaluated 1,520 patients with advanced heart failure (NYHA class III or IV) due to ischemic or nonischemic cardiomyopathy and QRS duration of 120 ms or more. In patients with advanced heart failure and a prolonged QRS interval, the use of CRT in combination with an ICD significantly reduced mortality. In this and other trials evaluating CRT, women appeared to have a better response to CRT than men. In MADIT-CRT, women assigned to CRT had consistently greater echocardiographic evidence of reverse cardiac remodeling than men. With the inclusion of a CRT study in this meta-analysis and a potentially greater benefit of CRT in women, this meta-analysis may have

A. Overall Mortality

Study or Subgroup	Weight, %	IV, Random (95% CI)
DEFINITE	21.2	0.89 (0.54–1.46)
MADIT II	16.9	1.37 (0.72–2.59)
MUSTT	30.8	1.19 (0.95–1.48)
SCD-HeFT	31.2	0.68 (0.55–0.84)
Total (95% CI)	**100.0**	**0.96 (0.67–1.39)**

Heterogeneity: $\tau^2 = 0.10$; $\chi^2 = 14.85$, df = 3 ($P = .002$); $I^2 = 80\%$
Test for overall effect: $Z = 0.21$ ($P = .84$)

Hazard Ratio IV, Random (95% CI): 0.2 — 0.5 — 1 — 2 — 5 (Lower women / Lower men)

B. Appropriate ICD Intervention

Study or Subgroup	Weight, %	IV, Random (95% CI)
SCD-HeFT	39.4	0.78 (0.52–1.17)
MADIT II	27.9	0.60 (0.37–0.97)
DEFINITE	7.1	0.39 (0.15–1.01)
COMPANION	25.6	0.56 (0.34–0.92)
Total (95% CI)	**100.0**	**0.63 (0.49–0.82)**

Heterogeneity: $\tau^2 = 0.00$; $\chi^2 = 2.32$, df = 3 ($P = .51$); $I^2 = 0\%$
Test for overall effect: $Z = 3.54$ ($P < .001$)

Hazard Ratio IV, Random (95% CI): 0.02 — 0.1 — 1 — 10 — 50 (Lower women / Lower men)

FIGURE 9.8. Meta-analysis of Primary Prevention Trials. Hazard ratio of overall mortality (A) and appropriate implantable cardioverter-defibrillator (ICD) intervention (B) in men and women. IV indicates inverse variance. (Adapted from Santangeli P, Pelargonio G, Dello Russo A, Casella M, Bisceglia C, Bartoletti S, et al. Gender differences in clinical outcome and primary prevention defibrillator benefit in patients with severe left ventricular dysfunction: a systematic review and meta-analysis. Heart Rhythm. 2010 Jul;7[7]: 876–82. Epub 2010 Apr 7. Used with permission.)

A. ICD Survival Benefit Among Men

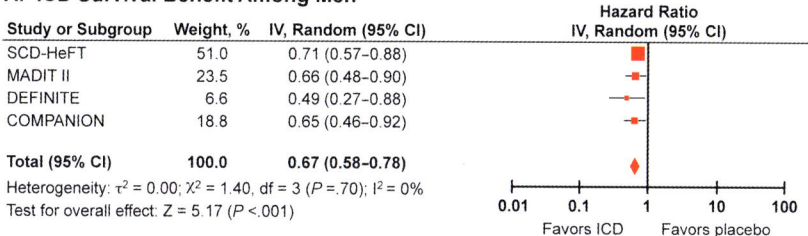

Study or Subgroup	Weight, %	IV, Random (95% CI)
SCD-HeFT	51.0	0.71 (0.57–0.88)
MADIT II	23.5	0.66 (0.48–0.90)
DEFINITE	6.6	0.49 (0.27–0.88)
COMPANION	18.8	0.65 (0.46–0.92)
Total (95% CI)	**100.0**	**0.67 (0.58–0.78)**

Heterogeneity: $\tau^2 = 0.00$; $\chi^2 = 1.40$, df = 3 ($P = .70$); $I^2 = 0\%$
Test for overall effect: $Z = 5.17$ ($P < .001$)

Hazard Ratio IV, Random (95% CI): 0.01 — 0.1 — 1 — 10 — 100 (Favors ICD / Favors placebo)

B. ICD Survival Benefit Among Women

Study or Subgroup	Weight, %	IV, Random (95% CI)
SCD-HeFT	44.3	0.90 (0.57–1.43)
MADIT II	18.9	0.57 (0.28–1.15)
DEFINITE	14.1	1.14 (0.50–2.58)
COMPANION	22.8	0.59 (0.31–1.12)
Total (95% CI)	**100.0**	**0.78 (0.57–1.05)**

Heterogeneity: $\tau^2 = 0.00$; $\chi^2 = 2.69$, df = 3 ($P = .44$); $I^2 = 0\%$
Test for overall effect: $Z = 1.63$ ($P = .10$)

Hazard Ratio IV, Random (95% CI): 0.01 — 0.1 — 1 — 10 — 100 (Favors ICD / Favors placebo)

FIGURE 9.9. Meta-analysis of Primary Prevention Trials. Hazard ratio of survival benefit associated with implantable cardioverter-defibrillator (ICD) use in men (A) and women (B). IV indicates inverse variance. (Adapted from Santangeli P, Pelargonio G, Dello Russo A, Casella M, Bisceglia C, Bartoletti S, et al. Gender differences in clinical outcome and primary prevention defibrillator benefit in patients with severe left ventricular dysfunction: a systematic review and meta-analysis. Heart Rhythm. 2010 Jul;7[7]:876–82. Epub 2010 Apr 7. Used with permission.)

actually overestimated the benefit of ICD therapy (without concomitant CRT) in women.

Alternatively, this meta-analysis, in which 22% (1,590) of the patients were women, may have been underpowered for showing a benefit of ICD therapy for women. In the SCD-HeFT analysis, the number of women needed to detect the same ICD benefit for women as for men (HR, 0.71) with 90% power (α=.05) was calculated: A study larger than SCD-HeFT would be required, with 1,585 women in each treatment arm (3,170 total women). The ICD benefit for women may also be less than that for men; sex differences in baseline characteristics and presentation of women at an older age with more comorbidities may also affect outcome.

Although not a randomized trial of ICD therapy, the INTRINSIC RV study enrolled 1,530 patients, including 293 women (19%). In this study, DDDR pacing with atrioventricular search hysteresis was compared with VVI backup pacing with ICDs implanted for primary or secondary prevention. Although unadjusted survival was better for men than for women, there were differences in baseline characteristics and medical therapy. Women were more likely to have had heart failure and less likely to have had CAD than men. Women were also more likely to have been treated with diuretics and less likely to be treated with angiotensin-converting enzyme inhibitors or β-blockers. During 11 months of follow-up, unadjusted mortality was higher for women than for men (6.8% vs 4.1%; P=.04). The percentages of patients hospitalized for heart failure were not significantly different for women (7.9%) and men (5.7%) (P=.13). After adjustment for differences in baseline characteristics and medical therapy, survival after ICD implantation did not differ between men and women (P=.34).

Important information can also be obtained from clinical registries, such as the Ontario ICD Database. A health payer–mandated, prospective study of patients referred for ICD implantation provided longitudinal follow-up for complications, deaths, and device outcomes. This study included 6,021 patients (4,733 men) referred for ICD implantation at 18 centers in Ontario, Canada, from February 2007 to July 2010. In this registry, total mortality after ICD implantation did not differ between men and women during 1-year follow-up (HR, 1.00; 95% CI, 0.64–1.55; *P*=.99).

Inducibility of Ventricular Arrhythmias

Previous studies have shown that women are less likely to have inducible sustained ventricular arrhythmias. These findings suggest that there is a sex difference in the arrhythmic substrate or in the triggering mechanism for arrhythmias. In MUSTT, which included only patients with underlying ischemic heart disease, women were less likely than men to have inducible sustained ventricular arrhythmias (24% vs 36%, *P*=.001) and were therefore less likely to be eligible for randomization in the trial.

Arrhythmic Events During Follow-up

Secondary Prevention

Even though population studies have shown that there are sex differences in the incidence of SCD, most studies have not identified sex differences in arrhythmia occurrence or appropriate defibrillator therapy after ICD implantation in patients presenting with sustained ventricular arrhythmias or syncope with inducible sustained ventricular arrhythmias. In contrast, 1 study has shown that female sex was an independent clinical predictor of shock therapy for cardiac arrest survivors.

Primary Prevention

Primary prevention studies examining sex differences in ventricular arrhythmic events have had variable results. In DEFINITE, after multivariable adjustment, women had somewhat fewer appropriate ICD shocks, but the difference was not significant (*P*=.06): 28 men (16.9%) and 5 women (7.9%) received appropriate ICD shock therapy for VT or VF (unadjusted *P*=.100) during a mean follow-up of 29 months. Findings were similar in MADIT II: The risk of appropriate ICD therapy for VT or VF was lower for women than for men (for women vs men,

HR, 0.60; 95% CI, 0.37–0.98; *P*=.04) after adjustment of clinical covariates (Figure 9.10).

In SCD-HeFT, 23% of men received appropriate ICD shock therapy, with a median time to shock of 14.7 months; 19% of women received appropriate ICD shock therapy, with a median time to shock of 15.5 months. There was no difference in the risk of appropriate shock therapy between men and women (*P*=.25). In the INTRINSIC RV study, no sex differences in appropriate or inappropriate ICD therapy were seen after a median follow-up of 11 months.

A meta-analysis of primary prevention trials (MADIT II, MUSTT, SCD-HeFT, DEFINITE, and COMPANION) showed that women received fewer appropriate

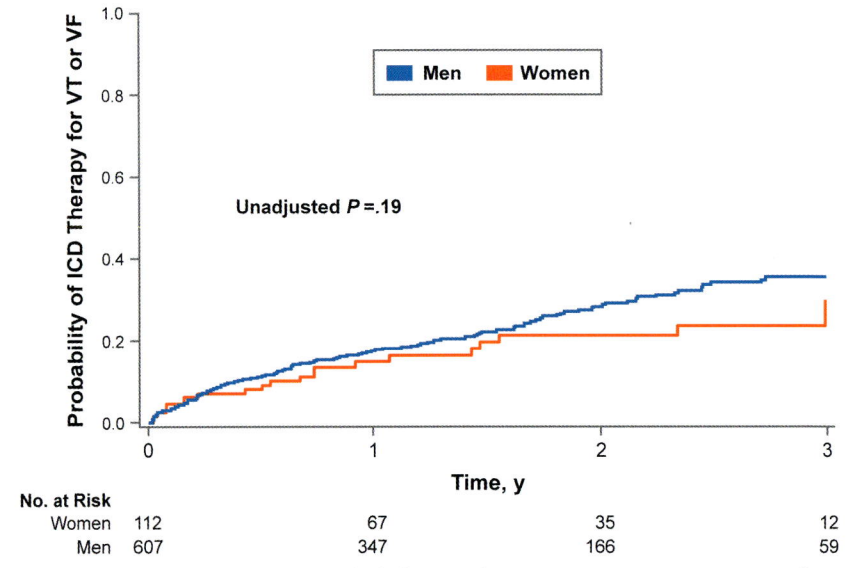

FIGURE 9.10. Cumulative Probability of First Appropriate Implantable Cardioverter-Defibrillator (ICD) Therapy in MADIT II. In multivariate analysis, the 2-year probability of appropriate ICD therapy for ventricular tachycardia (VT) or ventricular fibrillation (VF) was significantly lower for women than men (21% vs 28%). The difference was attributed to a higher frequency of VT episodes in men (hazard ratio, 0.60; 95% CI, 0.37–0.98; *P*=.04). (Adapted from Zareba W, Moss AJ, Jackson Hall W, Wilber DJ, Ruskin JN, McNitt S, et al; MADIT II Investigators. Clinical course and implantable cardioverter defibrillator therapy in postinfarction women with severe left ventricular dysfunction.J CardiovascElectrophysiol. 2005 Dec;16[12]:1265-70. Used with permission.)

ICD therapies for ventricular arrhythmias than men (HR, 0.63; 95% CI, 0.49–0.82; $P<.001$) (Figure 9.8B). This finding suggests that women with left ventricular dysfunction might benefit less from primary prevention ICD implantation than men. A sex difference in arrhythmic risk supports the concept that SCD has a smaller effect on total mortality for women.

Similarly, in a single-center study examining events in patients who underwent ICD implantation for primary or secondary prevention indications, women were less likely than men to experience VT or VF and had fewer VT or VF episodes during follow-up. Sustained VT or VF occurred in 52% of men and 34% of women ($P<.01$). These sex differences were greatest among patients presenting with sustained monomorphic VT and those with inducible VT at the electrophysiology study (ie, those with a more stable anatomical VT circuit). This study suggests that sex differences in susceptibility to arrhythmia triggering might underlie the known differences in SCD rates for men and women.

A retrospective study examining the effect of sex on appropriate ICD shock therapy for patients with nonischemic cardiomyopathy showed that men and women with ICDs had similar rates of appropriate shock therapy (36% for men and 38% for women; $P=.88$). The mean time to first appropriate shock was 11.9 months for men and 21.3 months for women ($P=.2$). Sex did not appear to be an important risk factor for arrhythmic events in this cohort with nonischemic cardiomyopathy.

An Italian registry, SEARCH-MI, enrolled patients after they had a myocardial infarction and evaluated the clinical and arrhythmic outcomes among patients who had received an ICD for primary prevention of SCD. Data on 556 patients showed that 30% of patients experienced sustained ventricular arrhythmias. Male sex was predictive of appropriate ICD therapy during follow-up (incidence, 25% for men and 5% for women; $P<.001$).

From the Ontario ICD Database, important data are now available from a health payer–mandated study of 6,021 patients (21% women) referred for ICD implantation. Women were less likely than men to receive appropriate ICD shock therapy (HR, 0.69; 95% CI, 0.51–0.93; $P=.02$) or appropriate shock or

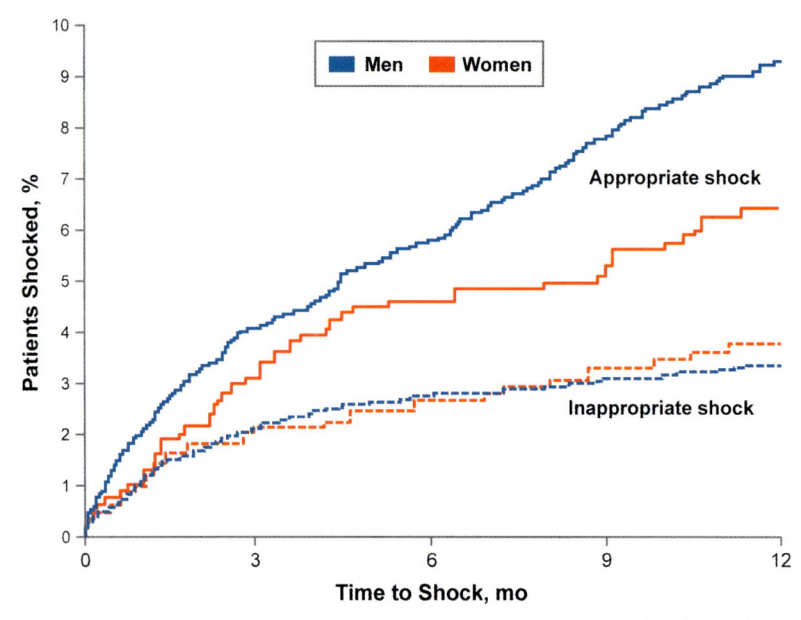

FIGURE 9.11. Time to First Appropriate or Inappropriate Shock in the Ontario Health Payer–Mandated Prospective Study. Women were less likely than men to receive appropriate shock therapy (hazard ratio, 0.69; 95% CI, 0.51-0.93; *P*=.02). (Adapted from MacFadden DR, Crystal E, Krahn AD, Mangat I, Healey JS, Dorian P, et al. Sex differences in implantable cardioverter-defibrillator outcomes: findings from a prospective defibrillator database. Ann Intern Med. 2012 Feb 7;156[3]:195-203. Used with permission.)

antitachycardia pacing therapy (HR, 0.73; 95% CI, 0.59-0.90; *P* =.003) during follow-up (Figure 9.11).

Potential Mechanisms for Differences in Arrhythmias

The incidence of SCD is lower for women than for men. Reasons for the lower incidence for women are unclear, but they may be related to hormonal influences, autonomic tone, ion channels, or sex differences in susceptibility to arrhythmia triggers.

As discussed earlier in this chapter, data suggest that the underlying pathophysiology and risk factors for SCD differ between men and women. The differences include a lower incidence of CAD and higher LVEF in women who survive out-of-hospital cardiac arrest. Thus, pathologic substrates underlying SCD seem to differ between women and men, which may help to explain sex differences in the incidence of sustained ventricular arrhythmias.

Sex differences in the inducibility of ventricular arrhythmias have also been noted among patients with underlying ischemic heart disease: Women are less likely to have inducible sustained ventricular arrhythmias at electrophysiology testing. This difference supports a theory related to potential sex differences in the triggering of arrhythmias. Previous investigation has shown that inducibility of ventricular arrhythmias is a powerful independent predictor of subsequent arrhythmia recurrence. One hypothesis is that this might lead to a reduced propensity for clinically occurring reentrant ventricular arrhythmias in women compared with men.

Some studies have shown that, among patients who have already received an ICD, women seem to experience fewer arrhythmic episodes than men, although other studies have shown no significant sex differences. In the meta-analysis by Santangeli and colleagues, the rate of malignant arrhythmia occurrence was lower for women than for men, without differences in overall mortality. This finding suggests that there are sex differences in arrhythmic risk for patients with left ventricular dysfunction. Since ICD therapy is expected to improve survival by preventing death due to malignant arrhythmias, these data may help to provide a mechanistic explanation for a smaller survival benefit associated with prophylactic ICD therapy for women.

ICD Complications

There are conflicting data on sex differences in complications related to ICD implantation. Several previous studies suggested that there were no apparent sex differences in ICD implantation complication rates for men and women undergoing implantation for secondary or primary prevention indications. However, more recent data from real-life clinical practice, including more recent information from the Ontario ICD Database and the NCDR ICD Registry, suggest otherwise.

The Canadian health payer–mandated prospective study evaluated patients referred for ICD implantation. Analysis of data from the Ontario ICD Database showed that women were significantly more likely than men to experience major complications by 45 days (odds ratio [OR], 1.78; 95% CI, 1.25–2.58; P=.002) and 1 year (HR, 1.91; 95% CI, 1.48–2.47; P<.001) after implantation. Women also had more occurrences of any major or minor complication at 45-day follow-up and 1-year follow-up.

Similar findings were also noted in the NCDR ICD Registry. In-hospital outcomes were examined in the NCDR ICD Registry for 161,470 patients (27%

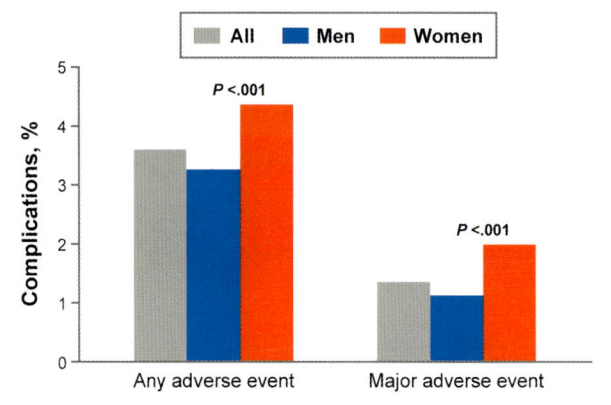

FIGURE 9.12. Unadjusted Rates of In-Hospital Adverse Events Related to Implantable Cardioverter-Defibrillator (ICD) Implantation by Sex. Data are from the National Cardiovascular Data Registry ICD Registry. In a multivariate analysis, women had a higher risk of any major adverse event. (Adapted from Peterson PN, Daugherty SL, Wang Y, Vidaillet HJ, Heidenreich PA, Curtis JP, et al; National Cardiovascular Data Registry. Gender differences in procedure-related adverse events in patients receiving implantable cardioverter-defibrillator therapy.Circulation. 2009 Mar 3;119[8]:1078-84. Epub 2009 Feb 16. Used with permission.)

women) undergoing ICD implantation between January 2006 and December 2007. In unadjusted analyses, women were more likely than men to experience any adverse event (4.4% vs 3.3%, $P<.001$) and major adverse events (2.0% vs 1.1%, $P<.001$) (Figure 9.12). After multivariable analysis, women had a significantly higher risk of any adverse event (OR, 1.32; 95% CI, 1.24–1.39) and major adverse events (OR, 1.71; 95% CI, 1.57–1.86).

ICD and Body Image

Although not specifically examined in clinical trials, women may express concern about the effect of an implanted device on body appearance. One small study did identify that women worried more than men about the effect of the implanted device on appearance, which was particularly notable among women who were younger (age <39 years). This may be less of an issue with smaller pulse generators. However, the device may be more visible in a pectoral location in women who have a smaller body size. One option may be to consider subpectoral implantation. Another option includes implantation of a totally subcutaneous device in the lateral chest, in a location that has a larger amount of subcutaneous tissue and is not typically visible while dressed. Although the recently approved subcutaneous ICD is larger than standard pulse generators, it still seems to result in a cosmetically acceptable appearance. In the future, pulse generators may be smaller. Although body image as it relates to acceptance of ICD therapy may be an issue for some women, personal experience suggests that this is not an issue for the vast majority of ICD recipients and should not be a limiting factor for acceptance of ICD therapy.

ICD USE

Sex disparities with ICD use have been noted. Real-life analysis of a clinical practice showed that women are less likely than men to undergo ICD implantation for primary or secondary prevention indications. In an analysis of a Medicare population, women were older and had more comorbidities than men when they presented for ICD implantation with LVEF of 35% or less.

Data were examined from a sample of Medicare beneficiaries who met criteria for ICD implantation from 1991 to 2005. For the primary prevention cohort, only 8.6 per 1,000 women received an ICD within 1 year of diagnosis compared with 32.3 per 1,000 men (HR, 3.15; 95% CI, 2.86–3.47). In multivariate analyses, men were more likely than women to receive ICD therapy (HR, 3.15; 95% CI, 2.86–3.47). In a secondary prevention cohort, 102.2 per 1,000 men and 38.4 per 1,000 women received ICD therapy. After controlling for demographics and comorbidities, men were more likely than women to receive ICD therapy for secondary prevention (HR, 2.44; 95% CI, 2.30–2.59).

In a study of 13,034 patients who had heart failure and LVEF of 30% or less and who were admitted to hospitals participating in the American Heart Association's Get With the Guidelines—Heart Failure quality improvement program, only 35.4% of patients had an ICD or a plan for ICD implantation at discharge. Compared with ICD use in white men, ICD use was less likely in black men (OR, 0.73), white women (OR, 0.62), and black women (OR, 0.56) after adjustment for patient characteristics and hospital factors. A significant increase in ICD therapy use was observed over time in all sex and race groups, although sex differences persisted.

In a retrospective cohort analysis of patients who appeared eligible for ICD implantation from review of administrative data in Ontario, Canada, men were more likely than women to receive an ICD for primary or secondary prevention indications. Sex bias for ICD use appeared greater for patients undergoing implantation for primary prevention indications. Age and comorbidities did not explain these sex differences. The patterns of ICD use in men and women over time were examined from the perspective of elapsed time before ICD implantation. For secondary prevention indications, time to ICD implantation was initially rapid for both sexes, but early implantation rates were approximately 2-fold higher for men (Figure 9.13A). For primary prevention indications, the time to implantation was initially higher for men, and subsequent ICD implantation rates continued to increase at higher rates for men (Figure 9.13B).

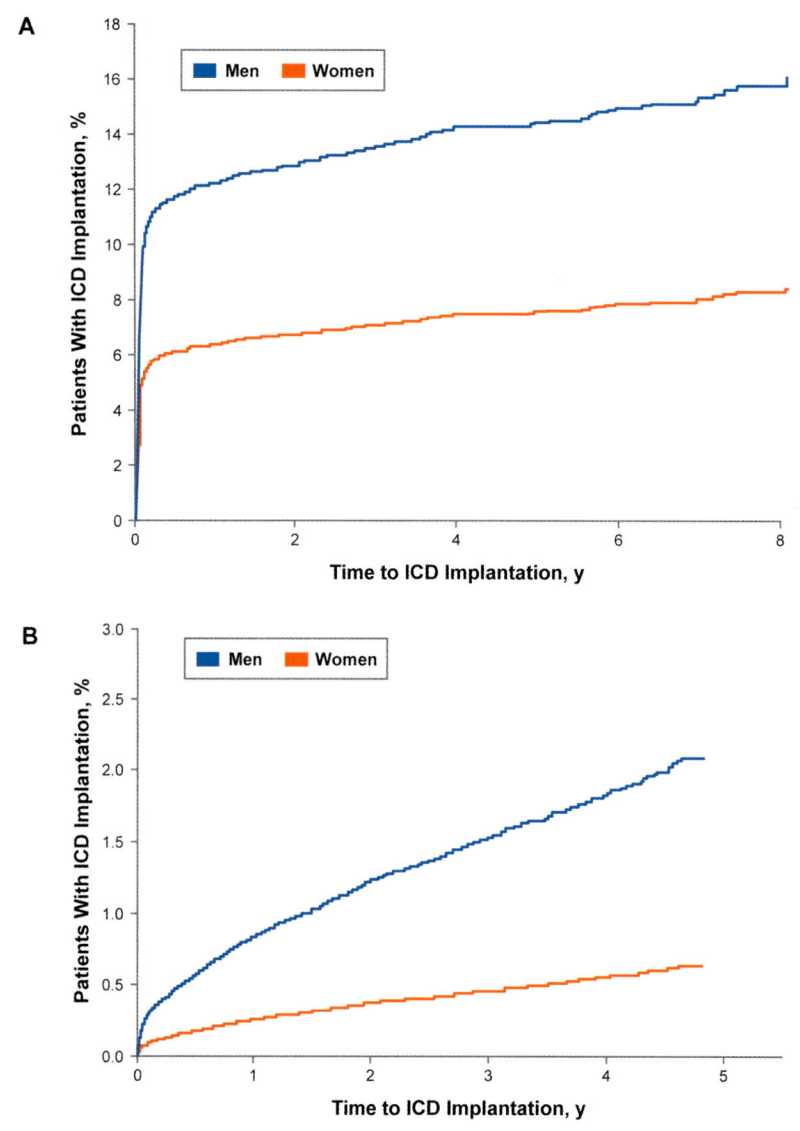

FIGURE 9.13. Time to Implantable Cardioverter-Defibrillator (ICD) Implantation by Sex for Secondary and Primary Prevention Indications. A, Time to ICD implantation for patients eligible for secondary prevention ICDs after cardiac arrest. B, Time to ICD implantation for patients eligible for primary prevention ICDs after myocardial infarction. (Adapted from MacFadden DR, Tu JV, Chong A, Austin PC, Lee DS. Evaluating sex differences in population-based utilization of implantable cardioverter-defibrillators: role of cardiac conditions and noncardiac comorbidities.Heart Rhythm. 2009 Sep;6[9]:1289-96. Epub 2009 May 18. Used with permission.)

The influence of sex on delivery of guideline-recommended heart failure therapy was also evaluated in IMPROVE HF. Baseline data from 15,381 eligible outpatients who had chronic heart failure and LVEF of 35% or less were collected at 167 outpatient cardiology practices. Women were less likely than men to receive guideline-recommended ICD therapy (43.2% vs 53.7%, *P*<.001) (Figure 9.14). This sex difference persisted with adjusted analyses that showed increased adherence with men (HR, 1.40; 95% CI, 1.22–1.61; *P*<.0001). The difference between men and women was not seen with the use of medical therapy, such as β-blockers, angiotensin-converting enzyme inhibitors, and angiotensin II receptor blockers.

The prospective ADVANCENT trial investigated the effect of sex and race on the rates of ICD and pacemaker implantation in 26,264 patients with LVEF of 40% or less from 106 centers in the United States. Female sex was independently associated with a decreased rate for implantation of any device (OR, 0.70; 95% CI, 0.66–0.76) and for any ICD (OR, 0.60; 95% CI, 0.55–0.64).

Several potential explanations for sex differences in ICD implantation rates may be considered. 1) This difference may be due to the possibility that

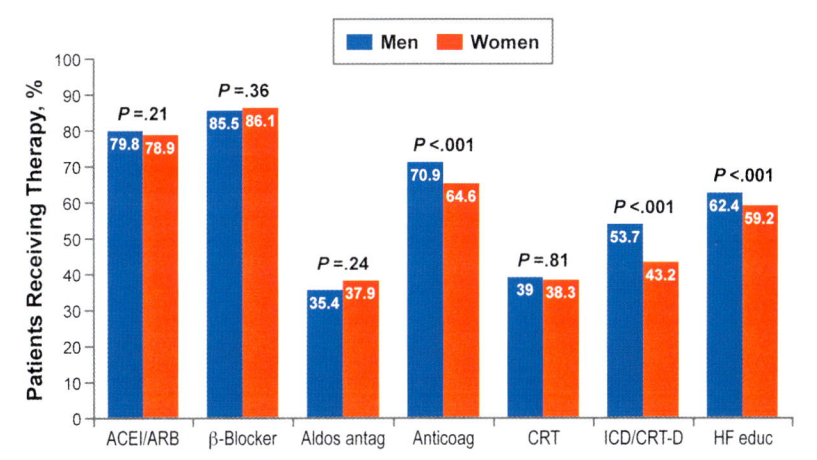

FIGURE 9.14. Heart Failure Therapy by Sex in IMPROVE HF. Sex differences in heart failure therapy are shown, including less use of ICDs in women (43.2%) compared with men (53.7%) (*P*<.001). ACEI indicates angiotensin-converting enzyme inhibitor; Aldos antag, aldosterone antagonist; Anticoag, anticoagulation for atrial fibrillation; ARB, angiotensin II receptor blocker; CRT, cardiac resynchronization therapy; CRT-D, cardiac resynchronization therapy device with defibrillation; HF educ, heart failure education; ICD, implantable cardioverter-defibrillator. (Adapted from Yancy CW, Fonarow GC, Albert NM, Curtis AB, Stough WG, Gheorghiade M, et al. Influence of patient age and sex on delivery of guideline-recommended heart failure care in the outpatient cardiology practice setting: findings from IMPROVE HF. Am Heart J. 2009 Apr;157[4]:754–62.e2. Used with permission.)

fewer women meet criteria for ICD therapy, or perhaps they are older with more comorbidities when criteria for ICD implantation are met. Although prior studies have examined the effect of baseline differences between men and women, with adjustments for baseline differences and comorbidities, it is possible that other, unexamined factors may have influenced the outcome. 2) Bias may be present, and fewer women might be offered ICDs while meeting criteria. However, 1 small study suggested that there was no evidence for a difference between men and women related to the rates of recommendation for ICD implantation. 3) The difference may represent patient preference, and fewer women may elect to undergo implantation when offered therapy. In 1 small study, women refused ICD implantation more often than men (19% vs 2%, $P=.02$).

CONCLUSIONS

There are sex-specific differences in the epidemiology of SCD. Reasons for the lower incidence of SCD among women are unclear, but sex differences in arrhythmia substrate or susceptibility to arrhythmia triggers may be contributory. Women are less likely to have inducible sustained ventricular arrhythmias at electrophysiology testing, supporting the hypothesis that there may be sex differences in the triggering mechanisms of arrhythmias.

ICD trials show differences in baseline characteristics and medical therapy for men and women. The benefit of ICD therapy for secondary prevention indications appears to be similar for men and women. For primary prevention indications, available data suggest a smaller ICD benefit among women, although smaller numbers of women were enrolled in clinical trials, and individual studies were underpowered for showing a benefit similar to men. With limited clinical trial data for women, efforts should be directed toward better risk stratification for both women and men.

Women are more likely to have adverse events related to ICD implantation, but the reasons for these differences are unclear. Care should be taken in extrapolating results of clinical trials to women when predominantly men were enrolled in the trials. More studies exploring the mechanisms of sex differences in arrhythmias are needed to enhance our understanding and to help ensure that women receive appropriate arrhythmia management.

Sex disparities are apparent with ICD use. The reasons for sex disparities in arrhythmia therapy are currently unclear and warrant further investigation.

SUGGESTED READING

Chen HA, Hsia HH, Vagelos R, Fowler M, Wang P, Al-Ahmad A. The effect of gender on mortality or appropriate shock in patients with nonischemic cardiomyopathy who have implantable cardioverter-defibrillators. Pacing Clin Electrophysiol. 2007 Mar;30(3):390–4.

Curtis LH, Al-Khatib SM, Shea AM, Hammill BG, Hernandez AF, Schulman KA. Sex differences in the use of implantable cardioverter-defibrillators for primary and secondary prevention of sudden cardiac death. JAMA. 2007 Oct 3;298(13):1517–24.

Gauri AJ, Davis A, Hong T, Burke MC, Knight BP. Disparities in the use of primary prevention and defibrillator therapy among blacks and women. Am J Med. 2006 Feb;119(2):167.e17–21.

Herlitz J, Rundqvist S, Bang A, Aune S, Lundstrom G, Ekstrom L, et al. Is there a difference between women and men in characteristics and outcome after in hospital cardiac arrest? Resuscitation. 2001 Apr;49(1):15–23.

Lampert R, McPherson CA, Clancy JF, Caulin-Glaser TL, Rosenfeld LE, Batsford WP. Gender differences in ventricular arrhythmia recurrence in patients with coronary artery disease and implantable cardioverter-defibrillators. J Am Coll Cardiol. 2004 Jun 16;43(12):2293–9.

Lin G, Meverden RA, Hodge DO, Uslan DZ, Hayes DL, Brady PA. Age and gender trends in implantable cardioverter defibrillator utilization: a population based study. J Interv Card Electrophysiol. 2008 Jun;22(1):65–70. Epub 2008 Mar 7.

MacFadden DR, Crystal E, Krahn AD, Mangat I, Healey JS, Dorian P, et al. Sex differences in implantable cardioverter-defibrillator outcomes: findings from a prospective defibrillator database. Ann Intern Med. 2012 Feb 7;156(3):195–203.

MacFadden DR, Tu JV, Chong A, Austin PC, Lee DS. Evaluating sex differences in population-based utilization of implantable cardioverter-defibrillators: role of cardiac conditions and noncardiac comorbidities. Heart Rhythm. 2009 Sep;6(9):1289–96. Epub 2009 May 18.

Mezu U, Ch I, Halder I, London B, Saba S. Women and minorities are less likely to receive an implantable cardioverter defibrillator for primary prevention of sudden cardiac death. Europace. 2012 Mar;14(3):341–4. Epub 2011 Nov 8.

Pires LA, Sethuraman B, Guduguntla VD, Todd KM, Yamasaki H, Ravi S. Outcome of women versus men with ventricular tachyarrhythmias treated with the implantable cardioverter defibrillator. J Cardiovasc Electrophysiol. 2002 Jun;13(6):563–8.

Russo AM, Day JD, Stolen K, Mullin CM, Doraiswamy V, Lerew DL, et al. Implantable cardioverter defibrillators: do women fare worse than men? Gender comparison in the INTRINSIC RV trial. J Cardiovasc Electrophysiol. 2009 Sep;20(9):973–8.

Russo AM, Poole JE, Mark DB, Anderson J, Hellkamp AS, Lee KL, et al. Primary prevention with defibrillator therapy in women: results from the Sudden Cardiac Death in Heart Failure Trial. J Cardiovasc Electrophysiol. 2008 Jul;19(7):720–4. Epub 2008 Mar 26.

Russo AM, Stamato NJ, Lehmann MH, Hafley GE, Lee KL, Pieper K, et al; MUSTT Investigators. Influence of gender on arrhythmia characteristics and outcome in the Multicenter UnSustained Tachycardia Trial. J Cardiovasc Electrophysiol. 2004 Sep;15(9):993–8.

Santangeli P, Pelargonio G, Dello Russo A, Casella M, Bisceglia C, Bartoletti S, et al. Gender differences in clinical outcome and primary prevention defibrillator benefit in patients with severe left ventricular dysfunction: a systematic review and meta-analysis. Heart Rhythm. 2010 Jul;7(7):876–82. Epub 2010 Apr 7.

Udell JA, Juurlink DN, Kopp A, Lee DS, Tu JV, Mamdani MM. Inequitable distribution of implantable cardioverter defibrillators in Ontario. Int J Technol Assess Health Care. 2007 Summer;23(3):354–61.

Wigginton JG, Pepe PE, Bedolla JP, DeTamble LA, Atkins JM. Sex-related differences in the presentation and outcome of out-of-hospital cardiopulmonary arrest: a multiyear, prospective, population-based study. Crit Care Med. 2002 Apr;30(4 Suppl):S131–6.

CHAPTER TEN

Pacing and Cardiac Resynchronization Therapy in Women

JUDITH A. MACKALL, MD, AND YONG-MEI CHA, MD

INTRODUCTION

Ongoing improvements and enhancements to cardiac pacing devices have expanded the indications for pacing therapy. Device therapy is now used for hemodynamic management as well as for rhythm management. Clinical trials have provided some insight into differences between men and women in indications for various pacing therapies and their responses to therapy. This chapter reviews important clinical trials that highlight differences in indications, implantation techniques, complications, outcomes, and survival among women who undergo pacing and cardiac resynchronization therapy (CRT).

CARDIAC PACING

Sex Differences in Pacemaker Selection and Survival

In the early 1990s, several studies reported differences in the use of cardiac procedures and the management of cardiac disease based on the sex of the patient.

Subsequently, several large databases were reviewed to determine whether sex differences existed for pacemaker selection, indications, and mortality.

In 1995, Lamas and colleagues analyzed 20% of Medicare beneficiaries (36,312 patients) who underwent permanent pacemaker implantation from 1988 through 1990. The authors looked at the relationship between pacemaker type and patient characteristics and found that 68.1% of patients received a ventricular single-chamber pacemaker, 30.5% received a dual-chamber pacemaker, and 1.4% received an atrial single-chamber device. Patients who received dual-chamber pacemakers were more likely to be younger and more likely to be male ($P<.001$). In addition, patients receiving dual-chamber pacemakers were more likely to have had complete atrioventricular (AV) block and significantly less comorbidity than patients who received ventricular single-chamber systems. This may in part contribute to the difference in mortality observed between patients who received a single-chamber device and those who received a dual-chamber pacing system. The 2-year mortality for patients with ventricular devices was 28.9% compared with 22.3% for patients with physiologic or dual-chamber devices ($P<.001$).

Brunner and colleagues analyzed 6,505 patients in a long-term longitudinal study with 30 years of follow-up. This study began in the 1980s; therefore, technologic advances and advances in medical treatment were in part responsible for improved survival among pacemaker patients as the years progressed, but there was a sex difference in survival. Even though women were older at the time of implantation (73.2 vs 71.0 years), they lived significantly longer than men (118.0 vs 91.7 months, $P<.001$). This difference in survival was present despite the indication for pacing, so that women with sick sinus syndrome, AV block, and atrial fibrillation (AF) had significantly longer median survival than men.

As the population ages, more patients are undergoing initial pacemaker implantation when they are older than 80 years. Udo and colleagues looked at long-term survival of patients older than 80 with data from the Dutch FollowPace study. For the 481 patients, the indications for pacemaker implantation were AV block in 45.9%, sinus node dysfunction in 32.2%, AF with slow ventricular rates in 20.2%, and other problems, including hypersensitive carotid sinus syndrome, in 1.7%. Although 53% of patients died during follow-up, more than half died of noncardiac causes. Survival among these patients was comparable to survival among age- and sex-matched controls from the general population. Male sex in addition to age, diabetes mellitus, coronary artery disease, and congestive heart failure at the time of implantation were independent predictors of all-cause mortality.

In an article published in 2000, Roeters van Lennep and colleagues reviewed data on 33,564 patients who underwent initial pacemaker implantation from 1988 through 1997. In this patient cohort, 52% (17,319) were women and 48% (16,245) were men. Women were older than men at the time of implantation (the difference between the mean ages was 3.6 years). There was no sex difference in pacemaker selection when patients were grouped by indication (AV block, sinus node dysfunction, or AF with slow ventricular response). Patients older than 80 years received fewer dual-chamber systems than younger patients. This finding was also observed in a review of 17,826 pacemaker implants from 2003 through 2006 in Germany (Figure 10.1).

The use of fewer dual-chamber systems in older patients may reflect a higher prevalence of AF. Veerareddy and colleagues retrospectively reviewed 274 patients who underwent pacemaker implantation from 2001 through 2003; 53.4% were men and 46.5% were women. Once again, the women were significantly older than the men at implantation (mean age, 64.1 years for women and 58.6 years for men). Findings from this study that agreed with findings from previous large

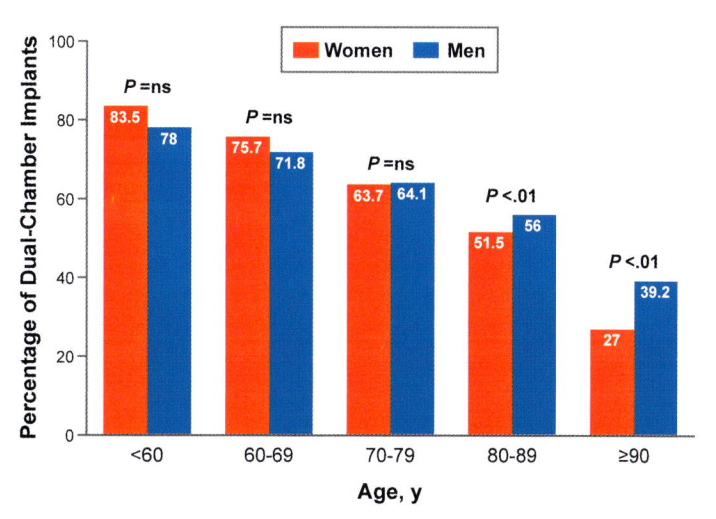

FIGURE 10.1. Percentage of Dual-Chamber Pacemakers Implanted in Patients According to Their Sex and Age. ns indicates not significant. (Adapted from Nowak B, Misselwitz B; Expert committee 'Pacemaker,' Institute of Quality Assurance Hessen, Erdogan A, Funck R, Irnich W, Israel CW, Olbrich HG, Schmidt H, et al. Do gender differences exist in pacemaker implantation? Results of an obligatory external quality control program. Europace. 2010 Feb;12[2]:210–5. Epub 2009 Oct 28. Used with permission.)

retrospective database studies included more women older than 65 years and sick sinus syndrome as the most common indication for pacing (55.6%) followed by complete AV block (29.0%). There were no sex differences in the indications for pacing. However, large registry data suggest that the indication for pacing in women is sinus node dysfunction more often than AV block. The less frequent use of dual-chamber pacing in older patients was due to the higher prevalence of AF.

Although several smaller studies and those that reported device use in the 1980s showed less use of dual-chamber devices in women, large databases from the past 20 years show no difference in device selection by sex. Women tend to be older at the time of initial implantation, but they tend to live longer than men.

Implant Considerations in Women

The size of a current-generation pacemaker or an implantable cardioverter-defibrillator (ICD) is small enough to permit prepectoral implantation in the majority of women. However, an alternative location should be considered if the patient is very thin (usually very young or elderly patients). In addition, some women prefer to have the device concealed as well as possible. In 1983, Belott and Bucko described an inframammary position for permanent pacemaker location. Subsequently, several approaches that provide a more cosmetically appealing result have been described.

Gillette and colleagues reported their experience with 56 pediatric patients whose pacemakers were implanted in a subpectoral pocket with excellent cosmetic results. The authors felt that this approach was preferred for children and young adults. A submammary approach has also been described. There have been no issues with device telemetry with submammary device placement. This approach minimizes a visible scar as well as a bulge from the device.

Giudici and colleagues reported their experience with a submammary-subpectoral approach in 51 patients. The cosmetic result was acceptable. In this report, the major drawbacks to this approach were that most of the devices were placed right-sided because of limited lead length (3 of the 51 patients had lead dislodgment) and that general anesthesia was necessary.

At University Hospitals Case Medical Center, a subpectoral position is used if it is suitable for the patient's physique and preference. This position yields a good cosmetic result, it minimizes the number of incisions, it avoids tunneling, and it can be performed under conscious sedation (Figure 10.2). As with any

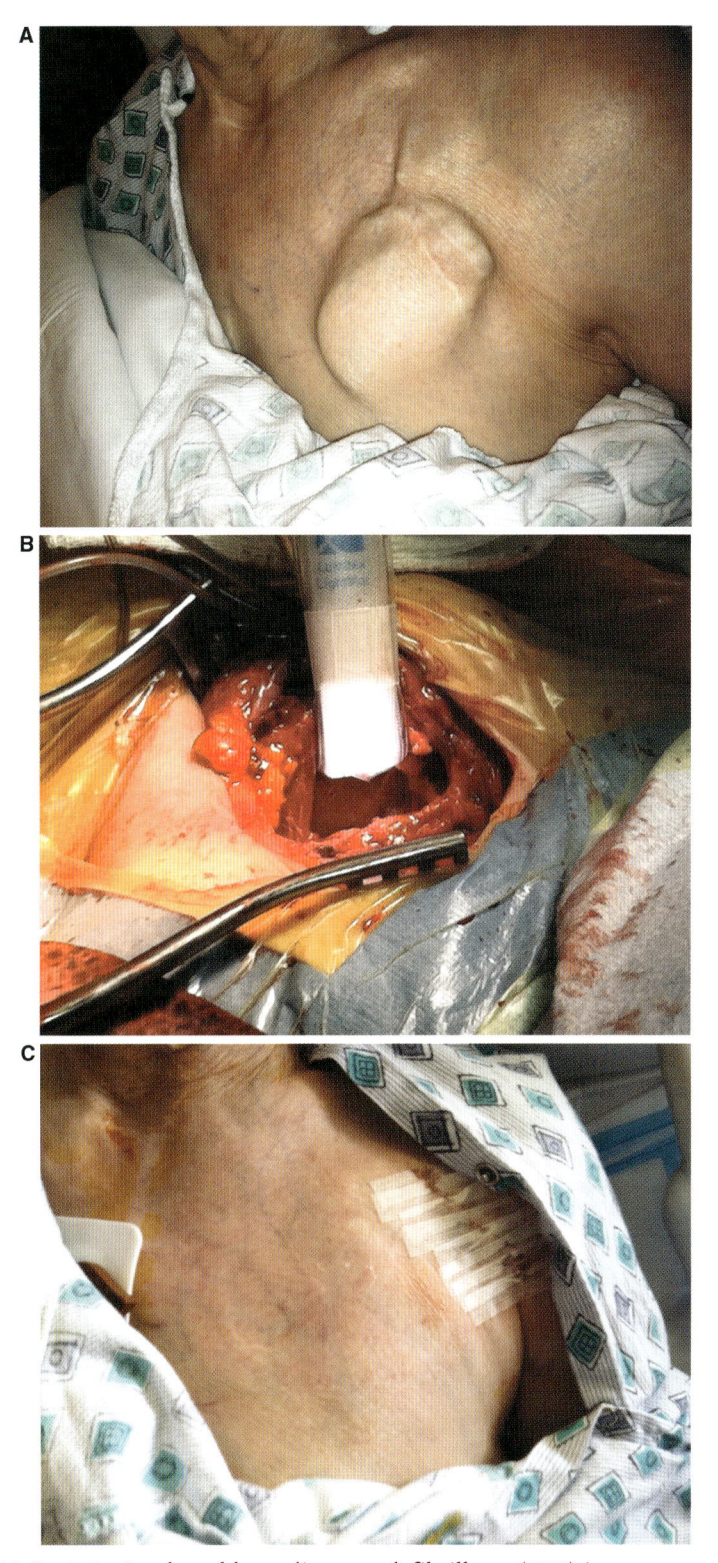

FIGURE 10.2. A, An implantable cardioverter-defibrillator (ICD) in a prepectoral pocket in a thin female patient. B, Subpectoral pocket fashioned from the deltapectoral groove. C, The ICD repositioned into the subpectoral pocket.

submuscular approach, patients should be informed to expect increased discomfort immediately postoperatively.

Women do have a higher risk of pneumothorax, and this risk is associated with subclavian vein access. To minimize the risk, either cephalic vein cutdown or axillary vein access should be attempted before subclavian puncture. In addition, a venogram can be obtained before subclavian vein puncture to help direct the needle.

Women do not appear to be at increased risk of venous thrombosis after device implantation. They also do not appear to be at increased risk of subclavian crush syndrome, a lead fracture that occurs when the lead is placed between the clavicle and first rib and through the costoclavicular ligament.

In addition, women with pacemakers should continue to undergo routine mammography. For patients with subpectoral implantation, there is no difficulty in interpretation. For prepectoral implants, however, 1 study reported that a portion of the breast tissue was obscured in 12% of studies.

Sex and Procedure-Related Complications

Women have a higher risk of complications with device implantation compared with men. Data from the NCDR ICD Registry published in 2009 showed a sex difference in adverse events related to ICD implantation. The registry of 161,470 patients, of which 27% were women, showed that women had significantly more adverse events than men (4.4% vs 3.3%, $P<.001$) (Figure 10.3). Age was not significantly different between men and women. The overall rate of any adverse event was 3.6%. Major adverse events included cardiac arrest, cardiac perforation, cardiac valve injury, coronary venous dissection, hemothorax, pneumothorax, deep vein thrombosis, transient ischemic attack, cerebrovascular accident, myocardial infarction, pericardial tamponade, and AV fistula. Women were twice as likely as men to have a major adverse event (2.0% vs 1.1%) (Figure 10.3). Even after adjusting for the higher comorbidity in women, the association of sex with adverse events persisted. Women were more likely to have a drug reaction, cardiac perforation, conduction block, coronary venous dissection, lead dislodgment, hemothorax, pneumothorax, pericardial tamponade, or deep vein thrombosis. Even though women were more likely to receive

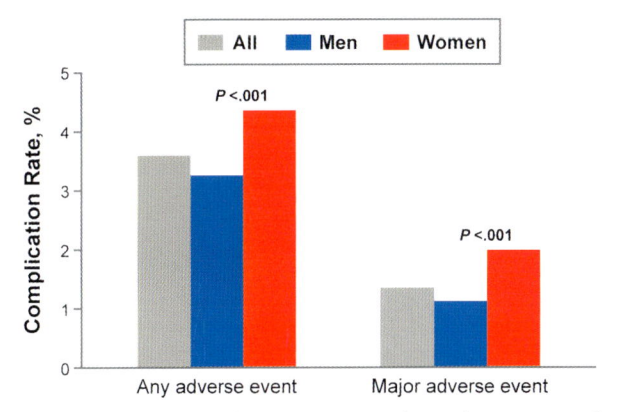

FIGURE 10.3. Complication Rate by Sex in Initial Implantation of an Implantable Cardioverter-Defibrillator. (Adapted from Peterson PN, Daugherty SL, Wang Y, Vidaillet HJ, Heidenreich PA, Curtis JP, et al; National Cardiovascular Data Registry. Gender differences in procedure-related adverse events in patients receiving implantable cardioverter-defibrillator therapy.Circulation. 2009 Mar 3;119[8]:1078-84. Epub 2009 Feb 16. Used with permission.)

CRT, the sex difference persisted across device types. In-hospital mortality was not different. The explanation proposed for the increased risk of mechanical complications in women was their smaller body habitus, thinner right ventricular wall, and smaller diameter vessels.

A sex difference was also found when data from the Ontario ICD Database were evaluated. The study evaluated 3,340 patients with new ICD implants; complications within 45 days and mortality were reported. Major complications occurred in 4.1% of patients. Patient characteristics that predicted increased risk of complication included female sex (hazard ratio [HR], 1.49), secondary prevention indication, dilated left ventricle (LV), and use of an antiarrhythmic drug other than amiodarone. The risk of a complication was also associated with the type of device implanted; CRT with defibrillator (CRT-D) implants carried the highest risk. Importantly, patients who experienced a complication had an increased mortality over the following 6 months.

The increased risk of periprocedural complications in women has been demonstrated in pacemaker implantation as well. Nowak and colleagues reviewed data from 17,826 patients (8,421 women) who underwent initial pacemaker implantation from 2003 through 2006 in Germany. Women, compared with men, had significantly more complications, specifically pneumothorax and pocket hematoma. While subclavian access has been associated with an increased risk of pneumothorax, the rate of subclavian access was similar between sexes, suggesting that smaller body habitus alone (lower body mass index) increases the risk of pneumothorax. In other studies, a lower body mass index has been associated with increased risk of pneumothorax.

Data were published in 2012 from the Danish Pacemaker Register on 28,860 patients (45% female) undergoing initial pacemaker implantation between 1997 and 2008. Overall, the pneumothorax rate was 0.66%. Women were almost twice as likely as men to have a pneumothorax (odds ratio, 1.9; 95% CI, 1.4–2.6). Other factors associated with increased risk of pneumothorax included age older than 80 years, history of chronic obstructive lung disease, implantation of a dual-chamber pacemaker, and subclavian vein puncture (odds ratio, 7.8; 95% CI, 4.9–12.5). These studies suggest that even though women are less likely to have cephalic access, cephalic or axillary venous access should be attempted before subclavian puncture because of its association with a higher complication rate of pneumothorax.

CARDIAC RESYNCHRONIZATION THERAPY

Heart failure (HF), a major cause of morbidity and mortality in the United States, has a prevalence of 5 million and claims nearly 300,000 lives annually. Despite advances in medical therapy that have significantly improved the management and outcome of this disease, HF still carries a high morbidity and mortality. One of the fundamental pathophysiologic findings in HF is dyssynchronous ventricular excitation and contraction mainly due to delayed electrical conduction to the LV lateral wall. CRT, a nonpharmacologic therapeutic approach, can resynchronize electrical and mechanical coupling by exciting the ventricular septum and lateral wall in a simultaneous, more efficient manner (Figure 10.4). The immediate hemodynamic benefit includes improvement in ventricular contractility and cardiac output and a reduction in mitral regurgitation and LV filling pressure.

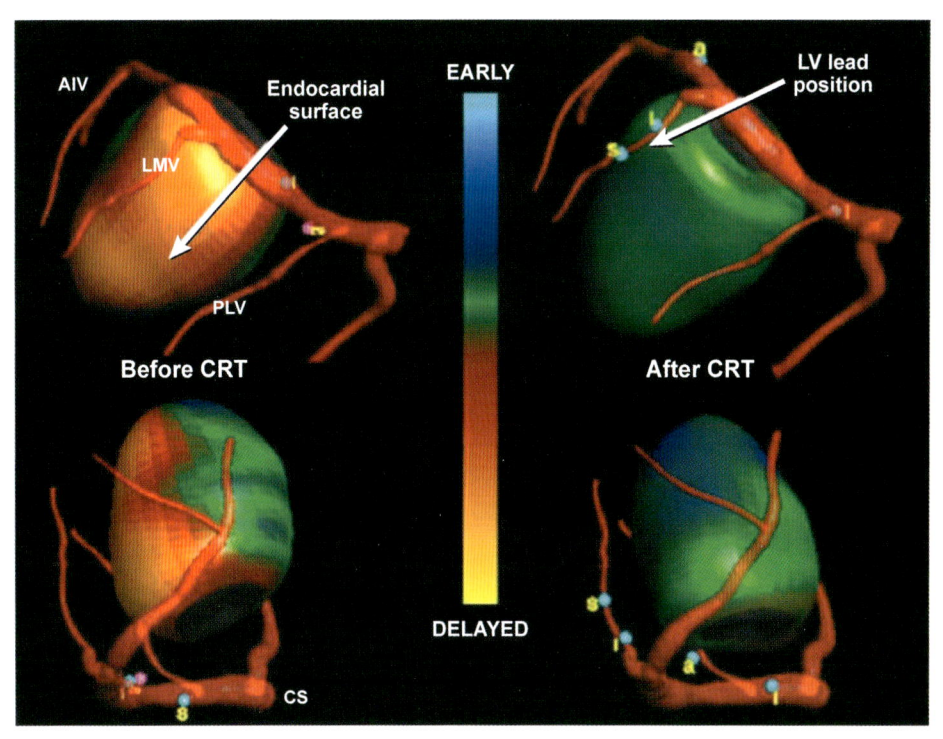

FIGURE 10.4. Integration of Functional (Mechanical Dyssynchrony) and Anatomical (Coronary Venous Anatomy) Information Before and After Cardiac Resynchronization Therapy (CRT) at End Systole. The red model shows branches of the coronary venous tree. The color difference indicates a mechanical contraction delay from red (septum) to green (lateral wall). AIV indicates anterior interventricular vein; CS, coronary sinus; LMV, lateral marginal vein; LV, left ventricular; PLV, posterolateral vein.

(Adapted from Tournoux FB, Manzke R, Chan RC, Solis J, Chen-Tournoux AA, Gerard O, et al. Integrating functional and anatomical information to facilitate cardiac resynchronization therapy. Pacing ClinElectrophysiol. 2007 Aug;30[8]:1021–2. Used with permission.)

Indication

Numerous randomized clinical trials and cohort studies have shown that CRT is an effective therapy for mild to severe HF in the majority of recipients. The indication for CRT initially included patients with advanced HF (New York Heart Association [NYHA] class III or IV), with evidence of severe LV systolic dysfunction (LV ejection fraction [LVEF] ≤35%), and with evidence of ventricular conduction delay (QRS duration ≥120 ms) despite having received optimal medical therapy as recommended in the American College of Cardiology (ACC)/American Heart Association (AHA)/Heart Rhythm Society (HRS) 2008 guidelines. The indication has been expanded to include patients in NYHA class I or II with mild or moderate HF symptoms as recommended in the 2012 ACC Foundation (ACCF)/AHA/HRS focused update of the 2008 guidelines for device-based therapy for cardiac rhythm abnormalities (Table 10.1). The hemodynamic benefit derived from CRT in patients with mild or moderate HF confers improvement in LV systolic function and reverse myocardial remodeling. Across

TABLE 10.1. Recommendations for Cardiac Resynchronization Therapy for Patients With Systolic Heart Failure

Patient Population	Class	Level of Evidence
NYHA class II, III, or ambulatory IV; LVEF ≤35%; QRS duration ≥150 ms; LBBB; sinus rhythm	I	A/B
NYHA class II, III, or ambulatory IV; LVEF ≤35%; QRS duration 120-149 ms; LBBB; sinus rhythm	IIa	B
NYHA class III or ambulatory IV; LVEF ≤35%; QRS duration ≥150 ms; non-LBBB; sinus rhythm	IIa	A
LVEF ≤35%; AVN ablation or medical rate control to allow 100% pacing in AF; anticipated device pacing >40%	IIa	B/C
NYHA class I; ischemic cardiomyopathy; LVEF ≤30%; QRS duration ≥150 ms; LBBB; sinus rhythm	IIb	C
NYHA class III or ambulatory IV; LVEF ≤35%; QRS duration 120-149 ms; non-LBBB; sinus rhythm	IIb	B
NYHA class II; LVEF ≤35%; QRS duration ≥150 ms; non-LBBB; sinus rhythm	IIb	B
NYHA class I or II; QRS duration ≤150 ms; non-LBBB	III	B
Comorbidities or frailty (or both) limit survival to <1 y	III	C

Abbreviations: AF, atrial fibrillation; AVN, atrioventricular nodal; LBBB, left bundle branch block; LVEF, left ventricular ejection fraction; NYHA, New York Heart Association.

Adapted from Tracy CM, Epstein AE, Darbar D, Dimarco JP, Dunbar SB, Estes NA 3rd, et al. 2012 ACCF/AHA/HRS focused update of the 2008 guidelines for device-based therapy of cardiac rhythm abnormalities: a report of the American College of Cardiology Foundation/American Heart Association Task Force on Practice Guidelines. J Am Coll Cardiol. 2012 Oct 2;60(14):1297–313. Epub 2012 Sep 10. Used with permission.

all NYHA classes, a greater benefit is seen in those with a QRS duration greater than 150 ms or the presence of left bundle branch block (LBBB). The new guideline has modified the CRT class indication on the basis of these electrocardiographic characteristics. The benefits translate into a decrease in hospitalization for HF and a decrease in mortality among patients who have severe HF, although for patients with mild to moderate HF, a survival benefit has not been shown in the follow-up to date.

Sex-Related Differences in HF

HF affects over 5 million Americans; of these, nearly 50% are women. The prevalence of HF increases with age for both sexes, but HF develops at an older age in more women than men. Women who have acute decompensated HF are almost twice as likely as their male counterparts to have HF with preserved LV function. Nonischemic cardiomyopathy is more common in women; an ischemic cause is more frequent in men. Compared with men, women who have HF are more likely to have hypertension. Community-based data have shown that from 1979 to 2000 the incidence of HF increased 8% in women and 5% in men; as a result, more women die every year of cardiovascular disease than of breast cancer. HF contributes 35% of the total cardiovascular disease mortality for women. Furthermore, women with HF have a lower quality of life than men, with more functional capacity impairment, and more hospital stays. However, HF in women has not achieved the same public awareness as in men.

CRT Implantation

The coronary venous tree serves as a host for LV lead placement, and the lateral veins are considered the optimal site for the LV lead. The anatomical features of the coronary vein are different between male and female patients. A study has shown that the presence of a lateral venous branch was equally distributed between men and women (95.7% vs 93.7%); however, inadequate size of a lateral branch for LV lead placement was more frequent in women (25.0% vs 10.9%, $P=.045$). In addition, the final mean (SD) LV lead pacing threshold was significantly higher in women compared with men (1.99 [1.17] V vs 1.51 [1.02] V, *P*=.02). Similarly, another study investigated coronary venous anatomy and showed that lateral veins were less prevalent in patients who had a history of lateral myocardial infarction than in patients who did not. Diameters were variable for the coronary sinus (7.3–18.9 mm) and its tributaries (1.3–10.5 mm). The coronary sinus was larger in men than in women, and it was larger in cases of ischemic cardiomyopathy than in cases of nonischemic cardiomyopathy (all *P*<.05). These findings suggest an anatomical challenge for LV lead placement in women. Yet, the success rate for LV lead placement is similar in both sexes.

Underrepresentation of Women in CRT Trials

Despite the fact that 50% of patients with HF are women, less than 30% of patients enrolled in ICD or CRT trials have been women. Figure 10.5 shows the proportion of men and women enrolled in each CRT clinical trial; Figure 10.6 shows

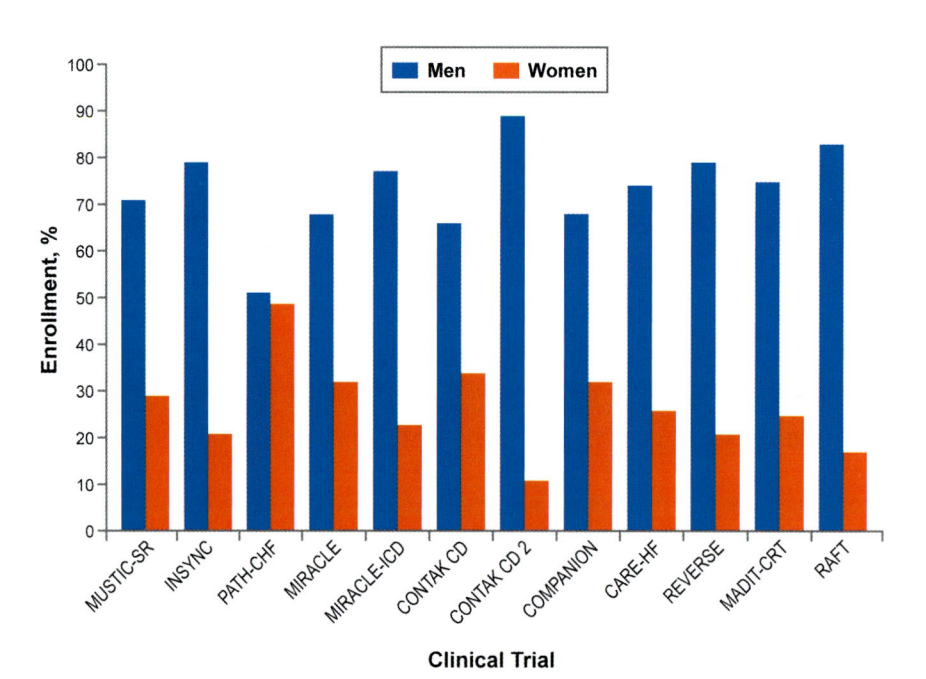

FIGURE 10.5. Proportion of Men and Women Enrolled in Cardiac Resynchronization Therapy Trials.

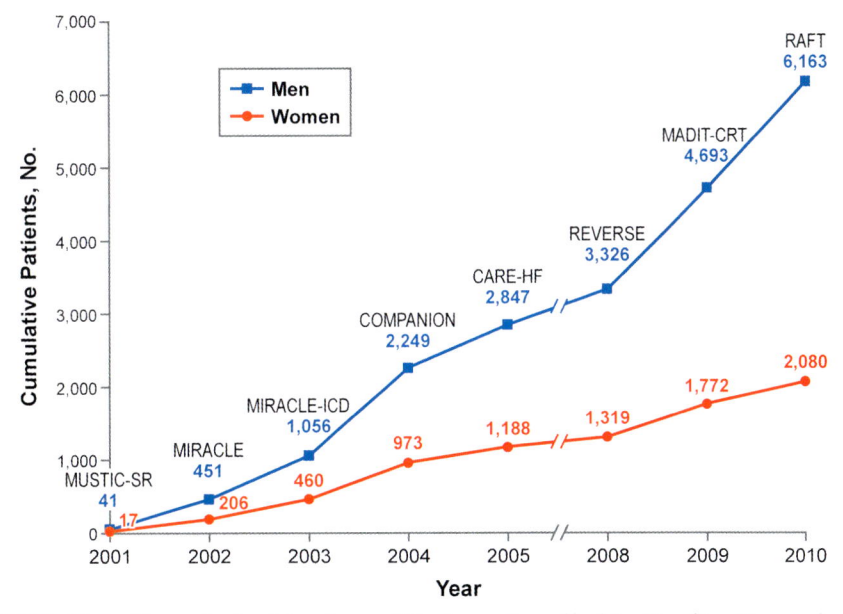

FIGURE 10.6. Cumulative Number of Patients Enrolled in Cardiac Resynchronization Therapy Trials by Sex.

the cumulative number of patients of each sex enrolled in CRT trials from 2001 through 2010.

Response of Women to CRT

Approximately 30% of patients do not respond clinically to CRT (so-called nonresponders). The nonresponse rate varies, depending in part on the criteria used for defining *nonresponder*, and multiple factors likely contribute to the failure of CRT. Before implantation, these factors are related to patient clinical characteristics, including sex, the nature of the cardiomyopathy, the width of the baseline QRS, the type of ventricular conduction delay, and the extent of the LV scar. After implantation, contributing factors (which may be modifiable) include LV lead position, percentage of biventricular pacing, and optimal atrioventricular and interventricular electrical coupling.

The characteristics of patients who are CRT responders and nonresponders are summarized in Table 10.2. Female patients are more likely to be

TABLE 10.2. Influence of Factors on Response to Cardiac Resynchronization Therapy

Factor	Response More Likely	Nonresponse More Likely
Clinical characteristics		
Cardiomyopathy	Nonischemic	Ischemic
Sex	Female	Male
QRS duration, ms	≥150	<150
QRS morphology	LBBB	RBBB, intraventricular conduction delay
Ventricular characteristics		
LV end-diastolic volume, mL	180-240	>240
Ventricular dyssynchrony	Present	Absent
Scar burden	Low, nontransmural	High, transmural
Right ventricular enlargement, dysfunction	Absent	Present
Device-modifiable factors		
Left ventricular lead position	Lateral, base, or mid	Anterior or inferior, apex
Biventricular pacing, %	99-100	<99
Atrioventricular and intraventricular optimization	Optimal	Not optimal

Abbreviations: LBBB, left bundle branch block; RBBB, right bundle branch block.

responders, but it is unclear as to whether this is due to their sex or to their associated characteristics, such as underlying cardiomyopathy and conduction abnormality.

The aggregate experience with CRT from 10 clinical trials involving more than 8,000 patients has provided undisputed proof that CRT is an effective therapy for patients with HF regardless of the severity of HF symptoms. The magnitude of the benefit is concordant, although the effects are heterogeneously distributed among different patient subtypes.

The MIRACLE trial, the first randomized controlled trial without crossover, showed the benefit of CRT. The 453 patients had an LVEF of 35% or less and a QRS duration of 130 ms or more. They were randomly assigned to the CRT group or to the control group. A significant symptomatic and functional (6-minute walk test) improvement in the CRT group was observed.

These improvements translated into a 40% reduction in death and HF hospitalization, a composite end point. In a subgroup analysis, women who received CRT, compared with women who did not, experienced statistically significant improvements in time to the first HF hospitalization and in mortality. However, a similar difference was not observed for men. The subsequent MIRACLE-ICD and CONTAK CD trials showed that women appeared to benefit to the same extent as men.

The COMPANION trial enrolled 1,520 patients who had either ischemic or nonischemic cardiomyopathy, NYHA class III or IV disease, LVEF of 35% or less, and a QRS duration of 120 ms or more. The patients were randomly assigned to 1 of 3 arms (optimal medical therapy alone, CRT with pacing alone [CRT-P], and CRT-D). Hospitalization for HF was significantly reduced in the CRT-P and CRT-D groups, but mortality was reduced in only the CRT-D group (likely because follow-up was relatively short). The efficacy of CRT-P and CRT-D was similar in men and women.

CARE-HF enrolled 813 patients who had an LVEF of 35% or less, NYHA class III or IV disease, and a QRS interval of 120 ms or more or a QRS interval of 120 to 150 ms in combination with echocardiographic evidence of dyssynchrony. The patients were randomly assigned to receive optimal medical therapy or CRT-P. In the CRT-P group, 39% of the patients reached the composite end point of hospitalization for HF or death from any cause as compared to 55% in the medical therapy group (HR, 0.63; 95% CI, 0.51–0.77; $P<.001$). The hazard ratios for the primary end points were similar for men and women, with patients of both sexes showing improved outcome with the CRT device.

The most recent MADIT-CRT trial expanded the CRT candidates to those with mild to moderate HF. The study enrolled 1,820 subjects who had NYHA class I (20%) or II (80%) symptoms, an LVEF of 30% or less, and a QRS duration of 130 ms or more (65% had a QRS duration ≥150 ms). Subjects were randomly assigned to receive either CRT-D or only an ICD. The CRT-D group had a substantially lower combined end point of death and HF hospitalization than the ICD group (17.2% vs 25.3%). Women had a significantly better result with CRT-D therapy than men for death or HF (HR, 0.31; $P<.001$), for HF only

(HR, 0.30; *P*<.001), and for death at any time (HR, 0.28; *P*=.02) (Figure 10.7). Furthermore, women had consistently greater improvements than men in reverse cardiac remodeling with CRT-D therapy (Figure 10.8).

Overall, multiple randomized trials have shown an unequivocal CRT benefit in women and men. Table 10.3 summarizes the clinical outcome and sex

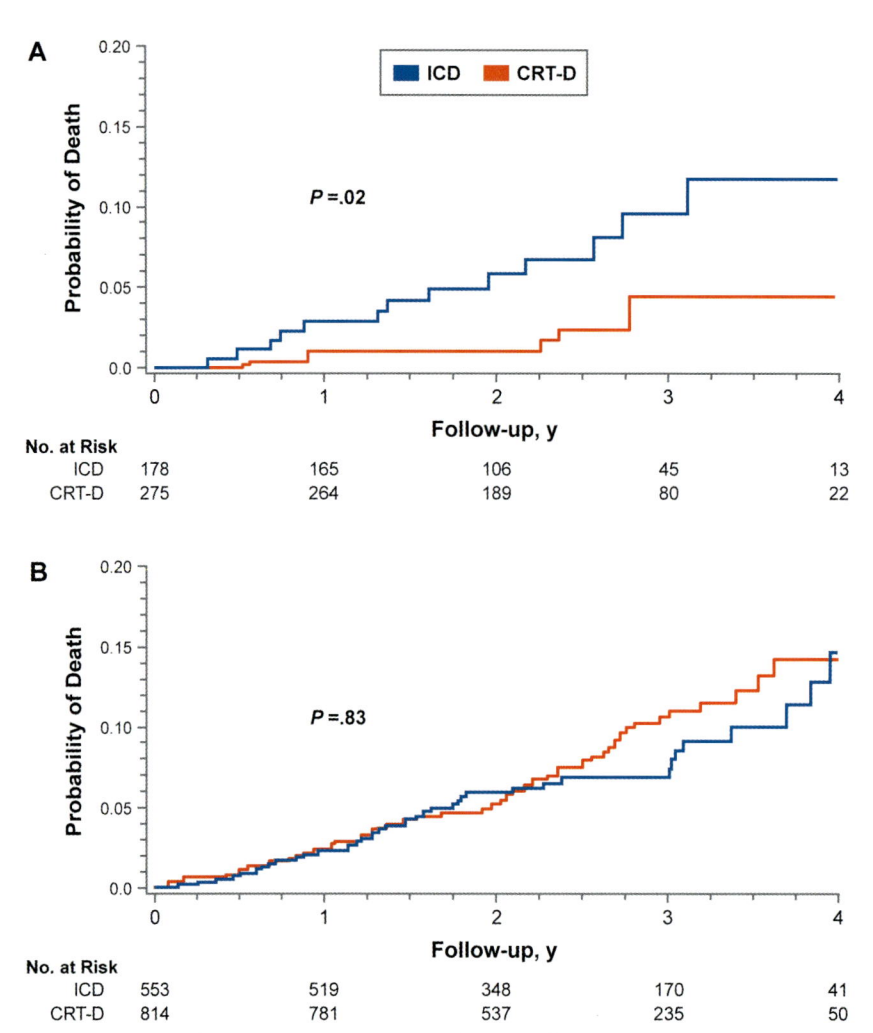

FIGURE 10.7. Kaplan-Meier Estimates of Cumulative Probability of Death in the MADIT-CRT Trial. A, For women, the probability of death was significantly less with cardiac resynchronization therapy with defibrillator (CRT-D) than with implanted cardioverter-defibrillator (ICD) therapy. B, For men, the probability of death was similar with CRT-D or ICD therapy. (Adapted from Arshad A, Moss AJ, Foster E, Padeletti L, Barsheshet A, Goldenberg I, et al; MADIT-CRT Executive Committee. Cardiac resynchronization therapy is more effective in women than in men: the MADIT-CRT [Multicenter Automatic Defibrillator Implantation Trial with Cardiac Resynchronization Therapy] trial. J Am CollCardiol. 2011 Feb 15;57[7]:813–20. Used with permission.)

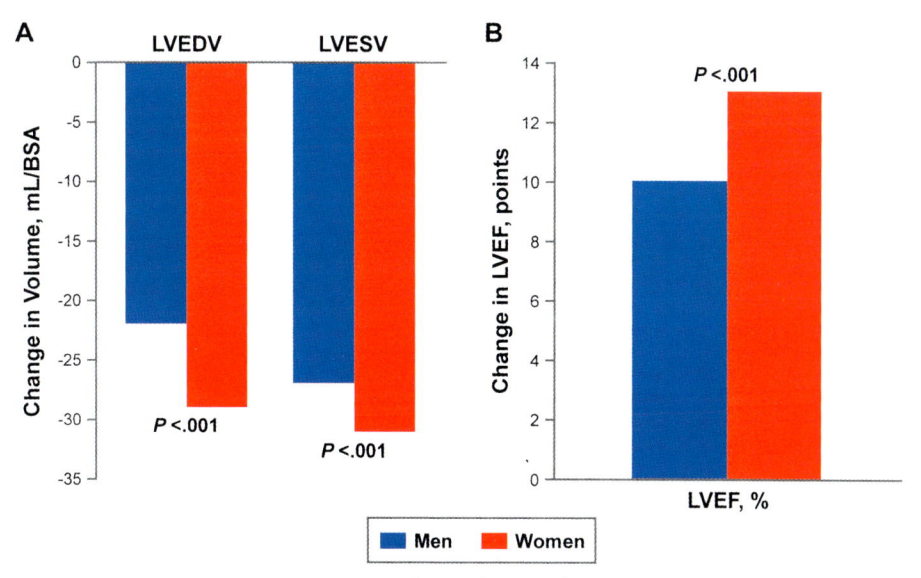

FIGURE 10.8. Improvement in Male and Female Patients in the MADIT-CRT Trial. A, Left ventricular end-diastolic volume (LVEDV) and left ventricular end-systolic volume (LVESV). B, Left ventricular ejection fraction (LVEF). BSA indicates body surface area.

comparison when the sex-related subanalysis is performed in randomized clinical trials. Women may benefit more from CRT with regard to mortality, HF events, or reverse LV remodeling, as shown in the MADIT-CRT and RAFT trials. Several retrospective cohort studies have compared CRT outcomes for men and women in real-life clinical practice (Table 10.4). The findings concur with the results from randomized trials.

The more favorable benefit with CRT for women may be associated with differences in baseline disease characteristics. A greater proportion of the female patients had a substrate of nonischemic cardiomyopathy and an LBBB pattern, factors that contribute to a favorable response to CRT, whereas a greater proportion of men had ischemic cardiomyopathy, a history of atrial fibrillation, and renal dysfunction, which are associated with a poor prognosis and a higher risk of death. A higher proportion of men had a right bundle branch block pattern, which is recognized as an unfavorable factor for CRT since, unlike an LBBB pattern, it is not associated with an electrical and mechanical delay in the LV lateral wall. These confounding differences between sexes, more than sex itself, may influence CRT outcome.

TABLE 10.3. Sex-Related Efficacy of Cardiac Resynchronization Therapy (CRT) in Randomized Trials

Trial (Publication Year)	Study Design	No. of Subjects; No. of Female Subjects (%)	Groups	NYHA Class	LVEF, Mean (SD), %	QRS Interval, Mean (SD), ms	Measures of HF Improvement	HF Admission CRT[a]	HF Admission Control[a]	RR (95% CI)	All-Cause Death CRT[a]	All-Cause Death Control[a]	RR (95% CI)	Sex-Related Differences in Efficacy
MIRACLE (2002)	Parallel, double-blind	453; 145 (32%)	CRT vs OMT	III or IV	22 (6)	166 (20)	6MWT NYHA QOL LVEF LVEDD	18/228	34/225	0.52 (0.3–0.9)	12/228	16/225	0.74 (0.36–1.53)	Benefit in HF hospitalization or death for women but not for men
MIRACLE-ICD (2003)	Parallel, double-blind	369; 86 (23%)	CRT-ICD vs ICD	III or IV	24 (6.2)	163 (22)	NYHA QOL	85/187	78/182	1.06 (0.84–1.33)	14/187	15/182	0.91 (0.45–1.83)	Not stratified by sex
CONTAK-CD (2003)	Parallel, open	490; 168 (34%)	CRT-ICD vs ICD	II-IV	21.5 (7)	158 (26)	Peak $\dot{V}o_2$ 6MWT NYHA QOL LVEF LV volume	32/245	39/245	0.82 (0.53–1.26)	11/245	16/245	0.69 (0.33–1.45)	Not stratified by sex
MIRACLE-ICD II (2004)	Parallel, double-blind	186; 20 (11%)	CRT-ICD vs ICD	I or II	24.5 (6.7)	165 (24)	NYHA LVEF LVEDV LVESV	…	…	…	2/85	2/101	1.19 (0.17–8.26)	Not stratified by sex
COMPANION (2004)	Parallel, open	1,520; 493 (32%)	CRT-ICD vs CRT vs OMT	III or IV	22	160	6MWT QOL NYHA	…	…	…	131/617	77/308	0.85 (0.66–1.09)	No significant difference

Study	Design	No.; No. (%) of Women	Intervention	NYHA Class	Age, Mean (SD), y	6MWT, m	Outcomes	Events, Treatment	Events, Control	RR (95% CI)	Sex-Specific Outcomes
CARE-HF (2005)	Parallel, open	813; 215 (26%)	CRT vs OMT	III or IV	25	160	NYHA QOL LVEF LVESV	72/409	133/404	0.64 (0.42–0.97)	Male: HR, 0.62 (95% CI, 0.49–0.79); Female: HR, 0.64 (95% CI, 0.42–0.97)
REVERSE (2008)	Parallel, double-blind	610; 131 (21%)	CRT vs OMT	I or II	27 (7)	153 (21)	LVEF LVEDV LVESV	17/419	15/191	0.51 (0.26–1.01)	9/419	3/191	1.37 (0.37–4.99)	Male: HR, 0.69 (95% CI, 0.43–1.11); Female: HR, 0.75 (95% CI, 0.26–2.19)
MADIT-CRT (2009)	Parallel, blinded	1,820; 453 (25%)	CRT-ICD vs ICD	I or II	24 (5)	65%≥150	LVEF LVEDV LVESV	136/1,089	140/731	0.65 (0.53–0.81)	74/1,089	53/731	0.94 (0.67–1.32)	Male: HR, 0.72 (95% CI, 0.57–0.92); Female: HR, 0.31 (95% CI, 0.19–0.50) P<.01
RAFT (2010)	Parallel, double-blind	1,798; 308 (17%)	CRT-ICD vs ICD	II or III	23 (5)	158 (24)	…	174/894	236/904	0.75 (0.63–0.89)	186/894	236/904	0.80 (0.67–0.94)	Somewhat better efficacy for mortality or hospitalization for women than for men

Abbreviations: HF, heart failure; HR, hazard ratio; ICD, implantable cardioverter-defibrillator; LV, left ventricular; LVEDD, left ventricular end-diastolic dimension; LVEDV, left ventricular end-diastolic volume; LVEF, left ventricular ejection fraction; LVESV, left ventricular end-systolic volume; 6MWT, 6-minute walk test; NYHA, New York Heart Association; OMT, optimal medical therapy; QOL, quality of life; RR, relative risk; $\dot{V}o_2$, oxygen consumption per unit time.

[a] Numerator is number of affected patients; denominator is number of patients in treatment group.

TABLE 10.4. Sex-Related Cardiac Resynchronization Therapy Outcomes in Observational Studies

Source	Design	No. of Subjects; No. of Female Subjects (%)	NYHA Class	LVEF, Mean (SD)	QRS Interval, Mean (SD), ms	Variable	Women vs Men[a]	Sex-Related Differences in Efficacy
Xu YZ et al. J Cardiovasc Electrophysiol. 2012;23:172–8	Retrospective study	728; 166 (23%)	III or IV	24 (7)	164 (31)	NYHA	−0.79 (0.78) vs −0.56 (0.85), P=.009	HR, 0.73 (95% CI, 0.48–1.09; P=.13)
Zabarovskaja S et al. Europace. 2012;14:1148–55	Retrospective study	619; 119 (19%)	II-IV	24 (9)	155 (32)	No sex difference	...	HR, 0.439 (95% CI, 0.214–0.903; P=.02)
Cheng A et al. Heart Rhythm. 2012;9:736–41	Retrospective study	846; 277 (33%)	II-IV	24 (7)	153 (21)	Change in LVESVi, mL/m²	13.4 vs 8.5, P=.002	...
Leyva F et al. Pacing Clin Electrophysiol. 2011;34:82–8	Prospective observational study	550; 122 (22%)	III or IV	24 (10)	155 (29)	LVESV LVEF	P=.04 P<.001	HR, 0.52 (95% CI, 0.34–0.79; P=.002)
Mooyaart EA et al. Am J Cardiol. 2011;108:63–8	Registry	578; 147 (25%)	III or IV	23 (7)	166 (25)	LVEDV, mL LVESV, mL	178 (73) vs 212 (78), P<.001 126 (63) vs 151 (67), P<.001	HR, 0.627 (95% CI, 0.405–0.969; P=.036)
Lilli A et al. Pacing Clin Electrophysiol. 2007;30:1349–55	Observational registry	195; 46 (26%)	III or IV	28 (7)	153 (22)	LVEDVi, mL/m² LVESVi, mL/m² LVEF, %	83.61 (36.48) vs 101.12 (33.95), P=.002 51.79 (32.38) vs 68.94 (31.33), P=.001 40.85 (12.35) vs 34.08 (10.15), P<.001	HR, 0.87 (95% CI, 0.48–1.58; P=.66)

| Zardkoohi O et al. Pacing Clin Electrophysiol. 2007;30:1344-8 | Longitudinal observational study | 117; 26 (22%) | III or IV | 20 (13) | 169 (47) | No sex difference | ... | P=.46 |
| Bleeker GB et al. Pacing Clin Electrophysiol. 2005;28:1271-5 | Retrospective study | 173; 36 (21%) | III or IV | 21 (9) | 173 (27) | No sex difference | ... | No sex difference |

Abbreviations: HF, heart failure; HR, hazard ratio; LVEDV, left ventricular end-diastolic volume; LVEDVi, left ventricular end-diastolic volume indexed to body surface area; LVEF, left ventricular ejection fraction; LVESV, left ventricular end-systolic volume; LVESVi, left ventricular end-systolic volume indexed to body surface area.

[a] *Nonparenthetical values that are not P values are means. Parenthetical values are standard deviations.*

SUMMARY

Cardiac implantable electronic device therapy has emerged as an important alternative in treating symptomatic bradycardia, tachyarrhythmia, and HF. However, for female patients, the recognition of a rhythm abnormality and initiation of appropriate therapy are often delayed. Procedure-related complication rates tend to be higher for female patients. Hence, precautions to avoid adverse effects associated with invasive procedures should be emphasized to the female population. Promoting awareness of the presence and consequence of bradyarrhythmia or tachyarrhythmia and of advancements in device technology and personalized medicine may yield significant improvements over current routine practice.

SUGGESTED READING

Bleeker GB, Schalij MJ, Boersma E, Steendijk P, van der Wall EE, Bax JJ. Does a gender difference in response to cardiac resynchronization therapy exist? Pacing Clin Electrophysiol. 2005 Dec;28(12):1271–5.

Brunner M, Olschewski M, Geibel A, Bode C, Zehender M. Long-term survival after pacemaker implantation: prognostic importance of gender and baseline patient characteristics. Eur Heart J. 2004 Jan;25(1):88–95.

Cha YM, Oh J, Miyazaki C, Hayes DL, Rea RF, Shen WK, et al. Cardiac resynchronization therapy upregulates cardiac autonomic control. J Cardiovasc Electrophysiol. 2008 Oct;19(10):1045–52. Epub 2008 May 9.

Cheng A, Gold MR, Waggoner AD, Meyer TE, Seth M, Rapkin J, et al. Potential mechanisms underlying the effect of gender on response to cardiac resynchronization therapy: insights from the SMART-AV multicenter trial. Heart Rhythm. 2012 May;9(5):736–41. Epub 2010 Sep 23.

Chung ES, Leon AR, Tavazzi L, Sun JP, Nihoyannopoulos P, Merlino J, et al. Results of the Predictors of Response to CRT (PROSPECT) trial. Circulation. 2008 May 20;117(20):2608–16. Epub 2008 May 5.

Giudici MC, Carlson JI, Krupa RK, Meierbachtol CJ, Vanwhy KJ. Submammary pacemakers and ICDs in women: long-term follow-up and patient satisfaction. Pacing Clin Electrophysiol. 2010 Nov;33(11):1373–5. Epub 2010 Aug 17.

Kirkfeldt RE, Johansen JB, Nohr EA, Moller M, Arnsbo P, Nielsen JC. Pneumothorax in cardiac pacing: a population-based cohort study of 28,860 Danish patients. Europace. 2012 Aug;14(8):1132–8. Epub 2012 Mar 19.

Knight BP, Curlett K, Oral H, Pelosi F, Morady F, Strickberger SA. Clinical predictors of successful cephalic vein access for implantation of endocardial leads. J Interv Card Electrophysiol. 2002 Oct;7(2):177–80.

Lee DS, Krahn AD, Healey JS, Birnie D, Crystal E, Dorian P, et al; Investigators of the Ontario ICD Database. Evaluation of early complications related to De Novo cardioverter defibrillator implantation insights from the Ontario ICD database. J Am Coll Cardiol. 2010 Feb 23;55(8):774–82.

Leyva F, Foley PW, Chalil S, Irwin N, Smith RE. Female gender is associated with a better outcome after cardiac resynchronization therapy. Pacing Clin Electrophysiol. 2011 Jan;34(1):82–8.

Lilli A, Ricciardi G, Porciani MC, Perini AP, Pieragnoli P, Musilli N, et al. Cardiac resynchronization therapy: gender related differences in left ventricular reverse remodeling. Pacing Clin Electrophysiol. 2007 Nov;30(11):1349–55.

Mooyaart EA, Marsan NA, van Bommel RJ, Thijssen J, Borleffs CJ, Delgado V, et al. Comparison of long-term survival of men versus women with heart failure treated with cardiac resynchronization therapy. Am J Cardiol. 2011 Jul 1;108(1):63–8. Epub 2011 Apr 27.

Nowak B, Misselwitz B; Expert committee 'Pacemaker,' Institute of Quality Assurance Hessen, Erdogan A, Funck R, Irnich W, Israel CW, Olbrich HG, Schmidt H, et al. Do gender differences exist in pacemaker implantation? Results of an obligatory external quality control program. Europace. 2010 Feb;12(2):210–5. Epub 2009 Oct 28.

Peterson PN, Daugherty SL, Wang Y, Vidaillet HJ, Heidenreich PA, Curtis JP, et al; National Cardiovascular Data Registry. Gender differences in procedure-related adverse events in patients receiving implantable cardioverter-defibrillator therapy. Circulation. 2009 Mar 3;119(8):1078–84. Epub 2009 Feb 16.

Roeters van Lennep JE, Zwinderman AH, Roeters van Lennep HW, van Hemel NM, Schalij MJ, van der Wall EE. No gender differences in pacemaker selection in patients undergoing their first implantation. Pacing Clin Electrophysiol. 2000 Aug;23(8):1232–8.

Tracy CM, Epstein AE, Darbar D, Dimarco JP, Dunbar SB, Estes NA 3rd, et al. 2012 ACCF/AHA/HRS focused update of the 2008 guidelines for device-based therapy of cardiac rhythm abnormalities: a report of the American College of Cardiology Foundation/American Heart Association Task Force on Practice Guidelines. J Am Coll Cardiol. 2012 Oct 2;60(14):1297–313. Epub 2012 Sep 10.

Udo EO, van Hemel NM, Zuithoff NP, Kelder JC, Crommentuijn HA, Koopman-Verhagen AM, et al. Long-term outcome of cardiac pacing in octogenarians and nonagenarians. Europace. 2012 Apr;14(4):502–8. Epub 2011 Oct 23.

Veerareddy S, Arora N, Caldito G, Reddy PC. Gender differences in selection of pacemakers: a single-center study. Gend Med. 2007 Dec;4(4):367–73.

Xu YZ, Friedman PA, Webster T, Brooke K, Hodge DO, Wiste HJ, et al. Cardiac resynchronization therapy: do women benefit more than men? J Cardiovasc Electrophysiol. 2012 Feb;23(2):172–8. Epub 2011 Sep 13.

Zardkoohi O, Nandigam V, Murray L, Heist EK, Mela T, Orencole M, et al. The impact of age and gender on cardiac resynchronization therapy outcome. Pacing Clin Electrophysiol. 2007 Nov;30(11):1344–8.

CHAPTER ELEVEN

Syncope and POTS: Are Women Really Faint of Heart?

CELINA M. YONG, MD, MSC, MBA, AND KAREN J. FRIDAY, MD

INTRODUCTION

Syncope is a symptom, not a diagnosis. It is characterized by a sudden loss of consciousness with quick recovery on supine positioning. Transient loss of cerebral perfusion is the common pathway for several mechanisms that cause syncope. Cardiac causes of syncope are associated with a markedly increased mortality and can be divided into arrhythmias or mechanical causes. Both tachycardia and bradycardia, including ion channel disorders, can produce syncope and are addressed in Chapter 5 ("Supraventricular Arrhythmias") and Chapter 6 ("Atrial Fibrillation in Women"). The differential diagnosis of syncope in women, particularly younger women, includes pulmonary processes such as pulmonary embolus and pulmonary hypertension. Syncope may be the presenting symptom of pulmonary hypertension in up to 25% of patients. Although pulmonary emboli are an infrequent cause of syncope, women using oral contraceptives have a 10-fold higher risk of fatal pulmonary emboli than women who do not use these medications. How contraceptive use influences the incidence of nonfatal, symptomatic pulmonary emboli has not been studied.

Excluding potentially life-threatening conditions is always the first priority in evaluating patients with syncope, since the mortality of cardiac-related syncope can be as high as 30% to 40% per year. However, this chapter focuses on more common causes of syncope: neurally mediated syncope (NMS), also known as vasovagal syncope or neurocardiogenic syncope, and orthostatic hypotension (OH). In various series, these conditions account for 35% to 60% of emergency department visits for syncope. These conditions have in common a component of orthostatic intolerance—the onset or worsening of symptoms with standing coupled with the autonomic responses to these hemodynamic changes. A third entity, postural orthostatic tachycardia syndrome (POTS), is also grouped in the category of orthostatic intolerance, although syncope is not typically a common complaint.

Each of these entities has distinct characteristics, but they share the common background physiology of orthostatic intolerance. Orthostatic intolerance may reflect a decreased central volume, altered volume distribution due to venous pooling, altered sympathetic outflow to maintain vascular tone, or altered vascular sensitivity to increased sympathetic tone. In symptomatic patients, several of these factors often combine to produce symptoms. Women experience these conditions more often than men (Table 11.1).

Tilt table testing (TTT) was developed to evaluate patients with frank syncope, but it has also become a tool for distinguishing the different types of orthostatic intolerance. With TTT, heart rate and blood pressure are continuously measured when the fasting patient is tilted to 60° to 80°, and that posture is maintained for 20 to 40 minutes or until symptoms develop. In NMS, an initial decrease in blood pressure is followed shortly by a slowing in heart rate and, typically, syncope if the posture is maintained. Patients may have predominantly a decrease in blood pressure (*vasodepressor response*), or they may have a greater decrease in heart rate, frequently progressing to the development of high-grade heart block or asystole (*cardioinhibitory response*), or they may have both a decrease in heart rate and a decrease in blood pressure (*mixed response*) (Figure 11.1). With OH, the blood pressure gradually decreases with little change in heart rate, and syncope may result if the position is maintained. For patients with POTS, the heart rate increases abruptly within the first 10 minutes, typically to rates greater than 120 beats per minute, with minimal decreases in blood pressure. Syncope rarely

TABLE 11.1. Comparison of Clinical Syncope Between Men and Women

Variable	Men (n=497)	Women (n=554)	P Value
Age at HUT, y			.22
Mean (SD)	35.6 (16.9)	36.3 (16.0)	
Median (IQR)	31 (21–50)	34 (23–49)	
Age at first syncopal episode, y			.78
Mean (SD)	28.1 (16.5)	27.5 (15.9)	
Median (IQR)	21 (16–38)	22 (15–38)	
Time between first and last syncopal episodes, y			.002
Mean (SD)	6.8 (9.2)	8.2 (9.5)	
Median (IQR)	3 (1–10)	4 (1–12)	
Total No. of syncopal episodes before HUT			.001
Mean (SD)	5.0 (6.4)	7.2 (9.4)	
Median (IQR)	3 (2–5)	3 (2–6)	
Micturition syncope, %	20.0	5.2	<.001
Defecation syncope, %	9.3	16.3	<.001

Abbreviations: HUT, head-up tilt table testing; IQR, interquartile range.

Adapted from Park J, Jang SY, Yim HR, On YK, Huh J, Shin DH, et al. Gender difference in patients with recurrent neurally mediated syncope. Yonsei Med J. 2010 Jul;51(4):499–503. Open Access article.

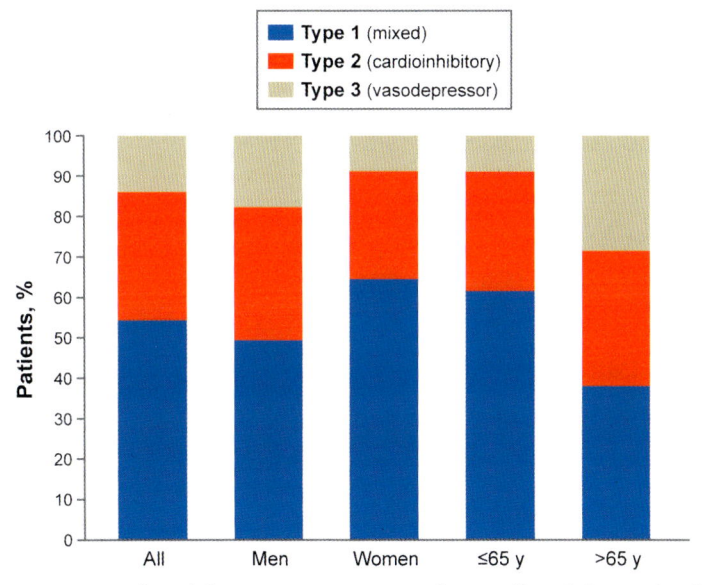

FIGURE 11.1. Type of Positive Response to Head-Up Tilt Table Testing by Age and Sex. (Adapted from McGavigan AD, Hood S. The influence of sex and age on response to head-up tilt-table testing in patients with recurrent syncope. Age Ageing. 2001 Jul;30[4]:295-8. Used with permission.)

occurs, but the tachycardia is sustained until the patient is placed in the supine position. With all these entities, after the patient is placed supine, the blood pressure and heart rate return to normal; if the patient has had syncope, consciousness is restored.

For patients who have experienced syncope, TTT can be an imperfect test, with limited specificity, sensitivity, and reproducibility. For some patients who have never had a clinical event, however, TTT can provoke syncope. Regardless, TTT may be useful for characterizing orthostatic intolerance if it is not found with routine vital signs and for helping patients identify prodromal symptoms before loss of consciousness.

NEURALLY MEDIATED SYNCOPE

Data from the Framingham study showed that the survival rate for people who had had at least 1 episode of NMS was identical to that for people who had never had a syncopal attack. However, the lack of mortality risk does not diminish the morbidity that can be associated with NMS. An estimated 30% to 40% of the population will have at least 1 syncopal episode in their lifetime, with many of these events unreported because people may not seek medical attention. A small minority of patients have recurrent syncope, which can impair their quality of life.

Most likely, NMS is not a single entity. Triggers include orthostatic changes, emotional stress, and physical maneuvers, including cough and defecation. As with any autonomic-related condition, a clinical event with NMS probably involves a combination of trigger and substrate.

In most series, NMS is more common in women than in men; typically, 50% to 60% of syncopal patients are women and 40% to 50% are men. Although popularized images show syncope occurring almost exclusively in women, this finding is not consistent with existing data.

The mechanism of NMS remains uncertain. Initially, the mechanism was thought to be simply increased vagal tone. However, as the entity has been studied more extensively, it seems unlikely that vagal tone could overcome sympathetic tone to the extent that it would predominate. Rather, the current leading hypothesis is that syncope is due primarily to decreased sympathetic tone rather than to increased parasympathetic tone. Why blood pressure decreases initially is also not clearly defined; studies suggest that sympathetic tone is maintained during the initial decrease in blood pressure, with abrupt withdrawal resulting in bradycardia and syncope.

When results of sympathetic nerve studies during TTT were compared between healthy asymptomatic adult men and women (mean ages, 30 and 26 years, respectively), the sympathetic outflow during TTT was reduced in women compared with men despite women having lower mean arterial pressures and narrower pulse pressures. Why asymptomatic women would have less sympathetic activation or baroreceptor responsiveness during TTT is unclear.

In studies that used lower body negative pressure to simulate orthostatic changes in healthy men and women who did not have a history of syncope, women had a lower tolerance than men to central hypovolemia: Lesser levels of lower body negative pressure were needed to produce symptoms of syncope. This difference was enhanced among patients who had a reduced blood volume. Reduced stroke volume was the key difference between the groups, with no differences in peripheral vasoconstriction or plasma norepinephrine levels, which suggested that orthostatic intolerance in women is related to decreases in cardiac filling rather than to a reduced responsiveness to vascular resistance. Venous pooling can be a factor in altered blood distribution, and the reduction in stroke volume seen in women when lower body negative pressure is applied may be due to a greater propensity for venodilation, resulting in venous pooling.

Hormonal fluctuations may also affect orthostatic intolerance. Increased progesterone levels in the luteal phase of the menstrual cycle may directly increase levels of aldosterone during high sodium intake. This may cause an antimineralocorticoid effect, resulting in a lower total blood volume.

Genetic predisposition to NMS has been identified by several groups. Frank syncope may have occurred in up to 25% of family members of patients treated for syncope, although the family members may never have received medical attention for the episodes. While NMS is more prevalent in women, the prevalence for men with fathers who fainted is 4-fold higher than for men without any parents who fainted. For women, the risk of syncope is greatest if both parents fainted. One debated issue with the studies of familial patterns of fainting is distinguishing how much fainting is biologically determined and how much is a pattern of coping skills learned in the family situation. Data suggesting a biologic basis for familial patterns of fainting were presented in a study of first-degree relatives of patients with NMS who underwent TTT. A positive TTT response, with a decrease in blood pressure or heart rate (or both), was seen in 100% of the relatives, independently of whether they had experienced syncope previously. A meta-analysis of reports suggesting genetic patterns for syncope concluded that there was not strong evidence for a genetic link, although the data were confounded by the high prevalence of NMS.

Psychologic testing of patients with recurrent syncope suggests that they have higher levels of anxiety and depression. Older studies also mentioned that a vasovagal response to the sight of blood or the fear of injury may trigger syncope in some people. If NMS is limiting a person's lifestyle, it is unclear whether the psychologic distress reflects the cause of the syncope or a response to life limitations. There seems to be no difference between men and women in the level of distress and psychologic impairment associated with syncope or with the response to blood or fear of injury.

Some studies suggest that for people who have rare episodes of NMS or obvious triggers (eg, having blood drawn), conservative measures such as avoiding triggers, increasing salt and fluid intake, and receiving education about syncope frequently result in no further syncopal episodes. One debate concerns whether the frequency of syncopal events predicts recurrences, but there appears to be no sex difference in the rates of recurrence or in the total number of syncopal episodes. For women who provide a history of symptoms that worsen around the time of their menses, a trial of oral contraceptives to reduce the hormonal variability may be helpful.

ORTHOSTATIC HYPOTENSION

Orthostatic hypotension is defined as a decrease in systolic blood pressure of more than 20 mm Hg or a decrease in diastolic blood pressure of more than 10 mm Hg upon standing at least 3 minutes. While OH tends to occur more commonly in the elderly, it is not uncommon in younger people, particularly with prolonged standing. In a study of Dutch military recruits, including men 18 to 25 years old, the incidence of orthostatic intolerance and fainting was 10%.

Among astronauts returning from extended space flights, 20% have OH or orthostatic symptoms of light-headedness, dizziness, or presyncope. One cause is the loss of plasma volume on space flights. In a study of male and female astronauts, women lost almost 3 times as much plasma volume in orbit as men did. Although all astronauts received fluid loading with 15 mL/kg of saline after their spacecraft returned, marked orthostatic intolerance and presyncope developed in all 5 of the women studied, whereas only 25% of the men were symptomatic. Changes in norepinephrine levels upon standing were markedly less in women than in men, even including men who were symptomatic. Orthostatic increases in epinephrine levels were present both in women and in symptomatic men. Compared with men who were asymptomatic, symptomatic men had markedly reduced orthostatic increases in norepinephrine and greater orthostatic increases in epinephrine levels. These differences were not present at baseline and resolved within 3 days after the astronauts returned to Earth.

OH is most commonly associated with older age groups, and the prevalence increases with advancing age. In the CHS, OH was present in 18% of all subjects who were older than 65 and living in the community, with no difference between men and women. Of the younger age group (65–69 years), 15% had orthostatic findings compared with 26% of the subjects older than 85. In the BWHHS, the prevalence of OH was 28% among women aged 60 to 80 years. Higher prevalence was noted among older women and those with hypertension. The number of antihypertensive medications used was associated with OH, but only β-blockers were independently associated with OH. The presence of multiple comorbidities was also associated with OH, although the association was with the total number of comorbidities rather than with any specific condition.

Parkinson disease is commonly associated with OH. Studies suggest that the incidence of Parkinson disease is lower among women than men and that if the disease does develop, it does so at a later age in women. The effects of estrogen on dopamine receptors have been postulated as a protective factor in promoting this sex difference since Parkinson disease is more common in nulliparous women than in those who have had children.

POSTURAL ORTHOSTATIC TACHYCARDIA SYNDROME

POTS is a heterogeneous condition characterized by an increase in heart rate when standing. The complexity of this disorder is reflected by the fact that in the mid 2000s, the National Institutes of Health (NIH) provided a "definition" of POTS, but now the NIH website provides a "description": POTS is described as being part of a family of conditions characterized by symptoms that worsen with standing and most often occur in women, frequently after pregnancy or a viral illness. The earlier diagnostic criteria included a standing norepinephrine level of more than 600 ng/mL, but this criterion is no longer included in the current description. An increase in the standing heart rate of more than 30 beats per minute or a standing heart rate of 130 beats per minute are generally accepted as criteria for the diagnosis of POTS. The complexity of the pathophysiology of POTS, and hence the challenges in managing patients, is reflected in the 20 clinical trials listed on the NIH website that address POTS pathophysiology and treatment protocols.

Fast heart rates, which can be over 200 beats per minute with minimal activity, are what often bring patients to the attention of cardiologists for evaluations. Although patients may clearly report that they are most symptomatic when standing, it is surprising how few physicians actually check orthostatic vital signs to identify the characteristic changes in heart rate. Fast heart rates should lead to a referral to a cardiologist for management, but POTS is a much more complex condition than the typical tachycardias.

Inevitably, any condition that manifests with tachycardia in young people, especially women, may be given an immediate and incorrect diagnosis of anxiety or panic attacks. Before the advent of electrophysiology testing, diazepam was the drug most often given to women with atrioventricular reciprocating tachycardia or atrioventricular nodal reentrant tachycardia, since those tachycardias were thought to be due to anxiety as well. Even patients whose heart rate markedly increases immediately after standing have received a diagnosis of anxiety attacks.

POTS is a condition primarily of women, although occasionally men may present with the same symptom complex. There are many reasons for heart rates to increase upon standing, leading to a spectrum of conditions that could be considered POTS. Some women have always had low blood pressure and some component of orthostatic intolerance. Others have never had any orthostatic issues, but they feel that they have never fully recovered after a viral illness and continue to have persistent symptoms of fatigue, dizziness, and orthostatic tachycardia.

POTS is also much more than a fast heart rate. Syncope is uncommon, but many patients do report presyncope or dizziness when standing. Other orthostatic symptoms include weakness, palpitations, chest pain, tremulousness, or dyspnea. However, several symptoms that occur in patients who meet the heart rate criteria for POTS are not particularly orthostatic. These symptoms include migraine headaches, nausea, abdominal pain, fatigue, myofascial pain, bloating, nausea, and constipation or diarrhea. This variety of symptoms suggests the presence of a more diverse autonomic dysfunction rather than a mechanism simply related to decreased blood pressure or increased heart rate.

There is an overlap between Ehlers-Danlos syndrome (EDS) hypermobility type and orthostatic intolerance, with orthostatic intolerance proposed as a minor criterion for EDS. In some series, a high proportion of patients presenting with POTS also have joint hypermobility. Women have greater hyperflexibility than do men, which could be a contributing factor to the prevalence of POTS in women. Increased muscular tension, which compensates for the joint laxity, may be a component of the myofascial pains reported by these patients. The greater joint mobility of the rib cage may also explain some of the nocturnal dyspnea or dyspnea on exertion since there may be a positional component to the thoracic mechanics.

Studies of women with POTS have shown decreases in blood volume, plasma volume, and stroke volume, with higher systemic vascular resistance compared with controls. Although blood and plasma volumes are lower in patients with POTS than in controls, aldosterone levels are also decreased and do not increase as greatly when standing. This finding suggests an altered neurohumoral response to position. A recent study also showed that patients with POTS have a smaller cardiac mass.

Management of orthostatic POTS symptoms is similar to management of other orthostatic intolerance conditions. Unique to POTS is the use of pyridostigmine as a neurotransmitter, which may be helpful in some patients, particularly those who have a more pronounced autonomic component to their symptoms.

In patients with a marked increase in standing norepinephrine levels, α-blockers, such as clonidine or possibly carvedilol, may be helpful in blunting the excess heart rate due to catecholamines. Although it may be tempting to use β-blockers in patients with an easily elicited tachycardia, β-blockers often make patients more symptomatic if a component of the heart rate response would otherwise help maintain blood pressure. Trials with β-blockers should start at the lowest possible dose, which is then titrated carefully. Anecdotal experience with verapamil and diltiazem has shown benefit for some patients. Ivabradine, a drug available in Canada but not in the United States, can slow the fast heart rate without decreasing the blood pressure.

Exercise is a well-studied therapeutic modality for POTS patients. It is beneficial in reducing or eliminating the POTS symptoms in many patients and in reversing some of the volume changes of POTS. However, this regimen does involve a slowly progressive build up to 20 to 30 minutes of aerobic exercise for up to 5 days weekly, which many patients cannot sustain.

ORTHOSTATIC INTOLERANCE: MECHANISMS AND THERAPEUTIC OPTIONS

All the above orthostatic intolerance conditions (NMS, OH, and POTS) occur more frequently in women. While these conditions have different manifestations, orthostatic intolerance seems to be a common thread. The tendency for women to have greater orthostatic intolerance is multifactorial.

Venous Pooling

Studies of healthy asymptomatic women have shown that women have less tolerance for lower body negative pressure than do men, a factor exacerbated by hypovolemia. Reasons for this are debated but may reflect a higher venous capacitance. Venous pooling is common in women with orthostatic intolerance and may be evident by acrocyanosis (purple hands or feet) on standing. Pooling of blood in the gut may be a significant factor in postprandial hypotension and may also be a factor for patients who report an increase in symptoms after meals, particularly large meals with a high carbohydrate load.

Management
- Determining triggers of venous pooling, such as being in a hot tub, standing for long periods, or eating large meals, may be the first step in avoiding situations in which the risk of orthostatic intolerance is highest.
- Eating frequent, small meals and avoiding eating large amounts of carbohydrates may reduce postprandial symptoms.
- Use of an abdominal binder (or body shaper in younger, more fashion-conscious patients) may reduce venous pooling in the abdomen. Compression stockings may also be useful, but studies suggest that two-thirds of venous pooling occurs in the splanchnic bed and pelvis.
- Exercise may help to maintain venous return and is recommended for all patients, although patients may need to begin with supine exercise. Pilates may also be useful in maintaining abdominal muscle tone, and many exercises can be done when supine.
- Tensing leg muscles has been shown to prolong standing time in patients with orthostatic intolerance.
- Midodrine probably most affects the venous system; patients with venous pooling already have a high systemic vascular resistance. Midodrine has an onset of action of 20 to 30 minutes, and the effect lasts 3 to 4 hours. It can be dosed on a regular basis or used as needed when patients are exposed to triggers of orthostatic intolerance, such as being in hot weather or needing to stand for long periods. Orthostatic hypertension can still occur with midodrine, particularly in elderly patients with orthostatic hypotension, but it is probably less likely to occur in younger people.

Reduced Blood Volume

Although reduced blood volume has been evaluated only in patients with POTS, measures to increase blood volume, such as increasing salt and water intake, are a mainstay of therapy for orthostatic intolerance. One factor may be the lower aldosterone levels in POTS patients, but there are no data suggesting why renal responses are not sufficient to maintain adequate fluid balance in otherwise healthy individuals, even in the face of relative hypotension.

Management
- Increase oral intake of sodium to 4 to 6 g daily and fluid intake to 4 to 6 L daily. Drinking 0.5 L of water over a short period has been shown to increase orthostatic blood pressures and reduce time to symptoms.
- Intravenous infusion of saline may also help patients maintain appropriate blood pressure, particularly if they are more dehydrated or less able to take in sufficient oral fluids.
- Fludrocortisone is often recommended and can be useful in expanding blood volume by increasing sodium retention, even if no specific endocrine abnormalities are identified. Potassium levels need to be monitored carefully during treatment.
- Desmopressin has shown some benefit, although many are reluctant to use this therapy in the absence of abnormal test results. It is also probably best used by practitioners with endocrinology training.
- Erythropoietin can be used to expand the red cell volume when appropriate.

Autonomic Function

Under controlled laboratory conditions, asymptomatic women, compared with men, tend to have a higher resting vagal tone and less robust sympathetic activation to the baroreceptor response when subjected to orthostatic stress. Venous (capacitance) vessels also tend to have higher responsiveness to sympathetic activation than the arterial (resistance) vessels.

Management
- Caffeine, nicotine patches, or decongestants can increase peripheral resistance and attenuate symptoms in some patients. The diuretic effects of caffeine need to be balanced with any positive effects on sympathetic activation.
- Higher vagal tone has been targeted in those susceptible to NMS. Pacemakers are an obvious choice to increase heart rate in patients with NMS, but previously the benefits were questionable. In the ISSUE-3 study, implanted loop recorders were used to record the heart rhythm during syncopal episodes. Pacemakers were useful in reducing recurrences only in patients who had syncopal episodes associated with marked bradycardia. OH is characterized by an inadequate heart rate response, which is difficult to control by current pacemaker technology but has been under evaluation.

Hormones

With fluctuating levels of estrogen and progesterone, women are uniquely subject to the hemodynamic effects of these changes. Progesterone enhances aldosterone elimination and can increase sodium excretion. Estrogen may affect vascular tone, particularly facilitating vasodilation.

Management
- Oral contraceptives may be useful in blunting hormonal swings, particularly if women report increased symptoms in the perimenstrual interval.

Hypermobility

Women's joints generally are more flexible than men's. Some of the difference may be related to the effects of estrogen, which can increase joint laxity. There is certainly overlap between hyperflexibility and the more extensive joint laxity associated with EDS hypermobility type. As noted, orthostatic intolerance is a proposed minor criterion for EDS hypermobility type, and many patients with POTS do have joint hypermobility. Patients with joint hypermobility have musculoskeletal pains related to muscle contraction in response to joint laxity, and they have headaches associated with craniocervical instability.

Management
- To date, there is no genetic test for EDS hypermobility type. However, a geneticist for adults may be able to provide patients with information and counseling about the disorder, including issues with pregnancy.
- Physical therapy with a therapist trained in evaluating patients with EDS may help with joint stability and musculoskeletal pains. The physical therapist may be able to optimize an exercise program, which may be one of the most useful management tools for orthostatic intolerance.

SUMMARY

Many physiologic components may predispose women to acute or chronic orthostatic intolerance. Key factors in management are recognizing how limiting orthostatic intolerance can be for the patient and recognizing the patient's frustration when the physiologic basis for these limitations is not appreciated by physicians, family, and peers.

SUGGESTED READING

Cheng YC, Vyas A, Hymen E, Perlmuter LC. Gender differences in orthostatic hypotension. Am J Med Sci. 2011 Sep;342(3):221-5.

Fu Q, Vangundy TB, Galbreath MM, Shibata S, Jain M, Hastings JL, et al. Cardiac origins of the postural orthostatic tachycardia syndrome. J Am Coll Cardiol. 2010 Jun 22;55(25):2858-68.

National Dysautonomia Research Foundation. [Website on the Internet]. [cited 2013 May 1]. Available from: http://www.ndrf.org/.

Strickberger SA, Benson DW, Biaggioni I, Callans DJ, Cohen MI, Ellenbogen KA, et al; American Heart Association Councils on Clinical Cardiology, Cardiovascular Nursing, Cardiovascular Disease in the Young, and Stroke; Quality of Care and Outcomes Research Interdisciplinary Working Group; American College of Cardiology Foundation; Heart Rhythm Society; American Autonomic Society. AHA/ACCF Scientific Statement on the evaluation of syncope: from the American Heart Association Councils on Clinical Cardiology, Cardiovascular Nursing, Cardiovascular Disease in the Young, and Stroke, and the Quality of Care and Outcomes Research Interdisciplinary Working Group; and the American College of Cardiology Foundation: in collaboration with the Heart Rhythm Society: endorsed by the American Autonomic Society. Circulation. 2006 Jan 17;113(2):316-27. Erratum in: Circulation. 2006 Apr 11;113(14):e697.

Task Force for the Diagnosis and Management of Syncope; European Society of Cardiology (ESC); European Heart Rhythm Association (EHRA); Heart Failure Association (HFA); Heart Rhythm Society (HRS), Moya A, Sutton R, Ammirati F, Blanc JJ, Brignole M, Dahm JB, et al. Guidelines for the diagnosis and management of syncope (version 2009). Eur Heart J. 2009 Nov;30(21):2631-71. Epub 2009 Aug 27.

CHAPTER TWELVE

The Road to a Successful Women's Heart Clinic

DARCY H. THEISEN, MSN, CNP, AND BOBBI L. HOPPE, MD

We don't sit around and talk about the plight of being a woman. We just get on with it and do things.

Meredith Whitney, founder and chief executive officer of Meredith Whitney Advisory Group LLC

The above quotation reflects our exact sentiment, especially related to building a women's heart clinic. It was not difficult to convince a group of female cardiologists and providers that a women's heart clinic would fill a niche like no other. Despite a growing body of scientific evidence highlighting the sex-associated differences in cardiac pathophysiology and a growing body of major randomized clinical trials, very few clinics are specifically dedicated to the care of women who have cardiovascular issues, including rhythm disorders.

Substantial scientific progress has been made. The myth that heart disease is a man's disease has been debunked, public awareness of cardiovascular disease as the leading cause of death among US women has nearly doubled since 1997, and the age-adjusted death rate resulting from coronary artery disease in women is one-third of what it was in 1980. Despite significant gains, no one can deny the grim reality that heart disease is still the leading cause of death among women in every major developed country and in most emerging countries.

What has prevented the increased awareness and the growing body of scientific literature from being translated into the advancement of women's cardiovascular health? Is it possible that a glass ceiling has been a limiting factor? Traditionally, the term *glass ceiling*, which refers to women's lack of advancement into leadership positions, has been applied to academic medicine but not to advancement of women's health. Carnes and colleagues argued that a historical link exists between advances in women's cardiovascular health and women's leadership in academic medicine. Furthermore, perhaps the slow progress of women into academic leadership has stalled the advancement of women's cardiovascular health. As long as women in leadership roles and issues associated with caring for women in general are marginalized and devalued, women's cardiovascular health will continue to be limited by this glass ceiling and not reach the lofty goal envisioned in the early 2000s by providers and patients.

The importance of developing clinics devoted to the advancement of women's cardiovascular health cannot be understated. Through the development of dedicated clinics, the advancement of women's cardiovascular health can continue. In this chapter, we share our experience and business plan that culminated in a successful women's heart clinic in the metropolitan area of Minneapolis-St Paul, Minnesota.

INITIAL PLANNING PHASE

As more physicians became interested in women's cardiovascular issues during the early 2000s, educational programs emerged to provide the blueprint for implementing women's cardiovascular programs. Although we found these programs incredibly resourceful, we also sought advice from business and design consultants, we visited regional screening programs, and we attended conferences focusing on women's health issues.

Business Plan

Objective

Our goal was to build a unique comprehensive program that offered screening, diagnostic testing, preventive services, and treatment options specifically tailored to women. To create the first freestanding women's heart clinic in the Minneapolis-St Paul market area, our private practice group entered into a joint partnership with our local hospital system. We believed that each system had attributes and resources that complemented each other and would ultimately result in a successful business venture.

Market and Environmental Assessment

SERVICE AREA

We identified and analyzed our service area and determined the number of women in targeted age brackets in that area. Household income in the service area was also considered, reflecting our understanding that patients would have some responsibility for out-of-pocket expenses. We also analyzed our current private practice model, tallying the number of female consultations and the number of patients undergoing stress tests and interventional procedures.

DIRECTED FOCUS GROUPS

We worked with a marketing consultant and developed the Focus Group Project to identify what women in the community thought about a stand-alone women's heart clinic. The purpose of the research was to understand reactions to our proposed service from women, aged 40 to 55, who had never used our institution's cardiology services. Specifically, the purpose of this project was to survey women about the following:

1. Expectations of a new clinic, including design and key elements of service
2. Reactions to a heart screening package and its price
3. Thoughts on patient education materials, communication, and marketing

We wanted to gain insight into women's overall reaction to the clinic concept. Participants were excited about the idea of a women's heart clinic that would be created by female cardiologists and would feature a screening specifically for women. The clinic was identified as a unique and important new service. We also found that even though women knew that heart disease was a top health concern, they lacked an understanding of the symptoms of heart disease in women. Interestingly, only half of the participants mentioned heart disease as a high priority. Participants recognized that there are sex differences related to health care delivery. Comments included the following:

- "The impression that women have is that it's more a man-related disease."
- "Heart disease is the number one killer over breast cancer, but there's very little research done—very little care for your heart."
- "You go in with symptoms, but they don't pay much attention to women like they do to men."

We asked whether women would be willing to get a heart screening if their doctor recommended it. Many agreed that they would, thus reinforcing the importance of a strong alliance between female cardiology providers and referring primary care physicians.

We then asked women about the clinic atmosphere—specifically, what they would want the clinic to look like. Overwhelmingly, participants wanted the clinic to feel more like a spa than a traditional clinic and provide a stress-free environment. They described "a quiet peaceful environment, a place to escape for a moment," where they could spend time by themselves. They preferred gowns and robes made of cloth, not paper, that provided excellent coverage. Participants wanted to have clean, comfortable waiting spaces with current reading materials that were interesting to women. Surprisingly, no one wanted a television in the waiting room; the women wanted a fireplace or a water feature.

In addition to asking participants about the physical characteristics of the clinic, we asked them about desirable attributes of health care providers. The participants said that it was important to have female providers, and many said that female providers were more compassionate and understanding. Some participants said that those who worked in the clinic needed to understand the unique aspects of women's health. One said, "I would like to have them trained [to understand] that women are not men. They have different bodies, different needs, different ways of being—different everything." Most important was the stipulation that the providers be highly skilled, knowledgeable, competent, and highly respected among their peers. The women said that they expected the entire clinic staff to be personable and treat each other respectfully and with kindness.

We also wanted to gain further insight into the components of a women's heart disease screening package, so we presented the concept of the MyHeart Book Screening to the focus groups. We developed this comprehensive screening and assessment tool for women to help determine and manage heart disease risk. The focus groups gave input on including certain elements in the screening, identifying a price, and creating a reproducible positive patient experience. We determined that the screening would include a 1-hour comprehensive clinical screening and a face-to-face interview with a cardiology nurse practitioner. For the MyHeart Book Screening, patients would be charged a nominal fee (a break-even price that would cover the costs of materials and professional time). Patients would receive the following:

1. Personalized MyHeart Book (a hardcover book with detailed heart health information and a printed name label on the cover)
2. Fasting lipid profile values
3. Fasting blood glucose value
4. Blood pressure measurement
5. Body mass index determination
6. Body fat analysis (with body fat caliper)
7. Ankle-brachial index determination
8. Waist circumference measurement
9. Pedometer walking program information (including a pedometer)
10. Personal wellness prescription (written instructions with exercise, nutrition, and weight management recommendations recorded in the MyHeart Book)
11. Calculated 10-year heart disease risk score based on test results
12. Letter to the patient's primary provider with screening results, the 10-year risk score, and any lifestyle change recommendations.

Since potential competitors in the Midwest could develop a women's heart clinic and personalized wellness screenings, we obtained a service mark for MyHeart Book Screening to protect our product. (A service mark is similar to a trademark but for a service instead of goods.) MyHeart Book was available only as part of the MyHeart Book Screening and could not be purchased separately.

Overall reactions to the proposed screening were positive, with the most appealing aspect being the individualized patient plans. Women agreed that the screening should take enough time to adequately document their full medical history, but they "didn't want it to take hours." They wanted the screener to highlight and clearly explain the differences between the heart screening and a regular yearly examination. The participants said that we needed to be transparent about the price and to offer the screening at an affordable price.

Discussions about price brought various reactions from the focus groups about health insurance in general. Their responses illustrated the large variance among insurance plans and what is actually covered under individual plans. Many participants had difficulty understanding why insurance would not pay for the heart screening. Interestingly, this discussion also identified potential concerns about the screening. Some focus group participants said that the screening would not be unique:

- "I think it sounds a lot like what happens at a routine physical. It doesn't sound that much different from what I've had done before."
- "Why would you need something like this? If you know the right questions, most doctors will answer your questions."

We addressed the participants' concerns by identifying the differences between the MyHeart Book Screening and a routine physical examination at a physician's office. We did this by highlighting the following screening components that are not usually provided during a routine physical examination:

1. Body mass index determination
2. Ankle-brachial index determination
3. Body fat analysis

4. Waist circumference measurement
5. Calculated 10-year heart disease risk score
6. Pedometer walking program information (including a pedometer)
7. A 1-hour face-to-face interview with a cardiology nurse practitioner to create a personal wellness prescription
8. Personalized follow-up telephone calls 6 weeks and 12 weeks after the screening

We asked the focus group participants to discuss the importance of take-home materials and the types of materials that interested them. Participants said that generic pamphlets and brochures were minimally useful. They said that they preferred individualized, specific plans and programs and were particularly interested in personalized exercise and nutrition programs, recipes, written goals, resource lists, and other educational tools. When we asked participants about the importance of website access, they said that a website would be valuable only if it filtered information and was not too overwhelming. They expressed interest in an online program for tracking their progress and chatting with other patients. Some participants said that they were looking for ways to make themselves accountable so that they would be more disciplined in following the exercise and nutrition recommendations. Conversely, others said that several medical websites already existed and they did not see the value of a specific website. Some women simply lacked computer knowledge and a genuine interest in any computer-related activity.

Not only did we find this focus group information extremely valuable, but we used this information to design our women's heart clinic and the MyHeart Book Screening.

Competitive Data

When we developed our business plan, no freestanding women's heart clinic existed in the local market. Although several competitors expressed interest in creating women's heart clinics, most groups were limited by an important rate-limiting step: the number and type of female cardiology providers.

We studied national data to understand referral trends and to determine which types of services should be offered. The majority of women were self-referred, with a small percentage of patients referred by their obstetrician-gynecologist. Of the programs we reviewed, most offered screening with limited diagnostic testing (mostly managed by nurse practitioners); a small percentage (10%-20%) of the patients required further diagnostic tests.

SWOT Analysis

As part of the business plan we analyzed the strengths, weaknesses, opportunities, and threats (SWOT analysis) related to opening the women's heart clinic (Box 12.1).

BOX 12.1.

ANALYSIS OF STRENGTHS, WEAKNESSES, OPPORTUNITIES, AND THREATS (SWOT ANALYSIS) DURING THE PLANNING STAGES OF A WOMEN'S HEART CLINIC

Strengths
- Female cardiology leadership
- Reputation of local hospital system
- Experienced all-female support staff
- All aspects of cardiology (noninvasive, electrophysiology, and interventional)
- Strong industry relationships

Weaknesses
- Moderate financial resources
- Limited market presence
- Buy-in from larger private practice group
- Variability in patient-physician interactions
- Unknown anticipated perception within community

Opportunities
- Capture the first-to-niche market
- Create a women-focused model clinic
- Promote women's health with education
- Strengthen the relationship with the local hospital

Threats
- Local competition
- Shifting business from current clinic to new clinic
- Concept is prone to being copied
- Ability to sustain success long-term

BUSINESS OBJECTIVES

Our goal was to develop a new cardiology clinic in our targeted service area while minimizing the risk of shifting patients from our existing practice to our new clinic. The focus groups confirmed our suspicion that women directed the health care decisions for their families, and we thought that those women might encourage more men to become patients in the larger current practice.

We set target numbers for screenings, consultations, echocardiograms, and stress testing for the first year and specific targeted growth levels for each subsequent year. Tracking and measuring patient satisfaction and adhering to American Heart Association (AHA) guidelines were also included in the original business objectives.

MARKETING STRATEGIES

The marketing strategies were developed to address the anticipated needs of 2 age groups. For younger patients (35–49 years), we tailored education about risk factor modification and emphasized screening. For the older group (50 years or older), we focused more on secondary prevention and disease management.

After we analyzed our focus group data, we created a unique name for our clinic, determined the days of service per week, and defined the services that would be offered as follows:

1. Preventive screening with a set fee (development of MyHeart Book Screening)
2. Consultative and diagnostic services (echocardiograms, nuclear stress testing, vascular imaging, and device follow-up)
3. Value-added offerings to provide a unique patient experience (retail products, books, stress management programs, and support groups)

Several factors helped determine the location of the clinic. Important ones included easy access to other primary providers, proximity to ancillary services (radiography, phlebotomy, and laboratory services), and parking availability.

We also developed tactics for promoting the women's heart clinic through various media (radio, newspaper, direct mail, and magazine ads). We also planned physician and nurse practitioner speaking engagements, we developed the website, we explored strategic alliances with key organizations, and we defined activities that would strengthen our relationships with referring physicians.

OPERATIONS STRATEGIES

We developed a timeline for configuring the clinic and implementing the services (Figure 12.1).

Clinic Location and Design

We estimated the approximate amount of physical space necessary for our clinic, determined staffing requirements, and determined the quantity and type of technical equipment required for the clinic. We budgeted for appropriate clinic furniture and furnishings to fit the décor. A 2,000-square-foot leasable office space in our target area was chosen for the location of the clinic. This space was in a large clinic building that was co-owned by our local hospital and a competing large hospital system.

Taking into account the information gathered through the focus groups, we hired a professional interior designer to lead the design layout, including furniture selection and wall decorations. All textiles, patterns, and artwork were chosen to create a soothing environment. The entrance opened into a small waiting area with modern comfortable furniture, soft lighting, and relaxing background music. A trickling water feature was added and framed by a small boutique retail section

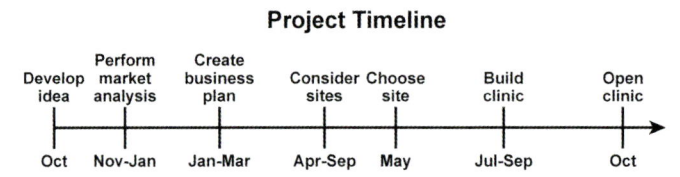

Project Timeline

Develop idea — Oct
Perform market analysis — Nov-Jan
Create business plan — Jan-Mar
Consider sites — Apr-Sep
Choose site — May
Build clinic — Jul-Sep
Open clinic — Oct

FIGURE 12.1. Timeline for Development and Implementation of a Women's Heart Clinic.

that sold educational books, recipe books for healthy eating, fitness videos, and relaxation aids.

The patient rooms were small but tasteful. To create a nonintimidating atmosphere, we purposely did not display providers' diplomas and certificates, heart models, and other medical equipment. Cloth gowns were stocked in each room. Special training for the nursing staff emphasized patient privacy. The stress test waiting area was a smaller version of the main waiting area and included a juice and coffee bar and healthy snacks. Men and children were invited to wait in the main waiting room; the stress test waiting room was exclusively for women.

Clinic Flow

Great effort was made to provide a smooth, courteous, and caring patient experience. The patient's first contact was with a well-trained, veteran staff member for appointment scheduling. Staffing consistency was valued, and the same compassionate scheduler greeted the patient at each contact. Priority was given to providing the patient with a well-designed, streamlined flow from check-in to examination to scheduling of follow-up visits.

MyHeart Book Screening Experience

From the focus group information, we designed screenings that included a face-to-face interview, specific screening components to assess heart disease risk (a computer-based risk assessment to generate a patient's 10-year heart disease risk score), a personalized copy of MyHeart Book, patient resource handouts, and a gift bag filled with heart health–related items, including a pedometer, dark chocolate, and refrigerator magnets listing heart attack warning signs and symptoms.

When a woman called to schedule a MyHeart Book Screening, she was instructed to arrive after fasting for the 12 hours before her visit. During a 75-minute face-to-face interview, a thorough personal and family history was taken and the patient was questioned about recent cardiac symptoms. Each patient then received her own copy of MyHeart Book, which included chapters on heart disease, associated risk factors, and cardiac testing. It also contained areas to document heart health goals, recommendations, test results, and the patient's 10-year heart disease risk score. In addition, it contained pages where the patient could write journal entries about her diet and weight loss, record her blood pressure readings, and review her personalized exercise prescription and pedometer walking program.

The following specific screening tests were performed during the visit:

1. Fasting lipid profile
2. Blood pressure measurement
3. Waist circumference measurement
4. Body mass index determination
5. Body fat analysis (with body fat caliper)
6. Ankle-brachial index determination

As part of the MyHeart Book Screening follow-up, all participants were contacted by telephone at 6 and 12 weeks to confirm that they were successful in implementing the personalized recommendations. Although under Medicare guidelines, the payment for MyHeart Book Screening was considered fee-for-service, some individual insurance plans covered this service through wellness program allocations.

Opening of the Clinic

To ensure a successful and timely opening of the women's heart clinic, the team worked diligently under the guidance of our business consultant and followed a Gantt chart timeline, which specified dates for completing key tasks.

While staff and managers worked to provide a smooth physical transition into our new space, the female cardiology providers shifted efforts toward mass marketing that included print ads, billboards, radio spots, direct mailers, television commercials, community events, and an open house.

Community partnerships were key to the successful opening of the clinic and helped to attract new patients on the first day. We partnered with a local fitness club to offer a community heart health screening, spoke at various women's clubs and senior citizen centers, and, most importantly, provided "lunch and learn" events for key referring providers in our service area.

We tracked marketing efforts and found that our biggest gain came from local newspaper ads, direct mailers to targeted zip codes, community talks, and physician referrals within our service area. Ads in local magazines and referrals from our website were less fruitful. We were surprised to learn that our program received national attention when several patients reported that they saw an article about the clinic in an inflight copy of *USA Today*.

Staff training before the clinic opened ensured that we could replicate the high-quality screening package on a daily basis. Subsequent patient feedback suggested that the most positive screening experiences were performed by nurse practitioners instead of other registered nurses or exercise physiologists.

OUTCOMES

Review of First-Year Results

MyHeart Book Screening visits, which occurred with a nurse practitioner, were tracked separately from cardiology consultations, which occurred with a cardiologist. The screening visit with the nurse practitioner was a 1-hour fee-for-service visit as described above, whereas the cardiology consultation included recommendations for lifestyle changes and for appropriate noninvasive or invasive testing according to a clinical assessment.

For each service, we identified volume goals for the first year. The goals were based on the idea that each service would generate a certain amount of income, and target volumes were identified from marketing strategies and a break-even point for the first-year financial objective. Over the next 5 years, we planned to expand all services except the MyHeart Book Screening. We heavily marketed the MyHeart Book Screening during the first year and identified it as our loss leader to attract new patients. Over the next few years, we purposely marketed consultations and other services more heavily and decreased the marketing emphasis on screenings. We knew that this marketing shift would follow the natural course of consumer interest, with women initially showing high interest in a preventive screening program and then identifying our clinic as their medical home for heart care. The goals were to generate growth at our women's heart clinic and to increase consultations at our larger cardiology clinic, which in turn would increase admission rates to our local hospital.

TABLE 12.1. Patient Volumes for Women's Heart Clinic Services

| | Year | | |
Service	1[a]	2[b]	3[b]
MyHeart Book Screenings	8	−80	−110
Cardiology consultations	240	188	189
Nuclear stress tests	185	59	37
Stress echocardiograms	47	20	−5
Resting echocardiograms	76	92	58

[a] *Values are percentages in relation to the first-year targets.*

[b] *Values are percentage changes in relation to the second-year targets.*

Our first-year volume estimates were conservative and were set at a financial break-even point. The actual total services volume was 80% higher than projected. Thus, the first year ended on a positive note from both financial and business strategy perspectives (Table 12.1).

Since we were in a committed partnership with our local hospital, we developed a basic database to track all patients seen in the women's heart clinic. We tracked the type of service that they received and their residence by zip code. Surprisingly, female admission rates with cardiac diagnoses to our local hospital increased by 25% during this time.

Review of Results for the Second and Third Years

In the second and third years, positive growth was strong for all services except MyHeart Book Screenings, for which we had expected a modest decrease in volume. Many primary physicians and obstetrician-gynecologists referred women for consultations and preferred that we order appropriate testing if indicated. Because of the decreasing number of primary care providers, many referrals from obstetrician-gynecologists were for management of hypertension, palpitations, and lipid levels. A very small percentage of providers referred patients for imaging only.

Patient Experiences

Although our results showed that our clinic volume was growing and we were meeting our short- and long-term objectives, we solicited patient comments to ensure that the experience was meeting patients' expectations. Those comments included the following:

- "Having an unpredictable and difficult-to-control arrhythmia is very stressful, and the women's heart clinic provided a nurturing and healing environment not present in the usual generic clinic."
- "The presence of books and products geared toward women's health, diet, and stress reduction conveyed an awareness that women have unique health concerns, often different from men."
- "When I had my heart problems, I felt extra comfortable and confident having a group of women cardiologists to turn to. When that circle includes caring, competent women doctors, it puts me at ease, raises my trust level, and speeds up my healing."

Providers' Perspectives

The initial marketing campaign for the new women's heart clinic was so successful that on the first day alone we received over 200 telephone calls from patients interested in MyHeart Book Screening. Patient surveys confirmed that we had indeed created the unique clinic environment that we intended. In addition, the clinic was staffed exclusively by female cardiology providers (noninvasive cardiologists, coronary interventionalists, and electrophysiology interventionalists) with no exceptions. Despite intermittent pressure from our male colleagues, male providers were never scheduled to work in the women's heart clinic. Equally important was the dedication of the ancillary staff. All providers had a strong interest in women's cardiovascular issues and promoted educational activities targeted toward colleagues, referring physicians, and the general public.

Numerous educational marketing events increased visibility and self-referrals; they also identified patients who shared a common interest in their own cardiovascular health. During the initial years, we emphasized marketing activities to increase awareness of MyHeart Book Screenings. As our reputation grew, more providers referred patients for initial consultations and more patients came as word-of-mouth referrals, so that we relied less heavily on referrals from MyHeart Book Screenings. We had more time to cultivate the clinic by adding additional services (a cardiac device clinic, nutrition services, MyHeart Book Screening rechecks, and a women's support group) and exploring research options. As stated above, we implemented a simple database in conjunction with the hospital to track marketing information, although in retrospect, a separate, more comprehensive clinical database would have been more valuable, especially from a research standpoint.

CONCLUSIONS

Building a successful women's heart clinic is dependent on a solid business plan created by business and marketing consultants with guidance from physicians and patients. Strategic planning with realistic short- and long-term goals is important, but flexibility is equally important to allow for implementing changes as necessary.

The emergence of women's heart clinics since the early 2000s is not a coincidence and reflects the endorsement of the AHA and patient demand. In 2007, the AHA expanded its focus on female-specific clinical recommendations and sponsored the preparation of the "Evidence-Based Guidelines for Cardiovascular Disease Prevention in Women: 2007 Update," which was updated in 2011. Through support from large national organizations and the development and continued success of women's heart clinics, an emphasis on women's cardiovascular health will be ensured. Many advances in women's health have been championed by female leaders, and the advancement of women's cardiovascular health will likely be no different.

One could argue that women's heart clinics are simply a marketing gimmick. To a small extent that may be true, but it is certainly a good gimmick. By increasing cultural awareness of women's cardiovascular health and creating a comfortable, nonthreatening environment where women can seek cardiovascular care, women's heart clinics have a positive effect on women's cardiovascular care.

Although substantial progress has been made in advancing women's cardiovascular care, in part by creating women's heart clinics, considerable challenges remain. Despite the absence of a visible barrier, the presence of a glass ceiling may limit progress. All who are concerned about women's cardiovascular care need to work collaboratively, sharing and learning from their experiences, to ensure continued success.

SUGGESTED READING

Carnes M, Morrissey C, Geller SE. Women's health and women's leadership in academic medicine: hitting the same glass ceiling? J Womens Health (Larchmt). 2008 Nov;17(9):1453–62.

Ford ES, Ajani UA, Croft JB, Critchley JA, Labarthe DR, Kottke TE, et al. Explaining the decrease in US deaths from coronary disease, 1980–2000. N Engl J Med. 2007 Jun 7;356(23):2388–98.

Gholizadeh L, Davidson P. More similarities than differences: an international comparison of CVD mortality and risk factors in women. Health Care Women Int. 2008 Jan;29(1):3–22.

Mosca L, Mochari-Greenberger H, Dolor RJ, Newby LK, Robb KJ. Twelve-year follow-up of American women's awareness of cardiovascular disease risk and barriers to heart health. Circ Cardiovasc Qual Outcomes. 2010 Mar;3(2):120–7. Epub 2010 Feb 10.

Weisman CS. Women's health care: activist traditions and institutional change. Baltimore (MD): Johns Hopkins University Press; 1998.

Xu JQ, Kochanek KD, Murphy SL, Tejada-Vera B. Deaths: final data for 2007. National vital statistics reports; vol 58 no 19. Hyattsville (MD): National Center for Health Statistics; c2010.

CHAPTER THIRTEEN

Taking a Look Around the World

UMA N. SRIVATSA, MBBS, MAS, AND AMPARO C. VILLABLANCA, MD

INTRODUCTION

The leading cause of death among men and women in the United States and globally is cardiovascular disease (CVD). According to World Health Organization estimates, 16.7 million people worldwide die of CVD each year, accounting for one-third of global deaths. Low- and middle-income countries bear disproportionate burdens, with 85% of the global CVD deaths occurring in those countries. Approximately 8.6 million women die of CVD annually (primarily from ischemic heart disease and stroke). CVD is the largest single cause of death among women, accounting for one-third of their deaths worldwide.

Conduction disturbances and arrhythmias are significant primary and secondary problems in women. Although no arrhythmias are exclusive and specific to women, there are sex differences in symptoms, etiology, incidence, treatment selection, and outcomes that are genetically determined or modified by sex hormones.

This chapter discusses coronary artery disease (CAD) and subsequent arrhythmias in women, with a focus on ethnic differences in South Asian populations; the global burden of arrhythmias in women, with an emphasis on ventricular arrhythmias, sudden cardiac death (SCD), and inflammatory arrhythmias due to Chagas disease among others; valvular and nonvalvular atrial fibrillation (AF); and channelopathies, including hypertrophic cardiomyopathy (HCM), arrhythmogenic right ventricular cardiomyopathy (ARVC), and long QT syndrome (LQTS). We hope to encourage a broader and sex-based approach to our understanding of the global perspective of conduction disorders and arrhythmias in women.

ARRHYTHMIA RELATED TO CAD

Ventricular arrhythmias are the most common cause of death from any cause and of cardiovascular death among patients with CAD. The prevalence of CAD is increasing to epidemic proportions worldwide. While there are quality measures in the United States for managing acute coronary syndrome (ACS) and congestive heart failure, these measures do not exist at a national level in many developing countries. Additionally, between and within countries, there are widely varying differences in access to preventive care, in acute management of ACS, and in prevention and treatment of SCD resulting from CAD.

Disparities in the prevalence of CAD and mortality rates are noted among various ethnic groups. Among these groups, the risk among South Asians—people with origins in India, Pakistan, Sri Lanka, Nepal, and Bangladesh—is disproportionately elevated, with a 40% higher risk compared to the risk for whites in Western society (Figure 13.1). The greater risk factor burden for South Asians has been long-standing, and the 30% prevalence of diabetes mellitus among Indians was initially reported in the 1920s. In a cohort study from Trinidad, comparing people of Indian, African, European, and mixed origins, the ethnic group with the highest risk of overall CVD mortality was Indian.

In a survey of patients older than 20 years who were residents of Fiji, total mortality was 16.8 per 1,000 patient-years for urban residents and 11.7 per 1,000 patient-years for rural residents. Among the female residents, ischemic electrocardiographic changes were associated with higher mortality among women of Indian origin, while higher diastolic blood pressure and lower body mass index were associated with higher mortality among Melanesian women.

In an analysis of South Asians living in the United Kingdom, mortality after acute myocardial infarction (MI) was higher among women (10.9%) than among men (5.1%). In that study, the South Asians of both sexes were more likely to have a delayed presentation to the hospital; South Asian ethnicity and female sex

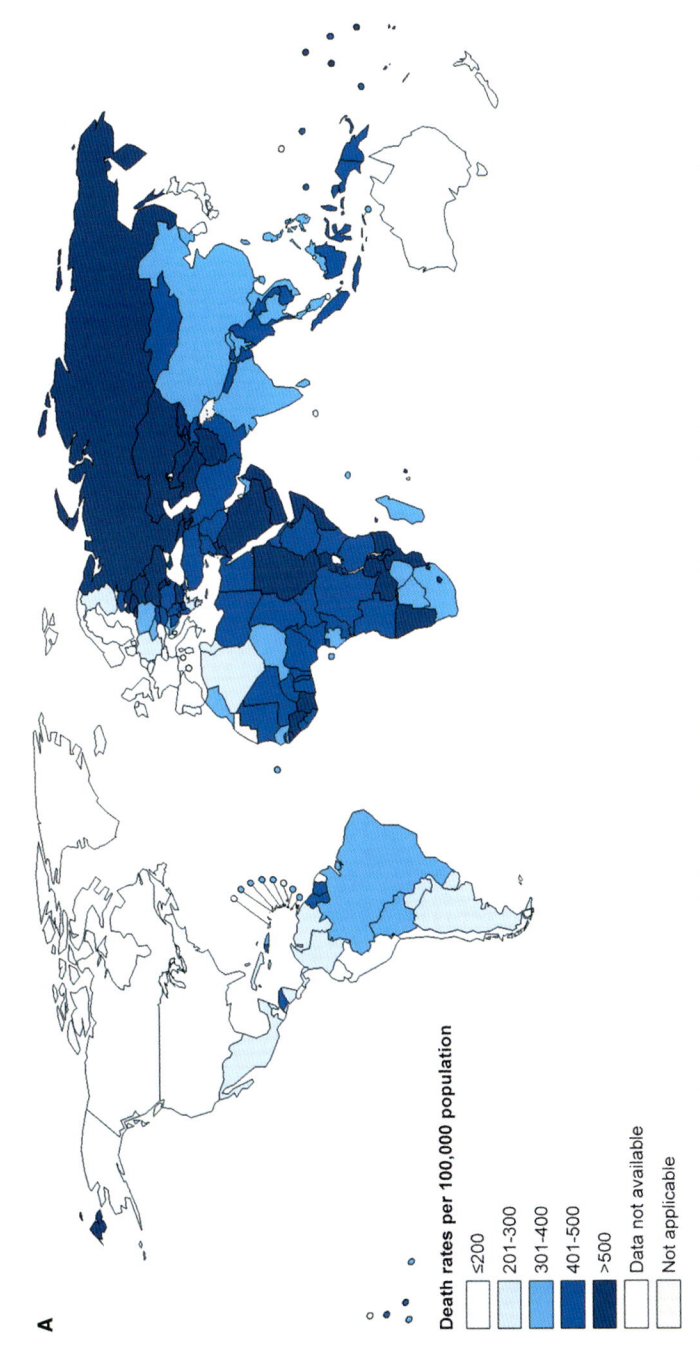

FIGURE 13.1. Global Mortality (2008) From Heart Disease and Diabetes Mellitus. A, Males. B, Females. (Adapted from Global health observatory map gallery. Geneva [Switzerland]: World Health Organization; c2006-2011. [cited 2013 May 9]. Available from: http://gamapserver.who.int/mapLibrary/. Used with permission.)

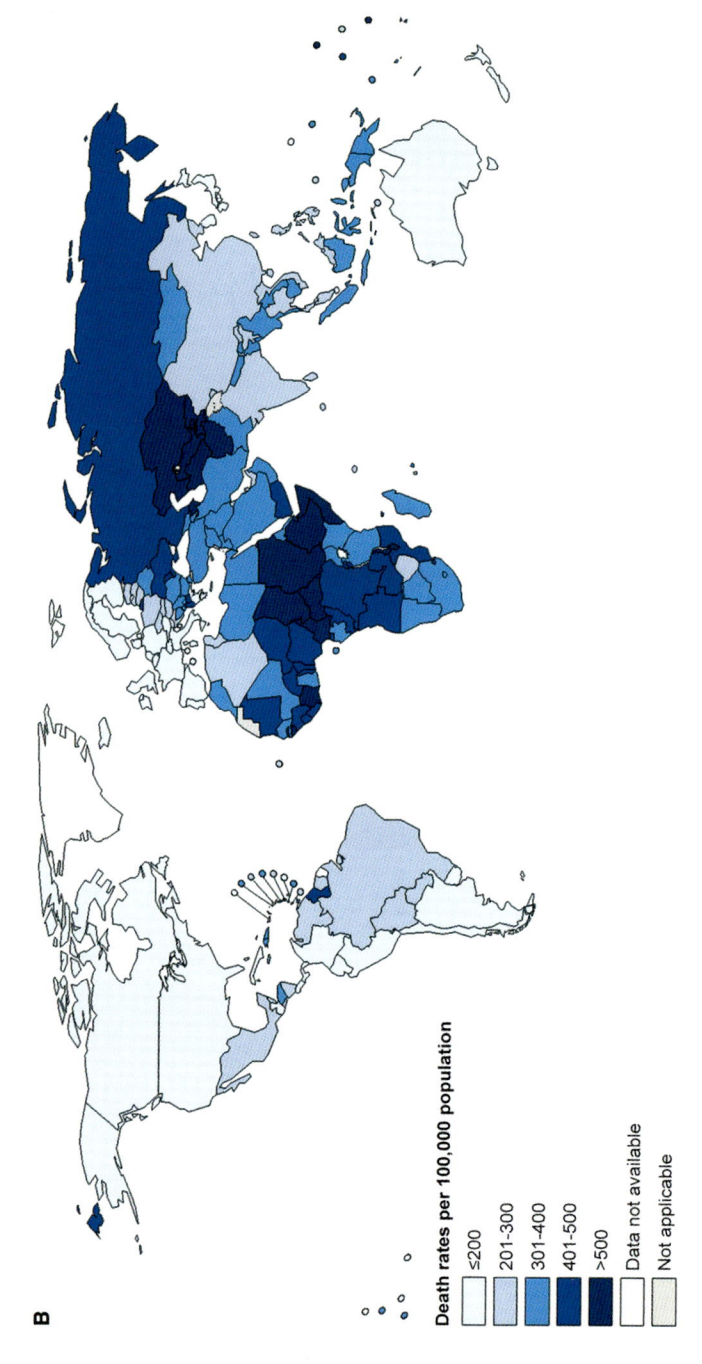

Death rates per 100,000 population
- ≤200
- 201–300
- 301–400
- 401–500
- >500
- Data not available
- Not applicable

FIGURE 13.1. (Continued)

were most likely associated with delayed revascularization after dismissal from the hospital.

The effect of late revascularization after ACS was assessed among patients (n=890) in a nonprofit hospital in South India that catered to patients of low socioeconomic status. Of the patients presenting with ACS, 91% were male. This observation raises the question of whether women were less likely to have an acute MI or less likely to use the health care system.

In summary, South Asian women have lower rates of presentation for ACS and MI and higher mortality when they do present, whether as residents in their native country or as immigrants. It is unclear whether this consistent observation is due to sex differences, cultural practices, or barriers for access to preventive and acute care. Since acute and chronic CAD are primarily responsible for the subsequent development of conduction system disease, ventricular arrhythmias, and SCD in many patients, addressing preventive and therapeutic measures will help to decrease the arrhythmic burden in both sexes.

SUDDEN CARDIAC DEATH

SCD is associated with various causes, including structural heart disease and channelopathies. In results from an autopsy questionnaire from South India to assess cause of death (cohort was 55% male), women were more likely than men to die at home, and 17% of the deaths were attributed to SCD. There was no sex difference in predictors, but for both sexes SCD was related to prior MI, hypertension, and age group (40–60 years).

The most important therapy for prevention of SCD after MI is medical management. In the CREATE registry of patients with acute MI from 89 centers in India, adherence with medication recommendations differed between high and low socioeconomic groups, respectively, as follows: use of a β-blocker, 58.8% vs 49.6%; use of a lipid-lowering agent, 61.2% vs 36.0%; and use of an angiotensin-converting enzyme inhibitor or an angiotensin II receptor blocker, 63.2% vs 54.1%. Aside from the differences between the socioeconomic groups, these percentages are significantly less than those for patients in Western societies. However, this study did not provide data broken down by sex for adherence to drug therapy.

In addition, in a review of industry data for the use of implantable cardioverter-defibrillators (ICDs) for primary and secondary prevention in India, less than 2,000 tachyarrhythmia devices were implanted annually (ie, <1 per 1 million people). Use of an ICD for primary prevention is generally not considered cost-effective and is rarely offered. Given that SCD is mainly due to acute or chronic CAD, the best primary prevention in this population is access to care and timely revascularization.

To assess ICD implantation for secondary prevention, we analyzed data from patients at a nonprofit tertiary care center. The patients presented with a history of ventricular arrhythmias (not reversible and not associated with acute MI). Among the 106 patients, 81% were men, mean (SD) age was 43 (12) years, and mean (SD) left ventricular ejection fraction (LVEF) was 48% (15%). At presentation, 84.9% had sustained ventricular tachycardia, 16% had nonsustained ventricular tachycardia (NSVT), 24.5% had syncope, and 1.9% had a family history of SCD. The patients' medications included β-blockers (53.8%), angiotensin-converting enzyme inhibitors (62.3%), and antiarrhythmics (29.2%). Structural heart disease was present in 79.2% (CAD in 46.2%, dilated cardiomyopathy in 14.1%, arrhythmogenic right ventricular dysplasia [ARVD] in 9.4%, HCM in 10.4%, and rheumatic heart disease [RHD] in 1.9%), channelopathy in 11.1%, and idiopathic ventricular tachycardia (VT) in 19.8%. Of the 59 patients deemed eligible, 17 received an ICD. More patients with syncope received an ICD compared with patients without syncope (58.8% vs 14.2%; $P<.001$); β-blocker use was less among those who had an ICD (29.4% vs 59.5%; $P=.04$). There was no sex variation among ICD recipients. These data are not generalizable in India since the practice patterns in for-pay hospitals are very different. An interesting observation is that in this cohort, only 46.2% of the patients had CAD even though CAD is widely prevalent in India. The low percentage could be explained by the low prevalence of systolic dysfunction after ACS; it may also reflect that most patients who have ventricular arrhythmias associated with ACS die before reaching the hospital.

In an autopsy study from South India, SCD accounted for more than 80% of the unexplained sudden deaths (80% of the cases of SCD were in men); 87% of these were due to MI (about one-third were old MIs), especially small and moderate-sized infarcts. These findings confirm that delayed therapy or lack of therapy, and most likely primary ventricular arrhythmias, caused these deaths since the autopsy data did not show any other mechanical explanations. The data support the case for consideration of increased use of β-blockers and primary prevention ICD implantation as outlined in the clinical guidelines—for both men and women.

ARRHYTHMIAS RELATED TO INFLAMMATORY OR INFECTIOUS DISEASES

Chagas Disease

While arrhythmias in South Asia are predominantly secondary to CAD, Chagas disease is responsible for the bulk of cardiac deaths in Latin American countries. Findings from paleoparasitologic studies of mummies from northern Chile have shown that Chagas disease has existed for thousands of years. Now it is a global problem as emigrants to North America and Europe have carried the parasite with them. An estimated 17 to 18 million people have Chagas disease worldwide. It is caused by *Trypanosoma cruzi*, a parasite with a complex life cycle and 4 morphologically distinct forms, and is transmitted by the reduviid bug (commonly known as the kissing bug). The vectors are most likely to be found in primitive dwellings. In addition to vector-borne transmission, Chagas disease can be transmitted through contaminated food or drink, blood transfusion, organ transplant, and vertical transmission through the placenta. Active vector control programs have been implemented by Latin American countries to prevent transmission.

Infection occurs in only some of the people who live where the disease is endemic, and symptoms develop in only one-third of those chronically infected. These observations have led to the suggestion that host genetic factors are responsible for the differences. Some single-nucleotide polymorphisms, such as those of tumor necrosis factor α, brown adipose tissue 1, monocyte chemoattractant protein 1, interleukin 12 β, and interleukin 10, have been associated with an intense immune response by the host and, hence, with the development of cardiomyopathy.

There is no sex difference in susceptibility to Chagas disease; however, special consideration is given to pregnant women, since the rate of vertical transmission is about 1% to 12% where the disease is endemic. The chance of cure is high for congenital Chagas disease, so screening is recommended for pregnant women. Benznidazole is contraindicated for pregnant women, and, for newborns, diagnosis is based on parasitologic testing; treatment is recommended for 30 to 60 days after birth. The criterion for cure is negative serologic test results.

The disease commonly involves conduction tissue, resulting in right bundle branch block, left anterior fascicular block, sinus node dysfunction, or atrioventricular nodal block. Patients with conduction tissue involvement are susceptible to ventricular arrhythmias. In 1 study, among patients who had Chagas disease and presented with nonsustained ventricular tachycardia or ventricular tachycardia, the only predictor for SCD was LVEF less than 40%; there was no sex difference for mortality. Ventricular arrhythmias are frequent; 1 study of patients who had Chagas disease and received an ICD showed that 50% had received appropriate shocks at an average of 45 months of follow-up, and 11% had received inappropriate shocks. Annual mortality was 7%. Predictors of death were New York Heart Association (NYHA) class III and LVEF, but not sex or age.

In the ICD-LABOR registry of patients from Brazil and Argentina with an ICD (75% were men), Chagas disease was the second most common indication after CAD (26.1% vs 39.7%). Male and female patients with Chagas disease seemed to benefit equally from an ICD. Predictors of death were age older than 70 years (hazard ratio [HR], 2.1), male sex (HR, 2.1), LVEF less than 30% (HR, 1.6), and NYHA class III or IV (HR, 2.9). As opposed to major secondary prevention trials such as AVID, this registry had a smaller proportion of patients with CAD and more females. The mortality data suggest that patients with Chagas disease, especially women, benefit from ICD therapy.

Lyme Disease

Lyme disease, also called Lyme borreliosis, is a multisystem disease caused by the spirochete *Borrelia* species. Clinical manifestations range from minor cutaneous erythema migrans to severe arthritis, neurologic manifestations, and heart block. Worldwide, about 250,000 cases are estimated to occur annually, with about 85,000 in Europe and 15,000 to 20,000 in the United States, especially in the Northeast. It is transmitted to humans by the bite of the ixodid tick. Cardiac involvement occurs in 0.5% to 10% of patients and includes myocarditis, pericarditis, and degenerative valvular disease, but most commonly it includes heart block that is reversible with treatment. There is no sex predilection for Lyme borreliosis; however, cardiac involvement is more prevalent in males by a 3:1 ratio. Heart block occurs at or above the atrioventricular node in about 50% of affected individuals, and it is reversible in 90% of patients receiving antibiotic therapy within 6 weeks of the tick bite. The mechanism has been attributed to a host immune reaction since scant organisms have been recovered in histopathology. Serology shows IgM antibodies in the acute phase and IgG antibodies in the chronic phase.

ATRIAL FIBRILLATION

Worldwide, stroke is the sixth most common cause of death, accounting for 6.15 million deaths annually. There is economic variability in the mortality rates; the percentages of death due to stroke are 4.9% in low-income countries, 8.7% in high-income countries, and 12.8% in middle-income countries. Cardioembolic stroke accounts for 14% to 30% of all cerebral infarctions, and AF is the most important cause of cardioembolic stroke. In a study of older adults in Singapore, women older than 75 had higher stroke risks than similarly aged men (8.3% vs 6.8%); however, the prevalence of AF varied between 2% and 10% and was not significantly different between men and women, suggesting that women are more susceptible to stroke.

AF, a widely prevalent arrhythmia, is associated in Western societies with aging, hypertension, diabetes mellitus, heart failure, obesity, and sleep apnea. In Asia, RHD is a leading cause of AF in addition to congestive heart failure, hyperthyroidism, aging, and hypertension. AF has a stronger association with female sex (odds ratio, 0.62 for men) in Asia. Unlike in Asia, in Western societies the prevalence of AF is lower among women, as shown by a population-based study in Germany in which the prevalence was 4.4 per 1,000 among men and 3.9 per 1,000 among women. Medical management with rate control or rhythm control is not associated with a difference in mortality; however, female patients who undergo ablation seem to have higher complication and mortality rates.

Rheumatic Heart Disease

The main cause of valve-related death and morbidity in developing countries is RHD, which is estimated to affect about 16 million people worldwide and to cause about 1.4 million deaths and 7.5% of all strokes in developing countries. In a population-based survey from Iran, 11.8% of ischemic strokes were cardio-embolic, and 45% of them were attributed to RHD. In a survey from Pakistan, the all-age prevalence of RHD was 5.7 per 1,000; the risk for girls was 1.7 times higher than for boys. The highest prevalence rate was at a younger age for women (45–54 years) than for men (55–64 years). AF is prevalent in about 40% of patients with RHD; a prevalence as high as 75% has been reported in surgical series. It is unclear whether the higher prevalence among girls is due to increased susceptibility or undertreatment of responsible infections.

The prevalence of RHD as the cardiac cause for hospitalization among pregnant women varies from 27% in Saudi Arabia to 88% in India. In Taiwan, about half of the 43 per 100,000 strokes occurring in pregnancy are attributed to RHD. Anticoagulant use is complicated by teratogenic effects, absence of organized follow-up of the international normalized ratio, and long-term cost.

Patients with AF in association with valvular disease are considered to have a high risk of stroke, with an approximate annual incidence of 8% per year; hence, warfarin is recommended for stroke prophylaxis in patients with AF. In a Brazilian study comparing aspirin and warfarin use in patients with AF in association with RHD, the incidence of stroke was 3.7% per year; there was no difference between the treatment groups. Of the 24 patients with stroke in the warfarin group, 21 received subtherapeutic levels of medication. Treatment adherence was 42% in the warfarin group and 72.7% in the aspirin group. Among patients who received therapeutic levels of warfarin, stroke risk was substantially decreased. Thus, adherence to medication and therapeutic anticoagulation are important modifiers of stroke risk for patients receiving warfarin therapy.

RHD carries high long-term morbidity and cost. The key to preventing RHD is public health measures targeting early diagnosis and treatment of streptococcal infections.

Rhythm Control Compared With Rate Control for AF

A study in India compared amiodarone (rhythm control) with placebo (rate control) for maintenance of sinus rhythm in 144 patients who had chronic rheumatic AF. Characteristics of the study population included a mean age of 38.6 years, predominantly female sex (55%), mean (SD) left atrial size of 47 (6) mm, mean (SD) AF duration of 6.1 (5.4) years, and history of prior valvular intervention (73%). Maintenance of normal sinus rhythm was higher among patients receiving rhythm control instead of rate control (69% vs 36%). The rhythm control group had better exercise time and improved NYHA class, quality of life, and mortality.

Small studies have evaluated AF ablation as a therapeutic option. In a study of 17 patients who had a history of RHD-associated AF and had undergone balloon valvotomy (mean age, 30.6 years; 53% women; mean left atrial size, 5.3 cm; mean [SD] duration of AF, 7 [1.2] years), the earliest activation was near the ostium of the coronary sinus and the left-sided interatrial septum; no early pulmonary vein activity was seen. At follow-up of 32 weeks after radiofrequency ablation, 59% of the patients remained in sinus rhythm. In another study by the same group (21 patients; 57% women; mean age, 44 years; left atrial size, 53 mm; mean AF duration, 3.8 years), patients underwent complex fragmentation mapping and pulmonary vein isolation. Early activation was widely distributed throughout the left atrium with a consistent pattern near the os of the coronary sinus. Organization of rhythm occurred in 71% and conversion in 14%; 14% remained in AF at the end of ablation. Patients were given amiodarone for 3 months after the procedure; at a mean follow-up of 10 months, 67% remained in normal sinus rhythm.

As in the group's earlier study, pulmonary vein activity was not significant in this predominantly young female population. These findings seem consistent with a wide area of early activity distributed in the left atrium. The consistent early activity in the coronary sinus is an interesting finding, perhaps related to elevated right-sided pressures. Maintenance of sinus rhythm in women of childbearing age without the use of amiodarone is a welcome paradigm shift in the management of AF, although failure rates were significant with relatively short follow-up, even with the use of amiodarone.

GENETIC DISEASES

SCD in the young during sports activities is an important public concern. In the United States, where the incidence is based on self-reporting, the prevalence is about 0.4 per 100,000, while in the Veneto region of Italy, where prospective data have been collected, the estimate is about 2.1 per 100,000. There is a significant sex predilection; the prevalence of HCM and ARVC among female athletes is one-tenth the prevalence among male athletes. This difference has been attributed to less participation in sports and less rigorous training among female athletes, but it may be related to genetic penetration as well. HCM and ARVC are the leading causes of SCD among adolescents and young adults.

Hypertrophic Cardiomyopathy

HCM is the most common cause of sudden death among the young and is also the leading cause of death among athletes worldwide. It is a disease of myofibrillar disarray due to defects in more than 11 genes (>1,400 variants) encoding contractile elements of the cardiac muscle. The population prevalence is about 1 in 500, with 6% phenotypic penetrance among families with positive mutations. The expression can be variable as well, manifesting later in life in some patients. HCM is truly a global disease and can affect men and women in all ethnic populations since it is predominantly transmitted by autosomal inheritance. Clinical recognition is earlier in men than in women, perhaps because more men than women participate in vigorous sports. In addition to ventricular arrhythmias causing SCD, patients are at risk of AF and embolic stroke.

Current data support the use of an ICD in patients who have 1 of the following risk factors: family history, syncope, septal thickness greater than 30 mm, documented ventricular arrhythmia, sudden cardiac arrest, and hypotensive response to exercise. Infants and children manifesting severe hypertrophy and heart failure have a poor prognosis. In patients older than 60 years, death seems to result mainly from non-HCM–related causes; hence, data do not support aggressive intervention with a defibrillator in this age group.

Since HCM carries a high risk of SCD with physical activity, patients are advised to avoid participating in competitive sports. Other recommendations include family screening of first-degree relatives and genetic screening if a sarcomeric mutation is known.

Japanese Type of HCM

Apical hypertrophy was initially described in Japan as a condition without a left ventricular outflow tract gradient, characterized by deep T wave inversions on the electrocardiogram and a spadelike appearance to the left ventricle during systole. This subset of HCM is characterized by hypertrophy of the left ventricular apex and is called the Japanese type of HCM. In a study from China, about 16% of patients with HCM had the apical type, with two-thirds having the pure form and one-third having the mixed form; more than 70% were men. Mortality with this subtype is considerably lower than with the other types.

Arrhythmogenic Right Ventricular Dysplasia

ARVD is a cardiac disease of the cardiac intercellular junctions. Mutations in genes encoding desmosomal proteins, such as those encoding desmoplakin, plakophilin-2, desmoglein-2, desmocollin-2, and lamin A/C, have been found in about 50% of the patients who have ARVC. Its prevalence is 1 per 2,000 to 1 per 5,000 of the general population; in North America, it affects 3 times as many males as females, although studies from Europe have shown equal prevalence between the sexes. Autosomal dominant and recessive forms with a cutaneous phenotype have been described (Naxos disease, Carvajal syndrome). Cardiomyocytes are progressively lost by apoptosis or necrosis and replaced by fibrofatty infiltrations.

ARVD is the second leading cause of sudden death in young athletes worldwide and the leading cause in northern Italy. Male and female patients with ARVD are equally susceptible to SCD. They should avoid participating in competitive athletics, and patients who satisfy the task force criteria should undergo ICD implantation since ARVD is a progressive disease.

In a study with long-term follow-up (mean [SD], 128 [92] months) study from Trieste, Italy, 65% of the patients had right ventricular dysfunction, and 25% had left ventricular dysfunction. Presence of both right ventricular and left ventricular dysfunction was an independent predictor of death or cardiac transplant (HR, 6.3). There was no sex difference for cardiac events.

Long QT Syndromes

Of all the arrhythmic genetic syndromes, LQTSs are uniquely more common in women than men. Female sex is an independent risk factor for drug-induced torsades de pointes. Endogenous and exogenous hormones affect the duration of the QT interval. Specifically, estrogen therapy alone increases the QT interval, which is mitigated by the addition of progesterone. At birth, there is no sex difference in the duration of the QT interval, but at puberty the QT interval shortens by 20% in adolescent boys compared with adolescent girls and then equalizes by about 50 years.

The strongest predictors of death with LQTS are female sex, corrected QT interval greater than 500 ms, and a history of previous syncope or aborted SCD. Silent carriers have normal QT intervals, but prolonged QT intervals and torsades de pointes can develop if the person is given noncardiac drugs that block the rapidly activating potassium current. The frequency varies from about 33% among patients with LQTS type 1 to less than 10% among those with LQTS type 3. Female sex, advanced age, electrolyte imbalance, bradycardia, and heart failure carry a high risk of drug-induced LQTS.

The worldwide prevalence of these genetic diseases is unknown, in part because of our evolving understanding of the various responsible genetic mutations, their phenotypic characteristics (including arrhythmic manifestations), and the role of hormonal and environmental factors. Diagnosis requires a high degree of awareness and, frequently, highly technical testing that is not uniformly available in many developing countries.

SUMMARY

SCD in South Asian populations is mainly attributable directly or indirectly to acute MI, with a small proportion of surviving patients having a residual LVEF of less than 30%. Considering the millions of patients affected, the rates of ICD use are extremely low; the primary limitation is cost. Thus, the best practical strategy for primary prevention of SCD for these populations is education, CAD risk factor reduction, rapid access to care, and timely revascularization.

In Latin America, Chagas disease is an important and common inflammatory cause of cardiomyopathy, contributing to death and disability with equal predilection in both men and women. Although survival is similar for both sexes because of the prolonged latent chronic infection phase, Chagas disease has additional implications for pregnant women and congenital disease transmission. Chagas cardiomyopathy is associated with an overall poor prognosis, and the ventricular arrhythmic burden and SCD burden are high.

AF, the most common arrhythmia in women, is a primary determinant of transient ischemic attack and stroke, representing the sixth leading cause of death globally. Anticoagulation therapy remains the mainstay of stroke prevention in high-risk populations, including those with valvular RHD and those with nonvalvular AF.

Because research ultimately informs clinical decisions and contributes to improved quality of care for patients, it is important to fill knowledge gaps. Herein we offer suggestions for 2 important areas in need of further study:

1. Outcomes after ICD placement are known to differ between men and women, and ICD therapy is a critical component in the management of several important arrhythmic conditions. Further research is needed to determine subpopulations in which ICD is more effective than pharmacologic treatment alone in preventing SCD among women.
2. Although the differences between men and women described in this report can be attributable to several factors, including geography, culture, ethnicity, sociocultural mores, and others, the genetic effects cannot be ignored. As medicine becomes increasingly more personalized, increasing importance will be given to identifying subpopulations with disease that will benefit

most from current and future diagnostics and therapeutics. For example, in sick sinus syndrome—a common disorder in the elderly and the most common indication for a permanent pacemaker—the *MYH6* α-myosin heavy chain single-nucleotide polymorphism, described with 38% frequency in the Icelandic population, confers a 50% increased lifetime risk of sick sinus syndrome compared with noncarriers. Thus, future investigations that use genome-wide association studies to identify single-nucleotide polymorphisms that are important in arrhythmic conditions, their global geographic prevalence or restriction, and populations most at risk should identify tailored diagnostic and therapeutic strategies and shed new information into mechanisms controlling cardiac conduction to optimize outcomes for men and women.

In summary, the genetic, hormone-mediated, and naturally occurring variations between the sexes represent potential opportunities to learn more about cardiovascular disease and its therapies, particularly when evidence derived from studies of men does not also hold for women, or when there is a paucity of data for women. Finally, it must be remembered that social, cultural, and economic barriers to health care access for women exist worldwide, even in developed countries; these barriers can skew research data and negatively affect the health and quality of life of women, their families, and their communities.

SUGGESTED READING

Andrade JP, Marin Neto JA, Paola AA, Vilas-Boas F, Oliveira GM, Bacal F, et al. I Latin American Guidelines for the diagnosis and treatment of Chagas' heart disease: executive summary. Arq Bras Cardiol. 2011 Jun;96(6):434–42. English, Portuguese, Spanish.

Biolo A, Ribeiro AL, Clausell N. Chagas cardiomyopathy: where do we stand after a hundred years? Prog Cardiovasc Dis. 2010 Jan-Feb;52(4):300–16.

Calkins H, Marcus F. Arrhythmogenic right ventricular cardiomyopathy/dysplasia: an update. Curr Cardiol Rep. 2008 Sep;10(5):367–75.

Carapetis JR. Rheumatic heart disease in Asia. Circulation. 2008 Dec 16;118(25):2748–53.

Dubner S, Valero E, Pesce R, Zuelgaray JG, Mateos JC, Filho SG, et al. A Latin American registry of implantable cardioverter defibrillators: the ICD-LABOR study. Ann Noninvasive Electrocardiol. 2005 Oct;10(4):420–8.

Joshi P, Islam S, Pais P, Reddy S, Dorairaj P, Kazmi K, et al. Risk factors for early myocardial infarction in South Asians compared with individuals in other countries. JAMA. 2007 Jan 17;297(3):286–94.

Kimura A, Harada H, Park JE, Nishi H, Satoh M, Takahashi M, et al. Mutations in the cardiac troponin I gene associated with hypertrophic cardiomyopathy. Nat Genet. 1997 Aug;16(4):379–82.

Lavitola Pde L, Sampaio RO, Oliveira WA, Boer BN, Tarasoutchi F, Spina GS, et al. Warfarin or aspirin in embolism prevention in patients with mitral valvulopathy and atrial fibrillation. Arq Bras Cardiol. 2010 Dec;95(6):749–55. Epub 2010 Oct 22. English, Portuguese, Spanish.

Nair M, Shah P, Batra R, Kumar M, Mohan J, Kaul U, et al. Chronic atrial fibrillation in patients with rheumatic heart disease: mapping and radiofrequency ablation of flutter circuits seen at initiation after cardioversion. Circulation. 2001 Aug 14;104(7):802–9.

Polin GM, Haqqani H, Tzou W, Hutchinson MD, Garcia FC, Callans DJ, et al. Endocardial unipolar voltage mapping to identify epicardial substrate in arrhythmogenic right ventricular cardiomyopathy/dysplasia. Heart Rhythm. 2011 Jan;8(1):76–83. Epub 2010 Nov 27.

Schwartz PJ. The congenital long QT syndromes from genotype to phenotype: clinical implications. J Intern Med. 2006 Jan;259(1):39–47.

Xavier D, Pais P, Devereaux PJ, Xie C, Prabhakaran D, Reddy KS, et al; CREATE registry investigators. Treatment and outcomes of acute coronary syndromes in India (CREATE): a prospective analysis of registry data. Lancet. 2008 Apr 26;371(9622):1435–42.

CHAPTER FOURTEEN

Pregnancy and Arrhythmias

LYNDA E. ROSENFELD, MD

INTRODUCTION

Pregnant women are usually relatively young and healthy, so the need to manage maternal arrhythmias during pregnancy is somewhat uncommon. Yet, young women with otherwise structurally normal hearts do have macroreentrant supraventricular tachycardias (SVTs), and as women delay childbearing and more women with congenital heart disease reach adulthood expecting to be mothers, familiarity with the management of arrhythmias during pregnancy becomes more important. In addition, the in utero identification of fetal arrhythmias may require using the mother to deliver lifesaving antiarrhythmic drugs to her unborn child. In all these situations, the cardiologist must consider 2 patients when making treatment decisions—the mother and her unborn child. Two pragmatic tenets are important in the management of these patients: 1) The best place for a fetus is generally in a healthy, hemodynamically stable mother. 2) Older drugs and treatments with a track record are usually better than the "newest and latest."

If a woman has heart disease, arrhythmias, a pacemaker, or an implantable cardioverter-defibrillator (ICD), planning for a pregnancy is always preferable to dealing with preventable problems that develop during an unexpected pregnancy. This is especially important when considering a change in medication or a procedure that can be scheduled before pregnancy, such as changing a pacemaker generator that is near the elective replacement indicator or performing an ablation.

INCIDENCE OF ARRHYTHMIAS DURING PREGNANCY

Sinus tachycardia is a normal consequence of pregnancy, especially during the third trimester, and, with a widened pulse pressure, may result in an increased sensation of palpitations. Further, atrial and ventricular premature contractions may be detected, but generally are of no clinical significance, during normal delivery and in more than 50% of women who have palpitations. Data are scarce and somewhat conflicting on the incidence of more important arrhythmias, such as sustained SVT, atrial fibrillation, and ventricular tachycardia or fibrillation. While some studies have suggested an increased incidence of first episodes of SVT during pregnancy, others have not confirmed this observation. No good data are available to document whether a consistent change in the frequency of SVT occurs during pregnancy or whether the incidence varies in a consistent way during pregnancy. In 1 series of women with preexisting arrhythmias, the majority of whom had structural heart disease, arrhythmia recurrence rates during pregnancy were 50% for SVT, 52% for paroxysmal atrial fibrillation or flutter, and 27% for ventricular tachycardia. Not unexpectedly, women often said that they were more symptomatic with episodes that occurred during pregnancy than with episodes that occurred before pregnancy.

TREATMENT OF ARRHYTHMIAS DURING PREGNANCY

Antiarrhythmic Drugs

Antiarrhythmic drugs are a mainstay of the treatment of arrhythmias. An informed clinician needs to consider not only what is known about the safety of using a drug during pregnancy but also how the physiologic and metabolic changes associated with pregnancy affect the drug's metabolism. The consideration of any antiarrhythmic therapy must include a calculus of the benefits of terminating or reducing the incidence of an arrhythmia and the risks to both the mother and the fetus.

Pregnancy results in changes that affect drug absorption, distribution, and excretion—changes that may alter the measured drug levels and the available therapeutically active drug. Many antiarrhythmic drugs cross the placental barrier and can affect the fetus. In fact, this is the basis for using maternal drug administration as a way to treat fetal arrhythmias. It is important to distinguish between drugs that are truly embryotoxic and have distinctly harmful effects and drugs that cross the placenta and have their predicted pharmacologic effects on the fetus.

Increased progesterone levels decrease intestinal motility, increase gastric and intestinal emptying time, and alter gastric pH; these changes can decrease or alter the absorption of oral medications. Since pregnancy results in about a 50% increase in plasma volume, a larger loading dose may be required to achieve significant drug levels rapidly. With the increase in plasma volume comes a progressive decrease in the plasma protein concentration. Along with altered binding of α_1-acid glycoprotein and hormonal changes, the proportion of unbound drug thus increases. This decreases the average total drug concentration at steady state, while the mean serum concentration of unbound or active drug remains unchanged. Thus, lower drug levels may be associated with therapeutic efficacy. Drug dosing is complicated even further because renal blood flow increases during pregnancy and results in a 50% increase in glomerular filtration rate and more rapid clearance of the many renally excreted antiarrhythmic drugs. Hepatic blood flow also increases, and hormonal induction of hepatic enzymes can further alter drug metabolism. The fetal liver and the placenta may contribute to drug metabolism as well.

Consideration must also be given to whether a mother is planning to breast-feed, since the drug choice may be affected by which drugs are less likely to appear in breast milk. Predominantly unbound, un-ionized drugs that are highly lipid-soluble achieve the highest concentrations in breast milk. For example, in picking a β-blocker during pregnancy, metoprolol would be a better choice than atenolol since metoprolol is not renally excreted and, post partum, it has low concentrations in breast milk.

TABLE 14.1. US Food and Drug Administration Categories for Drug Safety During Pregnancy

Pregnancy Category	Criteria
A	Controlled studies show no risk
B	There is no evidence of risk in humans; the chance of fetal harm is remote
C	Risk is not excluded; adequate studies are lacking; there is a chance of fetal harm, but the benefits outweigh the risks
D	There is positive evidence of risk; studies in humans show fetal risk, but the potential benefits in pregnant women may outweigh the risks
X	Contraindicated

The US Food and Drug Administration routinely grades pharmacologic agents according to a 5-point scale based on known and unknown effects that the agents may have on the fetus (Table 14.1). The majority of antiarrhythmic drugs are in pregnancy category C, largely based on a lack of evidence. Only a few drugs are in pregnancy category B: sotalol, lidocaine, and pindolol. Generally, the following drugs should be avoided during pregnancy: amiodarone (because of the potential for fetal thyroid toxicity), phenytoin (embryopathy), and dronedarone (teratogenicity in animals). Given the relatively uncommon use of all antiarrhythmic drugs during pregnancy and the absence of data from controlled trials, recommendations for most antiarrhythmic drugs are largely anecdotal. This lack of controlled trial data supports the concept that "older is better" because over time, more experience accrues with older drugs and older formulations of a particular drug.

The American Academy of Pediatrics has rated the safety of many drugs for use during lactation. These ratings, too, are often based on animal studies or individual case reports. The Thomson Lactation Rating is another scale for evaluating risk for the breast-feeding infant of a mother who is taking a specific medication. Table 14.2 summarizes information for the more commonly used antiarrhythmic drugs.

Cardioversion

The need for cardioversion during pregnancy is infrequent, but when it does occur, it raises certain practical and theoretical considerations. All the usual precautions for the procedure must apply, including monitoring electrolyte levels,

TABLE 14.2. Safety Ratings of Various Antiarrhythmic Drugs During Pregnancy and Breast-feeding

Vaughan-Williams Class	Drug	FDA Pregnancy Category	Comments	Crosses Placenta	Safety During Breast-feeding
IA	Disopyramide	C	Animal studies limited No increased malformations Possibly increased uterine contractions	Yes Fetal levels 40% of maternal	Usually compatible[a] Low levels in breast milk
	Procainamide	C	No apparent teratogenic effects	Yes Used to treat fetal arrhythmias	Usually compatible[a] Low levels in breast milk
	Quinidine	C	Relatively safe Fetal thrombocytopenia Cranial nerve VIII damage	Yes Used to treat fetal arrhythmias	Yes Usually compatible[a]
IB	Lidocaine	B	No risk demonstrated	Yes	Yes Usually compatible[a] Low levels in breast milk
	Mexiletine	C	Few studies No demonstrable toxic effects	Unknown	Yes Usually compatible[a] Low levels in breast milk Average plasma to milk ratio, 1.45:1
	Phenytoin	D	Clear risk Fetal hydantoin syndrome Increased fetal bleeding risk	Yes	Yes Usually compatible[a] Low levels in breast milk

(continued)

TABLE 14.2. (Continued)

Vaughan-Williams Class	Drug	FDA Pregnancy Category	Comments	Crosses Placenta	Safety During Breast-feeding
IC	Flecainide	C	Limited data No apparent teratogenic effects	Yes Used to treat fetal arrhythmias	Yes Usually compatible[a] Low levels in breast milk
	Propafenone	C	Limited data No known adverse effect	Probably	Yes Infant risk cannot be ruled out[b]
II	Atenolol	D	Evidence of human fetal risk Avoid in early pregnancy; give with caution in later stages	Yes	Yes Infant risk cannot be ruled out[b] Milk to maternal plasma ratio, 1.3:15.1
	Bisoprolol	C	Limited data	Unknown	Unknown Infant risk cannot be ruled out[b]
	Carvedilol	C	Limited data	Unknown	Yes, in rats Infant risk cannot be ruled out[b]
	Metoprolol	C	Animal studies: increased fetal loss at high doses	Yes Used to treat fetal arrhythmias	Yes Usually compatible[a] Concentrated in breast milk, but overall low levels

	Pindolol	B	Animal studies: adverse effects No human studies	Yes	Infant risk cannot be ruled out[b]
	Propranolol	C	Intrauterine growth retardation Neonatal bradycardia, hypoglycemia	Yes Used to treat fetal arrhythmias	Yes Usually compatible[a] Low levels in breast milk
III	Amiodarone	D	Evidence of human fetal risk Fetal thyroid abnormalities Weigh risks and benefits	Yes Amiodarone, 10%; metabolite, 25%	Infant risk cannot be ruled out[b]
	Dofetilide	C	Animal studies: fetal growth and survival adversely affected	Unknown	Infant risk cannot be ruled out[b]
	Dronedarone	X	Rats and rabbits: teratogenicity	Unknown	Infant risk cannot be ruled out[b] Contraindicated in nursing mothers
	Ibutilide	C	No human data Rats: teratogenicity at high doses	Unknown	Infant risk cannot be ruled out[b]
	Sotalol	B	No evidence of teratogenicity	Yes	Yes Usually compatible[a] Breast milk concentration higher than maternal plasma levels

(continued)

TABLE 14.2. (Continued)

Vaughan-Williams Class	Drug	FDA Pregnancy Category	Comments	Crosses Placenta	Safety During Breast-feeding
IV	Diltiazem	C	No reports of teratogenicity	Yes	Yes Usually compatible[a] Concentrations similar in breast milk and maternal serum
	Verapamil	C	No reports of teratogenicity	Yes Used to treat fetal arrhythmias	Yes Usually compatible[a] Low levels in breast milk
Other	Adenosine	C	No reports of fetal toxicity	Unknown	Unknown Infant risk cannot be ruled out[b]
	Digoxin	C	Long history of use Appears safe	Yes Used to treat fetal arrhythmias	Yes Usually compatible[a] Low levels in breast milk

Abbreviation: FDA, US Food and Drug Administration.

[a] American Academy of Pediatrics.

[b] Thomson Lactation Rating.

administering appropriate antiarrhythmic drug loading if indicated, and assessing the risk of thromboembolism and the need for anticoagulation.

Several factors can increase the risk and severity of aspiration during pregnancy: progesterone decreases the tone of the lower esophageal sphincter, the uterine contents push the lower portion of the esophagus into the thorax, the gastric pH is lower, and the gastric transit time is increased. Thus, for elective cardioversions, a generous period of fasting is advised with the use of proton pump inhibitors; sometimes metoclopramide is used to increase gastric pH and decrease transit time. Endotracheal intubation should be performed after the first trimester. With adhesive defibrillating patches, the procedure can be done with the patient in the upright position, especially to further decrease the risk of aspiration. Otherwise, the left lateral decubitus position is favored to increase uterine blood flow.

The short duration of anesthesia, especially in a hemodynamically stable patient, is generally safe for the fetus. The agents most commonly used (propofol, fentanyl, and midazolam) are generally considered safe during pregnancy.

During cardioversion, great care is taken to synchronize the delivered shock to the maternal QRS complex; thus, the shock is necessarily asynchronous to the fetal QRS complex. While this poses a theoretical risk of delivering an R-on-T and producing ventricular fibrillation in the fetus, the risk is quite small for several reasons. A critical mass of myocardium is necessary to sustain fibrillation, so the small size of the fetal heart makes it quite resistant to ventricular fibrillation. Also, the heart of the fetus is not physically located in the vector of the shock; hence, the energy delivered to the fetal heart is likely to be quite low. Despite these low risks, fetal monitoring should be performed before and immediately after cardioversion. Urgent delivery of a distressed viable fetus should be provided for but is rarely required.

Anticoagulation

A full discussion of anticoagulation during pregnancy is beyond the scope of this chapter; however, anticoagulation is important in managing various arrhythmias, especially atrial fibrillation and atrial flutter, and deserves special consideration during pregnancy. The use of warfarin during the first trimester, and possibly in weeks 6 through 12 specifically, has been associated with increased fetal loss and an embryopathy manifested as developmental abnormalities, midline neurologic defects, and nasal and epiphyseal malformations. Fetal risk may be partially related to the absolute dose of warfarin, and all management strategies must balance maternal thrombotic risk and fetal well-being. Weight-based full anticoagulation with low-molecular-weight heparin (LMWH), often with anti–factor Xa monitoring, has been used extensively during pregnancy.

The options for a woman contemplating pregnancy are to continue use of warfarin with frequent pregnancy tests and switch to LMWH if test results are positive or to switch to LMWH before attempting a planned pregnancy. Warfarin may be resumed during weeks 13 through 28 of gestation and then replaced with LMWH, which does not cross the placenta, until delivery; alternatively, LMWH may be continued for the entire pregnancy. Unfractionated heparin is also safe during pregnancy, and its short half-life may make it especially desirable around delivery, but its long-term use may be associated with a greater risk of osteoporosis when compared with LMWH. Warfarin is not found in appreciable quantities in breast milk and can safely be taken by a woman who is breast-feeding.

Aspirin is also frequently prescribed to patients with arrhythmias. Low-dose aspirin (ie, 75–100 mg) is thought to be generally safe during the second and third trimesters, but there is less certainty about its use during the first trimester. Higher doses of aspirin prevent closure of the ductus arteriosus and have been used therapeutically for that purpose. Otherwise, higher doses should be avoided, if possible.

Direct thrombin inhibitors do cross the placenta and should be used only in women with heparin-induced thrombocytopenia. Experience is limited with newer anticoagulants, such as apixaban, dabigatran, and rivaroxaban, during pregnancy and lactation, and this may be another situation in which the use of older drugs is preferable.

CARDIAC ARREST AND DEFIBRILLATION

Cardiac arrest during pregnancy is a rare event, occurring in about 1 in 30,000 deliveries, often in women with preexisting heart disease. Causes for the event include conditions specifically associated with pregnancy, such as aortic or coronary dissection and pulmonary or amniotic fluid embolus.

Until the fetus is viable, cardiopulmonary resuscitation (CPR) should be performed according to standard guidelines. After the age of fetal viability, emergent cesarean delivery should be considered to improve the outcomes for both the fetus and the mother. As always, a guiding principle is that the safest place for a fetus is in a hemodynamically stable mother, and if stability cannot be readily restored, the fetus should be removed from the mother.

Anatomical and physiologic considerations associated with pregnancy alter the standard recommendations for resuscitation. Classically, CPR is performed with the patient on her back, but in this position the gravid uterus compresses the major abdominal vessels. Thus, later in pregnancy the patient may be tipped on her left side and supported in this position during CPR. Alternatively, the uterine contents may be manually displaced to the left during supine CPR. The abdominal contents also shift the heart cephalad, so chest compressions should be performed a little higher than usual on the sternum. For similar reasons, the delivery of critical drugs by the femoral route should be avoided if at all possible.

As in cardioversion, the risk of fibrillating the fetus with defibrillating shocks is theoretical and low. Fetal dysrhythmia is more likely to be due to poor perfusion and metabolic changes related to maternal hemodynamic instability.

In an effort to improve neurologic recovery, current guidelines call for the induction of hypothermia in cardiac arrest patients who do not immediately have high levels of neurologic function. There are few data on the use of this procedure in women who have ongoing pregnancy. If emergency cesarean delivery is not performed in this situation, the fetus should be continuously monitored for bradycardia during maternal therapeutic hypothermia.

SUPINE HYPOTENSIVE SYNDROME

Supine hypotensive syndrome is a form of neurally mediated syncope that is unique to pregnancy. When a pregnant woman lies on her back, the gravid uterus compresses both her inferior vena cava and her aorta, causing a decrease in venous return and cardiac output. While these mechanical factors alone may result in hypotensive symptoms, their severity is often augmented by a secondary, reflex-mediated response to the reduced filling of the right ventricle, as is seen in other forms of neurocardiogenic syncope. This reflex leads to vasodilation and bradycardia. The treatment of these often dramatic, but generally benign, events entails aversive maneuvers, such as adequate hydration, the use of support stockings, perhaps increased salt intake, and, most importantly, avoidance of the supine position. Use of body pillows and appropriate positioning of the pregnant woman on her left side is often sufficient to minimize or prevent further episodes.

PACEMAKERS AND DEFIBRILLATORS

Patients with pacemakers and patients with ICDs can safely carry pregnancies to term. The major determinant of their ability to do so is the underlying cardiac condition that led to their device implantation. While most older patients receive ICDs because of ischemic and nonischemic cardiomyopathies with significant ventricular dysfunction, younger patients typically have various diagnoses, such as hypertrophic cardiomyopathy, long QT syndrome, and congenital heart disease. Often ventricular function is normal or nearly normal, and these women tolerate the hemodynamic changes of pregnancy well. Several reports have shown generally good outcomes for both the mother and the fetus, even when the mothers have received ICD shocks during the pregnancy. In these series, the presence of an abdominally located device has not resulted in any unusual or unexpected complications. The children of women with inherited cardiac conditions, such as channelopathies, should be screened for these conditions.

The need for urgent device implantation during pregnancy is relatively rare. Traditionally during pregnancy, lifesaving pacemakers have been implanted under fluoroscopic guidance with abdominal shielding and, if at all possible, the procedure has been deferred until after the first trimester. More recently, pacemakers and ICDs have been implanted with minimal or no fluoroscopy through the use of electrocardiographic and transthoracic or transesophageal echocardiographic guidance.

To avoid unplanned procedures during pregnancy, the timing of anticipated generator changes or device upgrades should be discussed with patients who are contemplating a pregnancy. These procedures should be done electively before the pregnancy.

ELECTROPHYSIOLOGY PROCEDURES DURING PREGNANCY

As with all the interventions described in this chapter, dealing with recurrent symptomatic arrhythmias before a planned pregnancy is preferable to having episodes occur during the pregnancy. Patients contemplating both pregnancy and radiofrequency ablation (RFA) for the management of SVT or other arrhythmias should generally be encouraged to have the RFA done before attempting to become pregnant. Usually with medical management, even if arrhythmias develop for the first time during pregnancy, RFA can be deferred until after delivery and the immediate postpartum period (when there is an increased risk of venous thromboembolism). Occasionally, life-threatening arrhythmias, such as recurrent hemodynamically unstable SVT or atrial fibrillation rapidly conducting over an accessory pathway, mandate more definitive treatment during pregnancy. In several studies, outcomes have been positive for both the mother and the fetus in women undergoing RFA during pregnancy. Minimal or no fluoroscopy was generally used in these cases in conjunction with abdominal shielding, ultrasonography, and noncontact electroanatomical mapping systems. In this instance, the "newest and latest" techniques have increased the safety of a treatment during pregnancy.

THE MOTHER AS A DRUG-DELIVERY SYSTEM FOR THE FETUS

Fetal echocardiography permits the intrauterine diagnosis of fetal arrhythmias. Prompt treatment of these arrhythmias, which often result in nonimmune fetal hydrops, may be lifesaving for the infant. These arrhythmias are diagnosed by using echocardiographic techniques to evaluate the fetal atrial and ventricular rates and their relationship (Figure 14.1). For example, an atrial rate of 400 beats per minute and a ventricular rate of 200 beats per minute suggest atrial flutter with 2:1 block, and a ventricular rate of 250 beats per minute with an atrial rate of 170 beats per minute may suggest ventricular tachycardia. Conversely, an atrial rate of 180 beats per minute with a ventricular rate of 80 beats per minute is consistent with heart block.

Recognition of the fetal arrhythmia is the first step in treatment. However, the challenge is how to deliver antiarrhythmic drugs to the fetus. The rather clever answer is to give them to the mother and monitor the fetal response. Medications that cross the placenta, including digoxin, verapamil, procainamide, and flecainide, have been used for this purpose. The cardiologist and electrophysiologist must ascertain that the mother's health is not jeopardized by this strategy. The mother should be monitored specifically for adverse drug effects, such as bradycardia and prolongation of the corrected QT interval, PR interval, or QRS complex.

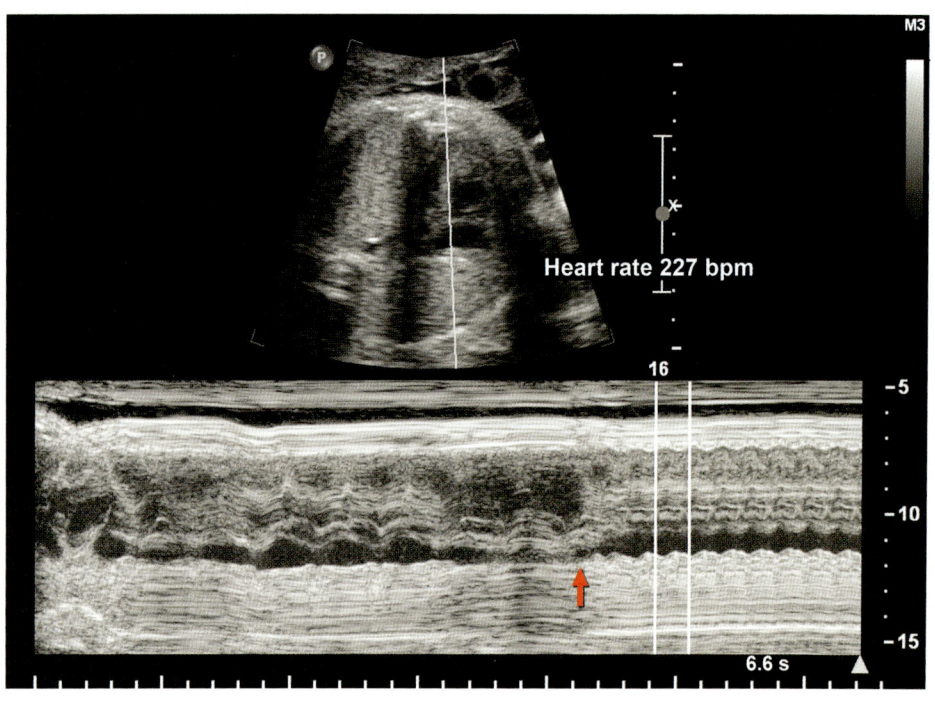

FIGURE 14.1. Two-Dimensional and M-Mode Fetal Echocardiograms. The arrow indicates the initiation of a fetal supraventricular tachycardia at a rate of 227 beats per minute (bpm). (Courtesy of the Yale Fetal Cardiovascular Center, New Haven, Connecticut. Used with permission.)

SUMMARY

The treatment of arrhythmias in pregnant women—and in their fetuses—should be guided by knowledge of the hemodynamic, physiologic, and pharmacokinetic changes during pregnancy. Two important tenets are that the safest place for a fetus is generally in a hemodynamically stable mother and that old drugs with a long track record, used wisely, are a better choice than new drugs with which there is relatively little experience.

SUGGESTED READING

Adamson DL, Nelson-Piercy C. Managing palpitations and arrhythmias during pregnancy. Heart. 2007 Dec;93(12):1630–6.

Barnes EJ, Eben F, Patterson D. Direct current cardioversion during pregnancy should be performed with facilities available for fetal monitoring and emergency caesarean section. BJOG. 2002 Dec;109(12):1406–7.

Bates SM, Greer IA, Pabinger I, Sofaer S, Hirsh J; American College of Chest Physicians. Venous thromboembolism, thrombophilia, antithrombotic therapy, and pregnancy: American College of Chest Physicians Evidence-Based Clinical Practice Guidelines (8th Edition). Chest. 2008 Jun;133(6 Suppl):844S-86.

DiCarlo-Meacham A, Dahlke J. Atrial fibrillation in pregnancy. Obstet Gynecol. 2011 Feb;117(2 Pt 2):489–92.

Duhl AJ, Paidas MJ, Ural SH, Branch W, Casele H, Cox-Gill J, et al; Pregnancy and Thrombosis Working Group. Antithrombotic therapy and pregnancy: consensus report and recommendations for prevention and treatment of venous thromboembolism and adverse pregnancy outcomes. Am J Obstet Gynecol. 2007 Nov;197(5):457.e1–21.

Kron J, Conti JB. Arrhythmias in the pregnant patient: current concepts in evaluation and management. J Interv Card Electrophysiol. 2007 Aug;19(2):95–107. Epub 2007 Aug 9.

Pedrinazzi C, Gazzaniga P, Durin O, Tovena D, Inama G. Implantation of a permanent pacemaker in a pregnant woman under the guidance of electrophysiologic signals and transthoracic echocardiography. J Cardiovasc Med (Hagerstown). 2008 Nov;9(11):1169–72.

Qasqas SA, McPherson C, Frishman WH, Elkayam U. Cardiovascular pharmacotherapeutic considerations during pregnancy and lactation. Cardiol Rev. 2004 Jul-Aug;12(4):201–21.

Silversides CK, Harris L, Haberer K, Sermer M, Colman JM, Siu SC. Recurrence rates of arrhythmias during pregnancy in women with previous tachyarrhythmia and impact on fetal and neonatal outcomes. Am J Cardiol. 2006 Apr 15;97(8):1206–12. Epub 2006 Mar 3.

Szumowski L, Szufladowicz E, Orczykowski M, Bodalski R, Derejko P, Przybylski A, et al. Ablation of severe drug-resistant tachyarrhythmia during pregnancy. J Cardiovasc Electrophysiol. 2010 Aug 1;21(8):877–82. Epub 2010 Feb 11.

CHAPTER FIFTEEN

Lead Extraction in Women

ULRIKA M. BIRGERSDOTTER-GREEN, MD, FHRS, AND MARGARET A. LLOYD, MD, MBA

INTRODUCTION

Expanding indications for cardiovascular implantable electronic devices (CIEDs) have resulted in an enormous increase in the number and complexity of these devices being implanted. More patients live for many years after their initial CIED is implanted, increasing the likelihood that they will outlive the lifespan of their original leads. Associated with increased patient longevity and device complexity is a trend toward an increase in device infections, further adding to the need for lead extraction. Lead recalls have also become increasingly common, and under some circumstances, the recalled lead may need to be extracted. Clinical circumstances change as well; after initial CIED implantation, many patients subsequently receive upgraded devices, such as implantable cardioverter-defibrillators (ICDs) and biventricular devices that require new or additional leads, necessitating the removal of nonfunctional leads. Few studies have specifically examined sex-related issues for lead extractions. This chapter reviews indications, procedural aspects, lead-related issues, and outcomes of lead extraction as they relate to women.

INDICATIONS AND PATIENT SELECTION

Indications for transvenous lead extractions are well described in the 2009 Heart Rhythm Society expert consensus document and do not differ between men and women (Box 15.1). However, male patients have consistently dominated extraction studies; 60% to 70% of the population in nearly all reports is male. This finding may reflect 1 or more of the following: a true higher rate of appropriate device implantation in men, a true higher risk of appropriate indications for lead extraction in men, or a male bias for implants or extractions (or both).

BOX 15.1.
INDICATIONS FOR TRANSVENOUS LEAD EXTRACTION

Recommendations for lead extraction apply only to patients for whom the benefits of lead removal outweigh the risks when assessment is based on individualized patient factors and operator-specific experience and outcomes. A level of evidence of B or C should not be construed as implying that the recommendation is weak. Many important clinical questions either do not lend themselves to experimentation or have not yet been addressed by high-quality investigations.

Infection

Class I

1. Complete device and lead removal is recommended in all patients with definite CIED system infection, as evidenced by valvular endocarditis, lead endocarditis, or sepsis. (*Level of evidence: B*)
2. Complete device and lead removal is recommended in all patients with CIED pocket infection as evidenced by pocket abscess, device erosion, skin adherence, or chronic draining sinus without clinically evident involvement of the transvenous portion of the lead system. (*Level of evidence: B*)
3. Complete device and lead removal is recommended in all patients with valvular endocarditis without definite involvement of the lead(s) and/or device. (*Level of evidence: B*)
4. Complete device and lead removal is recommended in patients with occult gram-positive bacteremia (not contaminant). (*Level of evidence: B*)

Class IIa

1. Complete device and lead removal is reasonable in patients with persistent occult gram-negative bacteremia. (*Level of evidence: B*)

Class III

1. CIED removal is not indicated for a superficial or incisional infection without involvement of the device and/or leads. (*Level of evidence: C*)

2. CIED removal is not indicated to treat chronic bacteremia due to a source other than the CIED when long-term suppressive antibiotics are required. (*Level of evidence: C*)

Chronic Pain

Class IIa

1. Device and/or lead removal is reasonable in patients with severe chronic pain, at the device or lead insertion site, that causes significant discomfort for the patient, is not manageable by medical or surgical techniques, and for which there is no acceptable alternative. (*Level of evidence: C*)

Thrombosis or Venous Stenosis

Class I

1. Lead removal is recommended in patients with clinically significant thromboembolic events associated with thrombus on a lead or a lead fragment. (*Level of evidence: C*)

2. Lead removal is recommended in patients with bilateral subclavian vein or SVC occlusion precluding implantation of a needed transvenous lead. (*Level of evidence: C*)

3. Lead removal is recommended in patients with planned stent deployment in a vein already containing a transvenous lead to avoid entrapment of the lead. (*Level of evidence: C*)

4. Lead removal is recommended in patients with superior vena cava stenosis or occlusion with limiting symptoms. (*Level of evidence: C*)

5. Lead removal is recommended in patients with ipsilateral venous occlusion preventing access to the venous circulation for required placement of an additional lead when there is a contraindication for using the contralateral side (eg, contralateral AV fistula, shunt or vascular access port, mastectomy). (*Level of evidence: C*)

Class IIa

1. Lead removal is reasonable in patients with ipsilateral venous occlusion preventing access to the venous circulation for required placement of an additional lead when there is no contraindication for using the contralateral side. (*Level of evidence: C*)

(continued)

Functional Leads

Class I

1. Lead removal is recommended in patients with life-threatening arrhythmias secondary to retained leads. (*Level of evidence: B*)
2. Lead removal is recommended in patients with leads that, due to their design or their failure, may pose an immediate threat to the patients if left in place (eg, Telectronics Accufix J wire fracture with protrusion). (*Level of evidence: B*)
3. Lead removal is recommended in patients with leads that interfere with the operation of implanted cardiac devices. (*Level of evidence: B*)
4. Lead removal is recommended in patients with leads that interfere with the treatment of a malignancy (radiation/reconstructive surgery). (*Level of evidence: C*)

Class IIb

1. Lead removal may be considered in patients with an abandoned functional lead that poses a risk of interference with the operation of the active CIED system. (*Level of evidence: C*)
2. Lead removal may be considered in patients with functioning leads that, due to their design or their failure, pose a potential future threat to the patient if left in place (eg, Telectronics Accufix without protrusion). (*Level of evidence: C*)
3. Lead removal may be considered in patients with leads that are functional but not being used (ie, right ventricular pacing lead after upgrade to ICD). (*Level of evidence: C*)
4. Lead removal may be considered in patients who require specific imaging techniques (eg, MRI) that cannot be performed because of the presence of the CIED system and for which there is no available imaging alternative for the diagnosis. (*Level of evidence: C*)
5. Lead removal may be considered in patients to permit the implantation of an MRI-conditional CIED system. (*Level of evidence: C*)

Class III

1. Lead removal is not indicated in patients with functional but redundant leads if patients have a life expectancy of <1 year. (*Level of evidence: C*)

2. Lead removal is not indicated in patients with known anomalous placement of leads through structures other than normal venous and cardiac structures (eg, subclavian artery, aorta, pleura, atrial or ventricular wall, or mediastinum) or through a systemic venous atrium or systemic ventricle. Additional techniques, including surgical backup, may be used if the clinical scenario is compelling. (*Level of evidence: C*)

Nonfunctional Leads

Class I

1. Lead removal is recommended in patients with life-threatening arrhythmias secondary to retained leads or lead fragments. (*Level of evidence: B*)
2. Lead removal is recommended in patients with leads that, due to their design or their failure, may pose an immediate threat to the patients if left in place (eg, Telectronics Accufix J wire fracture with protrusion). (*Level of evidence: B*)
3. Lead removal is recommended in patients with leads that interfere with the operation of implanted cardiac devices. (*Level of evidence: B*)
4. Lead removal is recommended in patients with leads that interfere with the treatment of a malignancy (radiation/reconstructive surgery). (*Level of evidence: C*)

Class IIa

1. Lead removal is reasonable in patients with leads that, because of their design or their failure, pose a threat to the patient that is not immediate or imminent if the lead is left in place (eg, Telectronics Accufix without protrusion). (*Level of evidence: C*)
2. Lead removal is reasonable in patients if a CIED implantation would require >4 leads on 1 side or >5 leads through the SVC. (*Level of evidence: C*)
3. Lead removal is reasonable in patients who require specific imaging techniques (eg, MRI) that cannot be performed because of the presence of the CIED system and for which there is no available imaging alternative for the diagnosis. (*Level of evidence: C*)

Class IIb

1. Lead removal may be considered at the time of an indicated CIED procedure in patients with nonfunctional leads if contraindications are absent. (*Level of evidence: C*)
2. Lead removal may be considered in patients to permit the implantation of an MRI-conditional CIED system. (*Level of evidence: C*)

(continued)

Class III

1. Lead removal is not indicated in patients with nonfunctional leads if patients have a life expectancy of <1 year. (*Level of evidence: C*)
2. Lead removal is not indicated in patients with known anomalous placement of leads through structures other than normal venous and cardiac structures (eg, subclavian artery, aorta, pleura, atrial or ventricular wall, or mediastinum) or through a systemic venous atrium or systemic ventricle. Additional techniques, including surgical backup, may be used if the clinical scenario is compelling. (*Level of evidence: C*)

Abbreviations: AV, atrioventricular; CIED, cardiovascular implantable electronic device; MRI, magnetic resonance imaging; SVC, superior vena cava.

Adapted from Wilkoff BL, Love CJ, Byrd CL, Bongiorni MG, Carrillo RG, Crossley GH 3rd, et al; Heart Rhythm Society; American Heart Association. Transvenous lead extraction: Heart Rhythm Society expert consensus on facilities, training, indications, and patient management: this document was endorsed by the American Heart Association (AHA). Heart Rhythm. 2009 Jul;6(7):1085–104. Epub 2009 May 22. Used with permission.

PROCEDURAL ASPECTS

Early attempts at lead extraction involved simple tools and techniques, such as locking stylets, telescoping sheaths, and traction. Success rates were suboptimal and complications were not uncommon; thus, lead extraction was typically performed only in cases of life-threatening systemic infection. The development of power extraction technology has paralleled the expansion of device indications and has made it possible to extract almost all leads with greater ease. The observed risk associated with lead extraction has decreased, especially in high-volume centers; however, it has not been eliminated.

Complications associated with lead extraction are related to the body's physiologic reaction to the presence of an intravascular foreign body. Materials that can be used in lead construction are limited; components must be nonallergenic, easy to handle, and able to withstand constant flexion and torsion in the hostile intravascular environment. Insulating materials consist of silicone

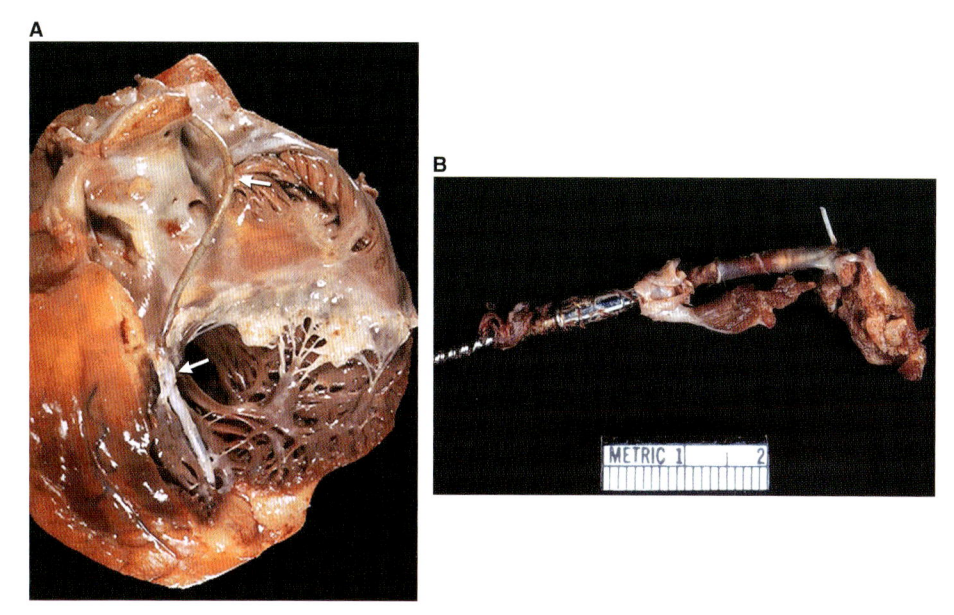

FIGURE 15.1. A, Explanted postmortem heart with ventricular lead in situ. Fibrosis can be seen along the length of the lead. Arrows indicate where the lead is adherent to myocardial tissue. B, Adherent fibrosis and cardiac tissue in an extracted ventricular lead.

and polyurethane variants; coil materials include specialty alloys (eg, Elgiloy and MP35N).

Within 4 to 5 days after implantation, the lead is encapsulated first by a thrombus and then by a fibrous sheath. The most robust fibrosis develops at the vascular entry site, along the superior vena cava, and at the electrode myocardial interface (Figure 15.1). In an autopsy series of 78 patients who died in the hospital (mean [SD] age, 77.9 [10.0] years; mean [SD] implantation duration, 4.0 [3.3] years), thrombi or fibrous tissue was found on 33% of 78 ventricular leads and on 48% of 21 atrial leads. There were connective tissue attachments to adjacent vascular and cardiac tissue in 87% of ventricular leads and in 71% of atrial leads. Ventricular leads were attached to tricuspid valve leaflets in 14% of patients and enmeshed in the subvalvular apparatus in 32%. Modern extraction techniques have not eliminated the tearing or perforation of vascular structures, tricuspid valve leaflets, and subvalvular tissue (Figure 15.2). Lead fibrosis tends to develop more intensely in younger patients. Calcification of adherent fibrous tissue can occur at any time, but it is more common in older patients, and it complicates even power-driven extraction methods. Leads may become tethered together, creating additional difficulty during extraction. The incidence and risk factors of traumatic tricuspid regurgitation after right ventricular lead removal have been evaluated in only small, single-center studies. However, the results suggest an increased occurrence in women, possibly related to an increased fibrotic reaction.

Byrd and associates reviewed lead extraction data from a prospective registry to which 315 physicians from 226 centers contributed data. Between January 1994 and April 1996, 3,540 leads were extracted from 2,338 patients. During this period, standard lead extraction techniques included traction, locking stylets, snares and baskets, and telescoping sheaths. The mean (SD) patient age was 64 (17) years; 59% were men and 41% were women. The mean (SD) duration of implantation was 47 (41) months; 53% were atrial and 46% were ventricular. Major complications were reported for 1.4% of patients, and minor complications for 1.7% of patients. The risk of major complications was significantly higher for women (2.3% for women vs 0.8% for men, $P<.005$); the highest-risk group was women undergoing extraction of 3 or more leads (8.6%, $P<.005$).

The US experience from 1995 to 1999 was reviewed in a study evaluating the early performance of the laser extraction system: 2,561 pacing and ICD leads were extracted from 1,684 patients. Major complications occurred in 1.9% of patients, and 0.8% of patients died. In that trial, only female sex was associated with an increased risk of complications in multivariate analysis.

In a retrospective review of all consecutive patients undergoing lead extraction from 2000 to 2007, Jones and colleagues reported their results for extracting 975 leads from 498 patients. Their high-volume referral center had an extremely low complication rate (0.2%) and no deaths. Because of the low complication rate in this series, the authors could not evaluate variables (including sex) associated with additional risk; however, they observed that important risk factors for extraction difficulty included long duration of lead implantation, use of ICD leads (versus pacing leads), and poor underlying health status.

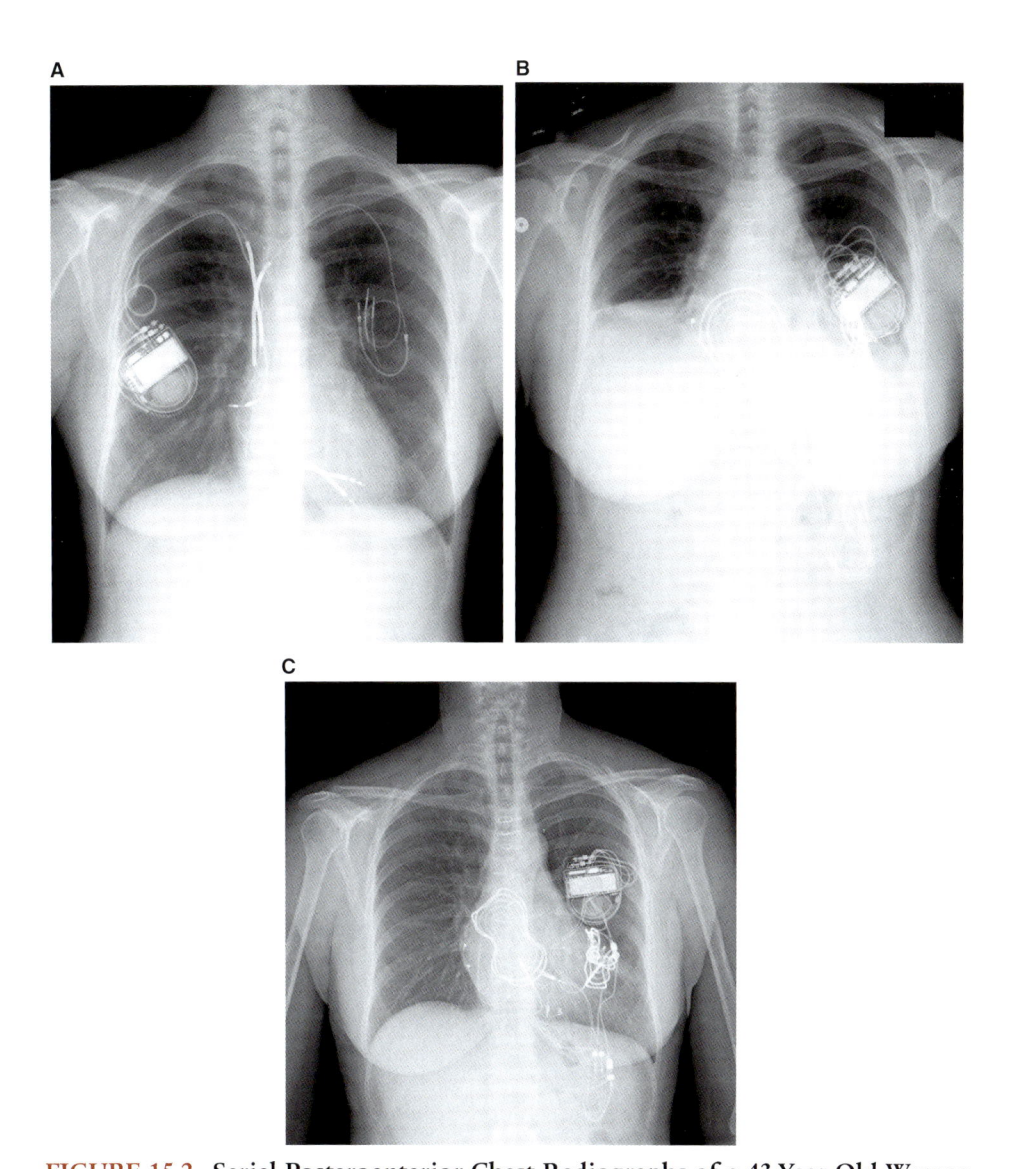

FIGURE 15.2. Serial Posteroanterior Chest Radiographs of a 43-Year-Old Woman With Arrhythmogenic Right Ventricular Dysplasia and Symptomatic Ventricular Arrhythmias. The radiographs show some of the difficulties encountered in long-term lead management and extraction. **A**, The patient initially had a single-chamber system with an implanted ventricular lead. Because of recurrent inappropriate shocks due to sinus tachycardia, the system was upgraded to a dual-chamber device 2 years later, when this radiograph was obtained. Extensive subclavian stenosis precluded advancement of an atrial lead; the left-sided ventricular lead was capped and abandoned, and a dual-chamber system was implanted in the right infraclavicular area. The patient required 2 atrial lead revisions over the ensuing 6 months for high atrial lead pacing thresholds and 1 pocket revision for painful lateral device migration. **B**, Four years later, severe symptomatic tricuspid regurgitation developed with both ventricular leads adhering to the valve leaflets. The right-sided lead was extracted without complication. Laser power tools were required to remove the left-sided lead; during the procedure, hypotension and pericardial effusion developed. The effusion was tapped, but it recurred, and the patient underwent surgery. Perforations were noted in the right ventricle and at the right atrial–right ventricular junction. The perforations were repaired, and the tricuspid valve was replaced with a bioprosthesis. A small section of the ventricular lead that was adherent to dysplastic right ventricular tissue was abandoned. Epicardial leads and patches were placed. A large right hemothorax is present, which was subsequently drained. **C**, Five years after lead extraction and tricuspid valve replacement, thresholds have remained satisfactory despite some deformation of the epicardial defibrillation leads, and the patient is doing well.

In the LExICon study, 1,449 consecutive patients at 13 sites in the United States and Canada underwent laser-assisted extraction of 2,405 leads (median implantation duration, 82.1 months). Extraction failure was highest at low-volume centers and among patients with body mass index (BMI) (calculated as weight in kilograms divided by height in meters squared) less than 25. Factors contributing to increased mortality included infection, endocarditis, diabetes mellitus, renal insufficiency, and BMI less than 25. Overall all-cause mortality was 1.86%; however, major adverse events associated with the procedure (including death) were 1.4%. In multivariate analysis, only BMI less than 25 was associated with an increased risk of major adverse events. The data did not encompass lead extractions that did not require laser assistance for successful extraction. In contrast to other studies, there was no association between sex and risk of adverse events.

LEAD-RELATED ISSUES

Accufix Atrial Lead

In the Accufix Multicenter Clinical Study and Worldwide Registry, 5,299 atrial lead extractions were recorded between 1994 and 1999; 4,023 were intravascular procedures. Life-threatening complications were noted in 0.5% of intravascular procedures, and fatal complications in 0.4%. The Accufix lead was unique in that the danger resulted from protruding J retention wires, which could also increase the risk of extraction. This experience occurred before the widespread use of power extraction tools, and cardiac surgical support was not uniform throughout the experience. The risk of extraction complications in this group was highest for longer duration of lead implantation, J wire protrusion, and female patients. Extraction risks for female patients were higher than for male patients at all durations of lead implantation (Figure 15.3).

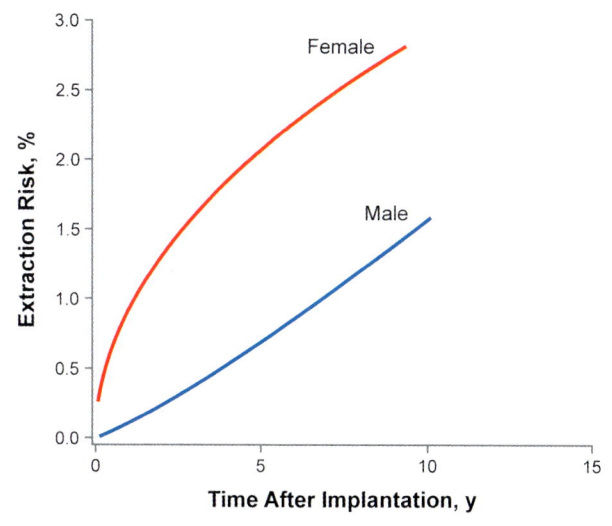

FIGURE 15.3. Extraction Risk With the Accufix Active Fixation Lead as a Function of Implantation Duration. Extraction risk for female patients was higher than for male patients at all lead implantation durations. (Adapted from Kay GN, Brinker JA, Kawanishi DT, Love CJ, Lloyd MA, Reeves RC, et al. Risks of spontaneous injury and extraction of an active fixation pacemaker lead: report of the Accufix Multicenter Clinical Study and Worldwide Registry. Circulation. 1999 Dec 7;100[23]:2344–52. Used with permission.)

ICD Leads

The long-term performance of ICD leads has been evaluated, with documentation of an increasing lead failure rate over time. A study of the annual rate of transvenous ICD lead defects in 900 consecutive patients with leads implanted between 1992 and 2005 showed that the failure rate increased progressively with time after implantation and reached 20% for 10-year-old leads. Patients with lead defects tended to be younger and female.

The Medtronic Sprint Fidelis lead was recalled in 2009, and the St Jude Riata ST lead was recalled in 2011. Early studies suggested that female sex was a predictor of Sprint Fidelis lead failure. The company's data showed that with lead model 6949, survival was statistically higher for male patients than for female patients ($P<.001$) (5-year survival: 91.9% for men [95% CI, 0.5 to −0.5]; 89.0% for women [95% CI, 0.9 to −1.0]). Comparable sex data were not available for the

Riata ST lead. The reasons for increased lead failure in women are unknown but may include a more restricted anatomy.

There is limited information on sex and risk with extraction of the Sprint Fidelis lead, but available data suggest that the Sprint Fidelis lead can be extracted safely by experienced operators and that the complication rate is lower than that reported for older-generation leads and with no sex-related differences in outcome. Case series of Sprint Fidelis and Riata ST extraction experience do, however, generally include few women, and no certain conclusions can be drawn from the available information.

Coronary Sinus Leads

Although coronary sinus leads are being increasingly used for biventricular pacing, the current extraction experience with these leads has not been examined in a controlled fashion. It is unknown whether extraction of these leads will confer a unique risk to women.

PROCEDURAL OUTCOMES

The assessment of complication risks associated with lead extraction has in some instances been compromised by the lack of a standardized classification of potential complications by which to compare studies. In the 2009 consensus document produced by the Heart Rhythm Society and endorsed by the American Heart Association, potential lead extraction complications were identified and classified in order to standardize lead management and extraction reporting (Box 15.2).

The development of power extraction systems has increased the number of successful extractions and reduced the time involved in lead extraction. These new tools have not, however, eliminated the risks involved in lead extraction, although overall complication rates in contemporary studies are less than those in early reports. There are no data to suggest that the new tools have improved safety for patients of either sex or in any age group; rather, the reduction in complication rates in reported studies is likely a result of operator experience in high-volume centers and of referral and reporting biases. The consensus document includes

> **BOX 15.2.**
> **RISKS OF CARDIAC LEAD EXTRACTION**
>
> Examples of Major Complications
>   Death
>   Cardiac avulsion or tear requiring intervention
>   Vascular avulsion or tear requiring intervention
>   Pulmonary embolism requiring surgical intervention
>   Anesthesia-related complications
>   Stroke
>   CIED infection propagation
> Examples of Minor Complications
>   Pericardial effusion not requiring intervention
>   Hemothorax not requiring chest tube
>   Pocket hematoma requiring drainage
>   Upper extremity thrombosis
>   Vascular injury requiring repair at insertion site
>   Hemodynamically significant air embolism
>   Migrated lead fragment without sequelae
>   Blood transfusion
>   Pneumothorax requiring chest tube
>   Pulmonary embolism not requiring surgical intervention
>
> Abbreviation: CIED, cardiovascular implantable electronic device.
>
> Adapted from Wilkoff BL, Love CJ, Byrd CL, Bongiorni MG, Carrillo RG, Crossley GH 3rd, et al; Heart Rhythm Society; American Heart Association. Transvenous lead extraction: Heart Rhythm Society expert consensus on facilities, training, indications, and patient management: this document was endorsed by the American Heart Association (AHA). Heart Rhythm. 2009 Jul;6(7):1085–104. Epub 2009 May 22. Used with permission.

recommendations for minimal levels of experience in training programs, a minimal annual extraction volume to maintain competency, and precautions that should be in place, such as emergency echocardiographic imaging and cardiovascular surgical capabilities.

Extraction studies to date have consistently included more men than women. Studies powered to examine differences, especially the early studies, have indicated that women have a higher risk of complications from lead extraction compared with men. In the LExICon study, conducted with a contemporary extraction toolbox, a sex difference in extraction risk was not observed, but smaller body size was associated not only with a higher risk of complications but also with a higher risk of extraction failure. The number of complications in this study was so low that it was difficult to draw further conclusions about risk. The higher risk for female patients, especially in historical studies, may be due to smaller body size, smaller vascular diameter, and smaller heart size rather than to female sex per se.

SUMMARY

Lead extraction for appropriate indications should not be deferred for female patients because of theoretical increased risk associated with lead removal; however, operators should be aware of the historical risk pattern, especially for small women with multiple leads being extracted. For all contemplated extractions, the patient's clinical situation may affect risk calculations, and recommendations may be modified depending on coexisting morbidities.

SUGGESTED READING

Byrd CL, Wilkoff BL, Love CJ, Sellers TD, Reiser C. Clinical study of the laser sheath for lead extraction: the total experience in the United States. Pacing Clin Electrophysiol. 2002 May;25(5):804–8.

Byrd CL, Wilkoff BL, Love CJ, Sellers TD, Turk KT, Reeves R, et al. Intravascular extraction of problematic or infected permanent pacemaker leads: 1994–1996: US Extraction Database, MED Institute. Pacing Clin Electrophysiol. 1999 Sep;22(9):1348–57.

Jones SO 4th, Eckart RE, Albert CM, Epstein LM. Large, single-center, single-operator experience with transvenous lead extraction: outcomes and changing indications. Heart Rhythm. 2008 Apr;5(4):520–5. Epub 2008 Jan 17.

Kay GN, Brinker JA, Kawanishi DT, Love CJ, Lloyd MA, Reeves RC, et al. Risks of spontaneous injury and extraction of an active fixation pacemaker lead: report of the Accufix Multicenter Clinical Study and Worldwide Registry. Circulation. 1999 Dec 7;100(23):2344–52.

Novak M, Dvorak P, Kamaryt P, Slana B, Lipoldova J. Autopsy and clinical context in deceased patients with implanted pacemakers and defibrillators: intracardiac findings near their leads and electrodes. Europace. 2009 Nov;11(11):1510–6. Epub 2009 Aug 14.

Wazni O, Epstein LM, Carrillo RG, Love C, Adler SW, Riggio DW, et al. Lead extraction in the contemporary setting: the LExICon study: an observational retrospective study of consecutive laser lead extractions. J Am Coll Cardiol. 2010 Feb 9;55(6):579–86. Erratum in: J Am Coll Cardiol. 2010 Mar 9;55(10):1055.

Wilkoff BL, Love CJ, Byrd CL, Bongiorni MG, Carrillo RG, Crossley GH 3rd, et al; Heart Rhythm Society; American Heart Association. Transvenous lead extraction: Heart Rhythm Society expert consensus on facilities, training, indications, and patient management: this document was endorsed by the American Heart Association (AHA). Heart Rhythm. 2009 Jul;6(7):1085–104. Epub 2009 May 22.

Index

Note: Page numbers followed by *f* or *t* indicate a figure or table.

AADs. *See* antiarrhythmic drugs
accessory pathway (AP)
   concealed, 66
   manifest, 66
Accufix atrial lead, 252, 253*f*
Accufix Multicenter Clinical Study and Worldwide Registry, 252
acquired long QT syndrome, 39–40
   in torsades de pointes, 40
adenosine
   for AVNRT, 62
   for AVRT, 68
   for sinus node reentry tachycardia, 75
   for WPW syndrome, 68
ADVANCENT. *See* National Registry to Advance Heart Health
AERP. *See* atrial effective refractory period
AF. *See* atrial fibrillation
AFFIRM. *See* Atrial Fibrillation Follow-up Investigation of Rhythm Management
AFL. *See* atrial flutter
alcohol intake, AF and, 88
amiodarone, 19*t*, 20*t*, 23*t*, 26, 27, 28, 29
   for AFL, 74
   for atrial tachycardia, 72
   for AVNRT, 64
   for AVRT, 68, 69
   in drug-induced LQTS, 108
   pacemaker implantation and, 109
   for rate control in AF, 91–92
   for rhythm control in AF, 92, 93*f*
   for sinus node reentry tachycardia, 75
   for WPW syndrome, 68, 69
androgens
   in drug-induced LQTS, 106
   QT interval and, 36
   sex-related electrophysiologic differences with, 52*t*, 54
   ventricular repolarization and, 50
ANDROMEDA. *See* Antiarrhythmic Trial With Dronedarone in Moderate to Severe CHF Evaluating Morbidity Decrease
angiotensin-converting enzyme inhibitors, for AF, 95
antiarrhythmic drug-mediated proarrhythmia, xi
antiarrhythmic drugs (AADs), 109*t*
   for fetal arrhythmias, 239–40
   during pregnancy, 228–30, 230*t*, 231–34*t*
   proarrhythmia and, 80*t*, 92
   randomized clinical trials of, 18, 19–22*t*, 26–29
Antiarrhythmics Versus Implantable Defibrillators (AVID), 10, 23*t*, 29, 132, 133*t*, 216
Antiarrhythmic Trial With Dronedarone in Moderate to Severe CHF Evaluating Morbidity Decrease (ANDROMEDA), 21*t*, 29
anticoagulant therapy
   for AFL, 74
   in atrial fibrillation, 6
   during pregnancy, 235–36
Anticoagulation and Risk Factors in Atrial Fibrillation (ATRIA), 6, 84

antithrombotic therapy, for stroke prevention in AF, 89–91
AP. *See* accessory pathway
apixaban
   pregnancy and, 236
   for stroke prevention in AF, 90
Apixaban for Reduction in Stroke and Other Thromboembolic Events in Atrial Fibrillation (ARISTOTLE), 90
Apixaban Versus Acetylsalicylic Acid to Prevent Stroke in Atrial Fibrillation Patients Who Have Failed or Are Unsuitable for Vitamin K Antagonist Treatment (AVERROES), 90
ARISTOTLE. *See* Apixaban for Reduction in Stroke and Other Thromboembolic Events in Atrial Fibrillation
arrhythmias
   fetal, 239–40, 240f
   genetic factors and, 35
   genetic testing for, 43–44
   hereditary factors and, 35
   during pregnancy, xii, 227–28
      antiarrhythmic drugs, 228–30, 230t, 231–34t
      anticoagulation, 235–36
      cardioversion, 230, 235
      incidence of, 228
      treatment of, 228
   related to global CVD, 210, 211–12f, 213
   sex-related electrophysiologic differences in, potential mechanisms, 51–55, 52t
      androgens, 52t, 54
      autonomic nervous system, 52–53, 52t
      estrogens, 52t, 54–55
      ionic basis, 52t, 53–54
arrhythmogenic right ventricular dysplasia (ARVD)
   global CVD and, 221–22
   SCD and, 120
aspirin, pregnancy and, 236
asystole, SCD and, 114, 115f
AT. *See* atrial tachycardia
ATRIA. *See* Anticoagulation and Risk Factors in Atrial Fibrillation
atrial effective refractory period (AERP), 82, 83
atrial fibrillation (AF), xi–xii, 5–7
   alcohol intake and, 88
   anticoagulant therapy in, 6
   birth weight and, 87
   bleeding events and, 5–6
   BMI and, 87
   caffeine intake and, 88
   cardioversion for, 6
   catheter ablation of, sex-related differences in clinical outcomes of, 13t
   clinical presentation of, 80t, 81–82
   electrophysiology of, 80t, 82–84
   genetic, 42
   in global CVD, 217–20
      RHD and, 218–19
      rhythm control compared with rate control for, 219–20
   hereditary, 41–42
   hypertension and, 87
   mortality and morbidity in, 80t, 86–87
   in pregnancy, 88–89
   prevalence of, 80–81
   pulmonary vein antrum isolation for, 7, 7f
   P-wave dispersion and, 83
   quality of life scores with recurrent persistent, 82, 83f
   radiofrequency ablation and, 6, 7
   rate control strategy for, 91–92
   rhythm control strategy for, 91, 92, 93f
   risk of, 81f
   sex differences that characterize, 79, 80t
   stroke risk and, 5–6, 84–86, 85f
   symptoms of, 80t, 81–82
   treatment of, 89–99
      adjuvant medical therapy, 94–96
      angiotensin-converting enzyme inhibitors, 95
      bisphosphonates, 95–96
      catheter ablation, 97–99, 98f
      DCCV, 96–97
      drug therapy, 91–94, 93f, 94f
      statins, 94–95
      stroke prevention, 89–91
      thyroid replacement, 96
Atrial Fibrillation Follow-up Investigation of Rhythm Management (AFFIRM), 93, 108
atrial flutter (AFL)
   anticoagulant therapy for, 74
   catheter ablation for, 74
   characteristic sex differences in, 67b
   DCCV for, 74
   incidence of, 73
   isthmus-dependent, 73
   management of, 73–74
   outcomes in, 74
   overdrive pacing for, 74
   reverse typical, 73
   typical, 73
atrial-His interval, sex-related differences in, 48t, 51

atrial tachycardia (AT)
  cardioversion for, 72
  catheter ablation for, 72
  characteristic sex differences in, 67b
  incidence of, 71
  management of, 71–72
  mechanism of, 70
  outcomes in, 72
  tachycardia-mediated cardiomyopathy secondary to incessant, 72
atrioventricular accessory pathway-mediated macroreentrant tachycardia, 66
atrioventricular nodal reentrant tachycardia (AVNRT), 4, 42–43, 61–66
  atypical, 61
  carotid sinus massage for, 62
  ECG for, 61, 62, 63f
  electrophysiologic characteristics in, 62, 64t
  ICD and, 62
  incidence of, 60f, 61–62
  management of, 62, 64–65
  outcomes in, 65–66
  typical, 61
  Valsalva maneuver for, 62, 64
atrioventricular reciprocating tachycardia (AVRT), 66–70
  antidromic, 66
  catheter ablation for, 69
  characteristic sex differences of, 67b
  DCCV for, 68
  electrophysiologic characteristics of accessory pathway in, 69–70, 69f
  EPS for, 68
  incidence of, 66–68
  management of, 68–70
  orthodromic, 66
  outcomes in, 70
  overdrive pacing for, 68
  SCD and, 70
autonomic function, orthostatic intolerance and, 188
autonomic nervous system, sex-related electrophysiologic differences in, 52–53, 52t
AVERROES. *See* Apixaban Versus Acetylsalicylic Acid to Prevent Stroke in Atrial Fibrillation Patients Who Have Failed or Are Unsuitable for Vitamin K Antagonist Treatment
AVID. *See* Antiarrhythmics Versus Implantable Defibrillators
AVNRT. *See* atrioventricular nodal reentrant tachycardia
AVRT. *See* atrioventricular reciprocating tachycardia

birth weight, AF and, 87
bisphosphonates, for AF, 95–96
bleeding events, atrial fibrillation and, 5–6
α-blockers, for POTS, 186
β-blockers
  for AFL, 74
  for arrhythmia during pregnancy, 229
  for atrial tachycardia, 72
  for AVNRT, 62, 64
  in cardiovascular mortality reduction and SCD, 74
  for inappropriate sinus tachycardia, 75
  for junctional tachycardia, 76
  OH and, 183
  for postural orthostatic tachycardia syndrome, 75
  for POTS, 186
  for rate control in AF, 91–92
  for sinus node reentry tachycardia, 75
  for sinus tachycardia, 75
blood volume, reduced, orthostatic intolerance and, 187–88
body mass index (BMI), AF and, 87
Borrelia species, 216
bradyarrhythmias, antiarrhythmic drug-induced, 108
bradycardia, SCD and, 114, 115f
breast cancer, endocrine therapy for, 111
British Women's Heart and Health Study (BWHHS), 183
Brugada syndrome, 121
  QT interval in, 40
BWHHS. *See* British Women's Heart and Health Study
bypass tracts, 43

CAD. *See* coronary artery disease
caffeine intake
  AF and, 88
  for autonomic function, 188
calcium channel blockers
  for atrial tachycardia, 72
  for AVNRT, 62
  for junctional tachycardia, 76
  for rate control in AF, 91–92
  for sinus node reentry tachycardia, 75
Canadian Amiodarone Myocardial Infarction Arrhythmia Trial (CAMIAT), 19t, 26
Canadian Implantable Defibrillator Study (CIDS), 23t, 29–30, 132
Canadian Registry of Acute Coronary Events (CANRACE), 118

Canadian Registry of Atrial Fibrillation (CARAF), 6, 90
cancer, of breast. *See* breast cancer
CANRACE. *See* Canadian Registry of Acute Coronary Events
captopril, 21*t*, 28
CARAF. *See* Canadian Registry of Atrial Fibrillation
cardiac arrest, during pregnancy, 236–37
Cardiac Arrhythmia Suppression Trial (CAST), 18, 19*t*, 124
Cardiac Arrhythmia Suppression Trial II (CAST II), 18, 19*t*
cardiac pacing
 implant location, 156, 157*f*, 158
 pacemaker selection, sex differences in, 153–56, 155*f*
 procedure-related complications, 158–60, 159*f*
 subpectoral pocket and, 156, 157*f*
 survival, sex differences in, 153–56, 155*f*
Cardiac Resynchronization-Heart Failure (CARE-HF), 24*t*, 30, 167, 171*t*
cardiac resynchronization therapy (CRT), 138, 161–69, 161*f*
 with defibrillator, 159
 ICD combined with, 12–13
 implantation, 163–64
 indication for, 162–63, 162*t*
 response to, 165–69, 166*t*, 168*f*, 169*f*, 170–73*t*
 sex-related differences in clinical outcomes of, 13*t*
 trials, underrepresentation of women in, 164–65, 164*f*, 165*f*
Cardiac Resynchronization Therapy Combined With Implantable Cardioverter Defibrillator Therapy (CONTAK CD), 167, 170*t*
cardiomyopathy
 dilated, SCD and, 116, 116*f*, 117*f*
 hypertrophic, SCD and, 119–20
 tachycardia-mediated, secondary to incessant atrial tachycardia, 72
cardiopulmonary resuscitation (CPR), 237
cardiovascular disease (CVD), xii
 "sex-blind" treatment of, viii
 sex differences in, vii–viii
 sex-specific evidence in, viii
 women's symptoms of, viii
cardiovascular disease (CVD), global, 209–10
 AF, 217–20
 RHD and, 218–19
 rhythm control compared with rate control for, 219–20

arrhythmia related to, 210, 211–12*f*, 213
Chagas disease, 215–16
genetic diseases, 220–22
 ARVD, 221–22
 HCM, 220–21
 Japanese type of HCM, 221
 LQTS, 222
Lyme disease, 216
SCD in, 213–15
 ICD for prevention of, 214
cardiovascular implantable electronic devices (CIEDs), 243
cardiovascular toxicity, of rhythm-control drugs, 108–9, 109*t*
cardioversion. *See also* direct current cardioversion
 for atrial fibrillation, 6
 for atrial tachycardia, 72
 for AVNRT, 62
 during pregnancy, 230, 235
 for AF, 89
CARE-HF. *See* Cardiac Resynchronization-Heart Failure
carotid sinus massage, for AVNRT, 62
carvedilol, 20*t*, 28
 for POTS, 186
Carvedilol or Metoprolol European Trial (COMET), 20*t*, 27–28
CASS. *See* Coronary Artery Surgery Study
CAST. *See* Cardiac Arrhythmia Suppression Trial
CAST II. *See* Cardiac Arrhythmia Suppression Trial II
catecholaminergic polymorphic ventricular tachycardia (CPVT), 41
catheter ablation
 for AF, 97–99, 98*f*
 for AFL, 74
 for atrial tachycardia, 72
 for AVNRT, 64, 65
 for AVRT, 69
 for inappropriate sinus tachycardia, 75
 for junctional tachycardia, 76
 for postural orthostatic tachycardia syndrome, 75
 for PSVT during pregnancy, 65
 for sinus node reentry tachycardia, 75
 for WPW syndrome, 69
Chagas disease, 215–16
channelopathies, SCD and, 120–21
CHF. *See* congestive heart failure
CHF-STAT. *See* Congestive Heart Failure: Survival Trial of Antiarrhythmic Therapy
CIDS. *See* Canadian Implantable Defibrillator Study

CIEDs. *See* cardiovascular implantable electronic devices
clinic, women's heart. *See* heart clinic, women's
clinical trials. *See* randomized clinical trials
clonidine, for POTS, 186
COMET. *See* Carvedilol or Metoprolol European Trial
Comparison of Medical Therapy, Pacing, and Defibrillation in Heart Failure (COMPANION), 24*t*, 30, 125, 138, 139*f*, 142, 167, 170*t*
complete atrioventricular nodal ablation, for rate control in AF, 91–92
congenital long QT syndrome, 37–38
congestive heart failure (CHF)
    atrial fibrillation and, 5
    ICD trial enrollment and, 10, 11–12
Congestive Heart Failure: Survival Trial of Antiarrhythmic Therapy (CHF-STAT), 20*t*, 26–27
CONTAK CD. *See* Cardiac Resynchronization Therapy Combined With Implantable Cardioverter Defibrillator Therapy
Copenhagen City Heart Study, 84, 86, 88
coronary artery disease (CAD)
    SCD and, 115–16, 116*f*, 117*f*, 118–19
    South Asian ethnicity mortality rates and, 210, 213
    sudden cardiac death and, 8
Coronary Artery Surgery Study (CASS), 118
coronary sinus leads, 254
corrected QT interval (QTc), 3
    age-associated sex differences in, 49–50, 50*f*
    exogenous testosterone administration and, 50
    during follicular phase of menstrual cycle, 36
    menstrual cycle and, 49*t*
    sex-related differences in, 48–50, 48*t*, 49*t*
CPR. *See* cardiopulmonary resuscitation
CPVT. *See* catecholaminergic polymorphic ventricular tachycardia
CREATE. *See* Treatment and Outcomes of Acute Coronary Syndromes in India
CRT. *See* cardiac resynchronization therapy
CVD. *See* cardiovascular disease
CYP2D6. *See* cytochrome P450 2D6 isozyme
CYP3A. *See* cytochrome P450 3A isozyme
cytochrome P450 2D6 isozyme (CYP2D6), 111
cytochrome P450 3A isozyme (CYP3A), in drug-induced LQTS, 107, 107*f*

dabigatran
    pregnancy and, 236
    for stroke prevention in AF, 90
Danish Investigations of Arrhythmia and Mortality on Dofetilide in Congestive Heart Failure (DIAMOND-CHF), 21*t*, 28, 92, 105
DCCV. *See* direct current cardioversion
decongestants, for autonomic function, 188
defibrillation, during pregnancy, 236–37, 238–39
Defibrillator in Acute Myocardial Infarction Trial (DINAMIT), 24*t*, 30
Defibrillators in Nonischemic Cardiomyopathy Treatment Evaluation (DEFINITE), 23*t*, 30, 125, 132*t*, 134, 136, 136*f*, 138, 139*f*, 141, 142
depression, SCD and, 121–22
desmopressin, for reduced blood volume, 188
diabetes mellitus, global mortality from, 210, 211–12*f*
DIAMOND-CHF. *See* Danish Investigations of Arrhythmia and Mortality on Dofetilide in Congestive Heart Failure
Digitalis Investigation Group (DIG), 109–10, 110*f*
digoxin
    for AF in pregnancy, 89
    for AFL, 74
    for AVNRT, 62
    in drug-induced LQTS, 107–8
    for fetal arrhythmias, 240
    mortality with, 109–11, 110*f*
    for rate control in AF, 91–92
dilated cardiomyopathy, SCD and, 116, 116*f*, 117*f*
diltiazem
    for AFL, 74
    for AVNRT, 64
    for POTS, 186
    for PSVT during pregnancy, 65
DINAMIT. *See* Defibrillator in Acute Myocardial Infarction Trial
direct current cardioversion (DCCV)
    for AF, 96–97
    for AFL, 74
    for AVRT, 68
    for WPW syndrome, 68
disopyramide, for atrial tachycardia, 72
dofetilide, 21*t*, 28
    for AFL, 74
    in drug-induced LQTS, 105–6
    for rhythm control in AF, 92, 93*f*
dronedarone, 21*t*, 22*t*, 28–29
    for rhythm control in AF, 92, 93*f*
D-sotalol, 18, 19*t*, 26
    in drug-induced LQTS, 104–5

dual-chamber pacemaker, 8
Dutch FollowPace, 154

E-4031, in drug-induced LQTS, 106, 106f
ECG. *See* electrocardiogram
echocardiography, fetal, during pregnancy, 239–40, 240f
Ehlers-Danlos syndrome (EDS) hypermobility type, 189
  orthostatic intolerance and, 185
electrocardiogram (ECG), for AVNRT, 61, 62, 63f
electrophysiology study (EPS)
  for AVRT, 68
  PSVT and, 60
  for WPW syndrome, 68
EMIAT. *See* European Myocardial Infarct Amiodarone Trial
encainide, 18, 19t
endocrine therapy, for breast cancer, 111
endoxifen, 111
EPS. *See* electrophysiology study
erythromycin, QT interval prolongation due to, 4
erythropoietin, for reduced blood volume, 188
estradiol-17β, 2
  in drug-induced LQTS, 104
estrogen
  in drug-induced LQTS, 106
  orthostatic tolerance and, 3
  potassium channel protein synthesis and, 2
  QT interval and, 36
  sex-related electrophysiologic differences in, 52t, 54–55
Euro Heart Survey on Atrial Fibrillation, 5, 6
European Myocardial Infarct Amiodarone Trial (EMIAT), 19t, 26
exercise
  hypermobility and, 189
  for POTS, 186
  for venous pooling, 187

fetal arrhythmias, 239–40, 240f
fetal echocardiography, during pregnancy, 239–40, 240f
Fibrillation Registry Assessing Costs, Therapies, Adverse Events, and Lifestyle (FRACTAL), 109
flecainide, 18, 19t
  for AF in pregnancy, 89
  for AFL, 74
  for atrial tachycardia, 72
  for AVNRT, 64
  for AVRT, 69

for fetal arrhythmias, 240
for junctional tachycardia, 76
for rhythm control in AF, 92, 93f
for WPW syndrome, 69
fludrocortisone, for reduced blood volume, 188
Focus Group Project, 193
follicular phase, of menstrual cycle, QTc during, 36
FRACTAL. *See* Fibrillation Registry Assessing Costs, Therapies, Adverse Events, and Lifestyle

genetic diseases, in global CVD, 220–22
  ARVD, 221–22
  HCM, 220–21
  Japanese type of HCM, 221
  LQTS, 222
genetic testing, role of, for arrhythmias, 43–44
GESICA. *See* Grupo de Estudio de la Sobrevida en la Insuficiencia Cardiaca en Argentina
Global Registry of Acute Coronary Events (GRACE), 118
Grupo de Estudio de la Sobrevida en la Insuficiencia Cardiaca en Argentina (GESICA), 20t, 26–27

HCM. *See* hypertrophic cardiomyopathy
Heart and Estrogen/Progestin Replacement Study (HERS), 94, 122, 123
heart clinic, women's
  business objectives for, 199
  initial planning phase for, 192–98
    analysis of strengths, weaknesses, opportunities, and threats (SWOT analysis), 198, 198b
    business plan, 193
    competitive data, 197–98
    directed focus groups, 193–97
    market and environmental assessment, 193–97
    objective, 193
    service area, 193
  marketing strategies for, 199–200
  operations strategies for, 200f
    clinic design, 200–201
    clinic flow, 201
    clinic location, 200–201
    clinic opening, 202–3
    MyHeart Book Screening experience, 201–2
  outcomes of
    first-year results review, 203–4, 204t
    patient experience, 205
    providers' perspectives, 205–6

second-year results review, 204
third-year results review, 204
heart disease
  global mortality from, 210, 211–12*f*
  screening package, 195
  sex-related differences in, 14
heart failure
  antiarrhythmic drug-induced, 108
  sex-related differences in, 163
heart rate
  menstrual cycle and, 48
  at rest, 2
  sex-related differences in, 47–48, 48*t*
heart rate variability (HRV), 122
hERG. *See* human ether-à-go-go-related gene
HERS. *See* Heart and Estrogen/Progestin Replacement Study
His-ventricular interval, sex-related differences in, 48*t*, 51
hormones
  effects on QT interval, 35–37, 37*f*
  myocytes and, 35
  NMS and, 181
  oral contraceptives and, 189
  orthostatic intolerance and, 189
  proarrhythmia and, 93
  PSVT and, 60
HRV. *See* heart rate variability
human ether-à-go-go-related gene (*hERG*), 107, 108
4-hydroxytamoxifen, 111
hypermobility, orthostatic intolerance and, 189
hypertension
  AF and, 87
  pulmonary. *See* pulmonary hypertension
hypertrophic cardiomyopathy (HCM), 220–21
  Japanese type of, 221
  SCD and, 119–20
hypotension, orthostatic. *See* orthostatic hypotension

ibutilide
  for AFL, 74
  in drug-induced LQTS, 103, 106
$I_{Ca,L}$. *See* L-type calcium current
ICD. *See* implantable cardioverter-defibrillator
ICD-LABOR. *See* Implantable Cardioverter-Defibrillator Latin American Bioelectronic Ongoing Registry
I_{Kr}. *See* rapid component of delayed rectifier potassium current

I_{Ks}. *See* slow component of delayed rectifier potassium current
Immediate Risk-Stratification Improves Survival (IRIS), 24*t*, 30
implantable cardioverter-defibrillator (ICD). *See also* cardiac pacing
  arrhythmic events during follow-up, 141–44
    primary prevention, 141–44, 142*f*, 144*f*
    secondary prevention, 141
  AVNRT and, 62
  body image and, 146–47
  complications, 145–46, 146*f*
  CRT combined with, 12–13
  difference in arrhythmias, potential mechanisms for, 144–45
  implantation studies, 9–12, 9*f*
    mortality reduction and, 10, 11
    shocks and, 10–11
  inducibility of ventricular arrhythmias, 141
  leads, 253–54
  during pregnancy, 238–39
  randomized clinical trials of, 23–25*t*, 29–31
  sex disparities with use of, 147–50, 148*f*, 149*f*
  trials
    as primary prevention, 132–41, 142*t*
    as secondary prevention, 132
Implantable Cardioverter-Defibrillator Latin American Bioelectronic Ongoing Registry (ICD-LABOR), 216
IMPROVE HF. *See* Registry to Improve the Use of Evidence-Based Heart Failure Therapies in the Outpatient Setting
inappropriate sinus tachycardia, 75
Inhibition of Unnecessary Right Ventricular Pacing With Atrioventricular Search Hysteresis in Implantable Cardioverter-Defibrillators (INTRINSIC RV), 132*t*, 140, 142
in-hospital cardiac arrests, 114
INTRINSIC RV. *See* Inhibition of Unnecessary Right Ventricular Pacing With Atrioventricular Search Hysteresis in Implantable Cardioverter-Defibrillators
ionic basis, for sex-related electrophysiologic differences, 52*t*, 53–54
IRIS. *See* Immediate Risk-Stratification Improves Survival
ISSUE-3. *See* Third International Study on Syncope of Uncertain Etiology
ivabradine, for POTS, 186

Japanese type of HCM, 221
junctional tachycardia, 76

KCNH2 mutations, 38
KCNQ1 mutations, 38

Lead Extraction in the Contemporary Setting (LExICon), 256
left ventricular dysfunction, SCD and, 119
levothyroxine, for AF, 96
lidocaine, for arrhythmia during pregnancy, 230
LMWH. *See* low-molecular-weight heparin
long QT syndrome (LQTS), 3–4
   global CVD and, 222
   acquired, 39–40
   congenital, 37–38
   drug-induced, 103–8
      amiodarone, 108
      androgens, 106
      CYP3A, 107, 107*f*
      digoxin, 107–8
      dofetilide, 105–6
      D-sotalol, 104–5
      E-4031, 106, 106*f*
      estradiol-17β, 104
      estrogens, 106
      hormone-mediated changes, 107
      ibutilide, 103, 106
      quinidine, 108
      testosterone, 104
      torsades de pointes and, 104, 105*f*
   in menopause, 38–39
   in postpartum, 38, 39*f*
   progesterone and, 37, 37*f*
   SCD and, 120–21
   shifts in sex hormones and, 38–39, 39*f*
low-molecular-weight heparin (LMWH), pregnancy and, 236
LQTS. *See* long QT syndrome
L-type calcium current ($I_{Ca,L}$), 53–54
luteal phase, of menstrual cycle, PSVT episodes in, 4
Lyme disease, 216

MADIT. *See* Multicenter Automatic Defibrillator Implantation Trial
MADIT-CRT. *See* Multicenter Automatic Defibrillator Implantation Trial With Cardiac Resynchronization Therapy
MADIT II. *See* Multicenter Automatic Defibrillator Implantation Trial II
Marshfield Epidemiologic Study Area (MESA), 73

M cells. *See* midmyocardium cells
Medtronic Sprint Fidelis lead, 253, 254
menopause, LQTS in, 38–39
menstrual cycle
   follicular phase of, QTc during, 36
   heart rate and, 48
   luteal phase of, PSVT episodes in, 4
   PSVT and, 60
   QTc and, 49*t*
MESA. *See* Marshfield Epidemiologic Study Area
metoprolol, 20*t*, 28
   for arrhythmia during pregnancy, 229
midmyocardium cells (M cells), 56
midodrine, for venous pooling, 187
MIRACLE. *See* Multicenter InSync Randomized Clinical Evaluation
MIRACLE-ICD. *See* Multicenter InSync ICD Randomized Clinical Evaluation
moricizine, 18, 19*t*
Multicenter Automatic Defibrillator Implantation Trial (MADIT), 119, 132*t*
Multicenter Automatic Defibrillator Implantation Trial II (MADIT II), 23*t*, 30, 119, 125, 132*t*, 134, 135, 135*f*, 138, 139*f*, 141, 142, 142*f*
Multicenter Automatic Defibrillator Implantation Trial With Cardiac Resynchronization Therapy (MADIT-CRT), 25*t*, 30–31, 138, 167, 168*f*, 169, 169*f*, 171*t*
Multicenter InSync ICD Randomized Clinical Evaluation (MIRACLE-ICD), 167, 170*t*
Multicenter InSync Randomized Clinical Evaluation (MIRACLE), 166, 170*t*
Multicenter Unsustained Tachycardia Trial (MUSTT), 114, 118, 119, 125, 132*t*, 134, 135, 135*f*, 138, 139*f*, 141, 142
MyHeart Book Screening, 195–96, 201–2, 203
myocytes, hormones and, 35

National Cardiovascular Data Registry (NCDR), 145, 158
National Institutes of Health (NIH) Revitalization Act of 1993, 17
National Registry to Advance Heart Health (ADVANCENT), 149
NCDR. *See* National Cardiovascular Data Registry
neurally mediated syncope (NMS), 178, 180–82
   causes of, 180
   genetic predisposition to, 181–82
   hormonal fluctuation and, 181
   incidence of, 180
   mechanism of, 180–81

mortality and morbidity of, 180
psychologic testing and, 182
treatment of, 182
TTT and, 178, 181, 182
neurocardiogenic syncope. *See* neurally mediated syncope
NHS. *See* Nurses' Health Study
NICM. *See* nonischemic cardiomyopathies
nicotine patches, for autonomic function, 188
NIH. *See* National Institutes of Health Revitalization Act of 1993
NMS. *See* neurally mediated syncope
nonischemic cardiomyopathies (NICM), SCD and, 119–20
Nurses' Health Study (NHS), 114, 115f, 123

OAC. *See* oral anticoagulation
OH. *See* orthostatic hypotension
OHCAs. *See* out-of-hospital cardiac arrests
Ontario Health Payer-Mandated Prospective Study, 144f, 145
Ontario ICD Database, 140, 143, 145, 159
oral anticoagulation (OAC), for stroke prevention in AF, 89–91
oral contraceptives, hormones and, 189
organic anion-transporting polypeptide OATP1B1, 108
orthostatic hypotension (OH), 178, 182–83
TTT and, 178
orthostatic intolerance. *See also* neurally mediated syncope; orthostatic hypotension; postural orthostatic tachycardia syndrome
autonomic function and, 188
EDS hypermobility type and, 185
hormones and, 189
hypermobility and, 189
reduced blood volume and, 187–88
venous pooling and, 186–87
orthostatic tolerance, sex-related differences and, 3
out-of-hospital cardiac arrests (OHCAs), 114
overdrive pacing
for AFL, 74
for AVNRT, 62
for AVRT, 68
for WPW syndrome, 68

pacemaker. *See also* cardiac pacing
for autonomic function, 188
dual-chamber, 8
implantation of
amiodarone and, 109

mode selection and, 8
for rate control in AF, 91–92
permanent, for junctional tachycardia, 76
during pregnancy, 238–39
rate-responsive, 8
selection, sex differences in, 153–56, 155f
PALLAS. *See* Permanent Atrial Fibrillation Outcome Study Using Dronedarone on Top of Standard Therapy
panic attacks, SCD and, 122
Parkinson disease, OH and, 183
paroxysmal supraventricular tachycardia (PSVT), 4–5
distribution of, 59–60, 60f
EPS and, 60
hormone effects on, 60
management of, sex-specific differences in, 61
menstrual cycle and, 60
morbidity and mortality in, 60
during pregnancy, 4, 65
prevalence of, 59
risk of, 59
PEA. *See* pulseless electrical activity
Permanent Atrial Fibrillation Outcome Study Using Dronedarone on Top of Standard Therapy (PALLAS), 22t, 29
P-glycoprotein, 107–8
"pill-in-the-pocket," 64
pindolol, for arrhythmia during pregnancy, 230
postpartum, LQTS in, 38, 39f
postural orthostatic tachycardia syndrome (POTS), 75
management of, 185–86
symptoms of, 184–85
TTT and, 178, 180
potassium channel protein synthesis, estrogen and, 2
POTS. *See* postural orthostatic tachycardia syndrome
pregnancy
AF in, 88–89
arrhythmias during, xii, 227–28
antiarrhythmic drugs, 228–30, 230t, 231–34t
anticoagulation, 235–36
cardioversion, 230, 235
incidence of, 228
treatment of, 228
cardiac arrest during, 236–37
defibrillation during, 236–37, 238–39
electrophysiology procedures during, 239
fetal echocardiography during, 239–40, 240f
ICD during, 238–39

pregnancy (*Cont.*)
    pacemaker during, 238–39
    PSVT episodes during, 4, 65
    RFA during, 239
    supine hypotensive syndrome during, 237–38
premature ventricular contractions, sex-related differences in, 3
proarrhythmia
    antiarrhythmic drugs and, xi, 80*t*, 92
    hormonal fluctuations and, 93
procainamide
    for AF in pregnancy, 89
    for AFL, 74
    for AVRT, 68
    for fetal arrhythmias, 240
    for WPW syndrome, 68
progesterone
    LQTS and, 37, 37*f*
    PSVT episodes and, 4
    QT interval and, 36–37
propafenone
    for AFL, 74
    for atrial tachycardia, 72
    for AVNRT, 64
    for AVRT, 69
    for rhythm control in AF, 92, 93*f*
    for WPW syndrome, 69
propranolol, for AF in pregnancy, 89
PSVT. *See* paroxysmal supraventricular tachycardia
pulmonary embolus, syncope and, 177
pulmonary hypertension, syncope and, 177
pulmonary vein antrum isolation, for atrial fibrillation, 7, 7*f*
pulseless electrical activity (PEA), 8–9
    SCD and, 114, 115*f*
P-wave dispersion, AF and, 83
P-wave duration, sex-related differences in, 48*t*, 51

QRS complex, sex-related differences in, 2
QTc. *See* corrected QT interval
QT interval
    in Brugada syndrome, 40
    corrected. *See* corrected QT interval
    hormone effects on, 35–37, 37*f*
    prolongation, xi
quinidine, in drug-induced LQTS, 108

RACE. *See* Rate Control Versus Electrical Cardioversion for Persistent Atrial Fibrillation
radiofrequency ablation (RFA)
    atrial fibrillation and, 6, 7

    during pregnancy, 239
    for supraventricular tachycardia, 5
RAFT. *See* Resynchronization/Defibrillation for Ambulatory Heart Failure Trial
randomized clinical trials
    of AADs, 18, 19–22*t*, 26–29
    enrollment barriers, 17–18, 31–32
    of ICD therapy, 23–25*t*, 29–31
Randomized Evaluation of Long-term Anticoagulant Therapy: Dabigatran vs Warfarin (RE-LY), 90
rapid atrial flutter, antiarrhythmic drug-induced, 108
rapid component of delayed rectifier potassium current (I_{Kr}), 36, 37, 38
Rate Control Versus Electrical Cardioversion for Persistent Atrial Fibrillation (RACE), 93–94, 108
rate-responsive pacemaker, 8
Registry to Improve the Use of Evidence-Based Heart Failure Therapies in the Outpatient Setting (IMPROVE HF), 149, 149*f*
regular narrow complex tachycardia, 42–43
RE-LY. *See* Randomized Evaluation of Long-term Anticoagulant Therapy: Dabigatran vs Warfarin
renin-angiotensin system blockers, in cardiovascular mortality reduction and SCD, 74
repolarization reserve, 36
Resynchronization/Defibrillation for Ambulatory Heart Failure Trial (RAFT), 25*t*, 30–31, 169, 171*t*
Resynchronization Reverses Remodeling in Systolic Left Ventricular Dysfunction (REVERSE), 25*t*, 30–31, 171*t*
RFA. *See* radiofrequency ablation
rheumatic heart disease (RHD), 218–19
rhythm-control drugs, cardiovascular toxicity of, 108–9, 109*t*
rivaroxaban
    pregnancy and, 236
    for stroke prevention in AF, 90
Rivaroxaban Once Daily Oral Direct Factor Xa Inhibition Compared With Vitamin K Antagonism for Prevention of Stroke and Embolism Trial in Atrial Fibrillation (ROCKET AF), 90
ryanodine receptor, mutation in, 41

SAFIRE-D. *See* Symptomatic Atrial Fibrillation Investigative Research on Dofetilide

SCD. *See* sudden cardiac death
SCD-HeFT. *See* Sudden Cardiac Death in Heart Failure Trial
SCN5A mutations, 38, 40
SEARCH-MI. *See* Survey to Evaluate Arrhythmia Rate in High-Risk Myocardial Infarction Patients
sex bias, 1
sex disparities, 1
SF-36. *See* 36-Item Short Form Health Survey
short QT syndrome (SQTS), 41
sick sinus syndrome, drug-induced, 92–93, 108
sinus node reentry tachycardia, 75
sinus tachyarrhythmias, 75
sinus tachycardia, 75
slow component of delayed rectifier potassium current (I_{Ks}), 36, 37, 38
sotalol
    for AFL, 74
    for arrhythmia during pregnancy, 230
    for atrial tachycardia, 72
    for AVNRT, 64
    for AVRT, 68, 69
    for PSVT during pregnancy, 65
    for rhythm control in AF, 92, 93f
    for WPW syndrome, 68, 69
South Asian ethnicity, CAD and mortality rates in, 210, 213
SPAF I-III. *See* Stroke Prevention in Atrial Fibrillation I-III
SQTS. *See* short QT syndrome
statins, for AF, 94–95
St Jude Riata ST lead, 253, 254
stroke
    prevention of, in AF, 89–91
    risk of
        AF and, 84–86, 85f
        atrial fibrillation and, 5–6
Stroke Prevention in Atrial Fibrillation I-III (SPAF I-III), 84
subpectoral pocket, cardiac pacing and, 156, 157f
sudden cardiac death (SCD), 8–9
    AVRT and, 70
    causative rhythm of, 114
    depression and, 121–22
    epidemiology of, 129–30, 130f, 131f, 132
    etiologies of, 115–21
        ARVD, 120
        CAD, 115–16, 116f, 117f, 118–19
        channelopathies, 120–21
        dilated cardiomyopathy, 116, 116f, 117f
        hypertrophic cardiomyopathy, 119–20
        left ventricular dysfunction, 119
        LQTS, 120–21
        NICM, 119–20
        valvular heart disease, 116, 116f, 117f
    in global CVD, 213–15
        ICD for prevention of, 214
    ICD therapy for prevention of, sex-related differences in clinical outcomes of, 13t
    ICD trials
        as primary prevention, 132–41, 142t
        as secondary prevention, 132
    incidence of, 113
    panic attacks and, 122
    risk reduction in, 124–25
    risk stratification in, 123–24
    sex differences in epidemiology, 114–15, 115f
    sex differences in triggering of ventricular arrhythmias, 121–23
    WPW syndrome and, 68, 70
Sudden Cardiac Death in Heart Failure Trial (SCD-HeFT), 20t, 23t, 27, 30, 119, 125, 132t, 134, 136–38, 137f, 139f, 140, 142
supine hypotensive syndrome, during pregnancy, 237–38
supraventricular tachycardia, xi
    catheter ablation of, sex-related differences in clinical outcomes of, 13t
    paroxysmal. *See* paroxysmal supraventricular tachycardia
    radiofrequency ablation for, 5
Survey to Evaluate Arrhythmia Rate in High-Risk Myocardial Infarction Patients (SEARCH-MI), 143
Survival With Oral D-Sotalol (SWORD), 18, 19t, 92, 104–5
Symptomatic Atrial Fibrillation Investigative Research on Dofetilide (SAFIRE-D), 21t, 28
syncope. *See also* neurally mediated syncope
    causes of, 177–78
    in men compared to women, 179t
    TTT and, 178, 179f, 180
systole, duration of, 2

tachycardia
    atrial. *See* atrial tachycardia
    atrioventricular nodal reentrant, 4
    inappropriate sinus, 75
    junctional. *See* junctional tachycardia
    paroxysmal supraventricular. *See* paroxysmal supraventricular tachycardia
    regular narrow complex, 42–43

tachycardia (*Cont.*)
  sinus, 75
  sinus node reentry, 75
  supraventricular. *See* supraventricular tachycardia
  ventricular, SCD and, 114, 115*f*
tachycardia-mediated cardiomyopathy, secondary to incessant atrial tachycardia, 72
tamoxifen, for breast cancer, 111
testosterone
  administration of, QTc and, 50
  in drug-induced LQTS, 104
  QT interval and, 36
Third International Study on Syncope of Uncertain Etiology (ISSUE-3), 188
36-Item Short Form Health Survey (SF-36), 82, 83*f*
Thomson Lactation Rating, 230
thromboembolic event
  antiarrhythmic drug-induced, 108
  warfarin and, 84
thyroid replacement, for AF, 96
tilt table testing (TTT), syncope and, 178, 179*f*, 180, 181, 182
torsades de pointes
  acquired LQTS and, 40
  antiarrhythmic medication-induced, 4, 108
  in drug-induced LQTS, 104, 105*f*
transvenous lead extractions
  fibrosis and, 249–50, 249*f*, 251*f*
  indications for, 244–48*b*
    functional leads, 246*b*–247*b*
    infection, 244–45*b*
    nonfunctional leads, 247*b*–248*b*
    thrombosis, 245*b*
    venous stenosis, 245*b*
  lead-related issues, 252–54
    Accufix atrial lead, 252, 253*f*
    coronary sinus leads, 254
    ICD leads, 253–54
  patient selection for, 244
  procedural aspects, 248–52
  procedural outcomes, 254–56
  risk of, 255*b*
Treatment and Outcomes of Acute Coronary Syndromes in India (CREATE), 213
Trypanosoma cruzi, 215
TTT. *See* tilt table testing

vagal maneuvers, for sinus node reentry tachycardia, 75
VALIANT. *See* Valsartan in Acute Myocardial Infarction Trial
Valsalva maneuver, for AVNRT, 62, 64
valsartan, 21*t*, 28
Valsartan in Acute Myocardial Infarction Trial (VALIANT), 21*t*, 28
valvular heart disease, SCD and, 116, 116*f*, 117*f*
vasovagal syncope. *See* neurally mediated syncope
venous pooling, orthostatic intolerance and, 186–87
ventricular fibrillation (VF), SCD and, 114, 115*f*
ventricular repolarization
  androgens and, 50
  sex-related differences in, 48–50
ventricular tachycardia (VT), SCD and, 114, 115*f*
verapamil
  for AFL, 74
  for atrial tachycardia, 72
  for AVNRT, 64
  for fetal arrhythmias, 240
  for POTS, 186
VF. *See* ventricular fibrillation
VT. *See* ventricular tachycardia
VVI devices, 8

warfarin
  pregnancy and, 235–36
  for stroke prevention in AF, 90
  thromboembolic event and, 84
WHI. *See* Women's Health Initiative
WHS. *See* Women's Health Study: A Randomized Trial of Low-Dose Aspirin and Vitamin E in the Primary Prevention of Cardiovascular Disease and Cancer
WISE. *See* Women's Ischemia Syndrome Evaluation
Wolff-Parkinson-White (WPW) syndrome, 66
  catheter ablation for, 69
  DCCV for, 68
  electrophysiologic characteristics of accessory pathway in, 69–70, 69*f*
  EPS for, 68
  incidence of, 66–68
  management of, 68–70
  outcomes in, 70
  overdrive pacing for, 68
  SCD and, 68, 70
Women's Health Initiative (WHI), 85, 122
Women's Health Study: A Randomized Trial of Low-Dose Aspirin and Vitamin E in the Primary Prevention of Cardiovascular Disease and Cancer (WHS), 86–87, 88
women's heart clinic. *See* heart clinic, women's
Women's Ischemia Syndrome Evaluation (WISE), 118
WPW. *See* Wolff-Parkinson-White syndrome